Science Has No Sex

STUDIES IN SOCIAL MEDICINE

Allan M. Brandt and Larry R. Churchill, editors

Arleen Marcia Tuchman

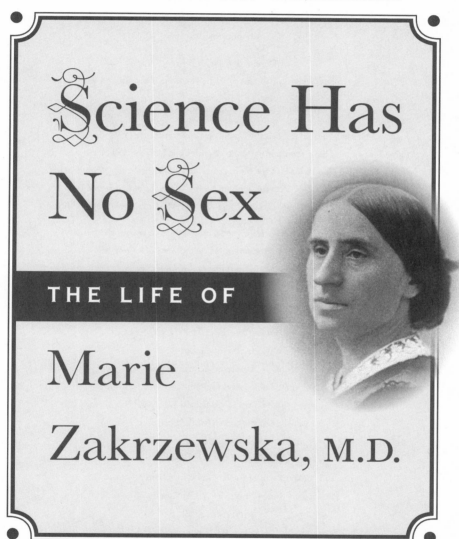

Science Has No Sex

THE LIFE OF

Marie
Zakrzewska, M.D.

The University of North Carolina Press • Chapel Hill

Designed by Heidi Perov

Set in Baskerville and Copperplate by Keystone Typesetting, Inc.

Manufactured in the United States of America

This volume was published with the generous assistance of Vanderbilt University and of the Greensboro Women's Fund of the University of North Carolina Press. Founding Contributors of the fund: Linda Arnold Carlisle, Sally Schindel Cone, Anne Faircloth, Bonnie McElveen Hunter, Linda Bullard Jennings, Janice J. Kerley (in honor of Margaret Supplee Smith), Nancy Rouzer May, and Betty Hughes Nichols.

The paper in this book meets the guidelines for permanence and durability of the Committee on Production Guidelines for Book Longevity of the Council on Library Resources.

Library of Congress Cataloging-in-Publication Data

Tuchman, Arleen, 1956–

Science has no sex : the life of Marie Zakrzewska /

Arleen Marcia Tuchman.

p. cm. — (Studies in social medicine)

Includes bibliographical references and index.

ISBN-13: 978-0-8078-3020-8 (cloth: alk. paper)

ISBN-10: 0-8078-3020-8 (cloth: alk. paper)

1. Zakrzewska, Marie E., 1829–1902.

2. Women physicians—United States—Biography.

[DNLM: 1. Zakrzewska, Marie E. (Marie Elizabeth), 1829–1902.

2. Physicians, Women—history—Massachusetts—Biography.

WZ 100 Z218t 2006]

I. Title. II. Series.

R692.T83   2006

610.92—dc22   2005036098

10 09 08 07 06   5 4 3 2 1

To my family and friends,
for reminding me of what is important in life

CONTENTS

ILLUSTRATIONS AND TABLES

ACKNOWLEDGMENTS

The day has finally arrived when I get to thank everyone who has helped me to bring this book to fruition. This would never have happened without the support of funding institutions, research assistants, librarians, archivists, colleagues and friends near and far, and my family. It is with great pleasure that I now acknowledge them all.

Many funding institutions expressed their confidence in this project. I wish to thank the American Philosophical Society, the German Academic Exchange Service (DAAD), the National Endowment for the Humanities (RH-21250-95), and the National Institutes of Health (R01-LM06859-01) for their generous financial support. My own institution, Vanderbilt University, provided sabbatical leave and research grants at critical moments in the development of this book. I particularly appreciate the year I spent as a Fellow at Vanderbilt's Robert Penn Warren Center for the Humanities in 1994–95. Thanks to the members of the Seminar on Science and Society for stimulating conversations that were especially valuable in the early stages of this book. I wish to express my gratitude as well to the National Humanities Center in Research Triangle Park, North Carolina, for the wonderful fellowship year I spent there in 1995–96.

The research for this book benefited greatly from two research assistants: Marla Connelly, now Dr. Marla Doehring, spent a summer doing bibliographic research for me; and Daniel Sargent, a graduate student at Harvard University, helped me to compile the demographic information on hospital patient populations contained in Tables 1–9 in Chapter 9. I also appreciate the assistance of the archivists and librarians at the following institutions: the Geheimes Staatsarchiv Preussischer Kulturbesitz, the Universitätsarchiv der Humboldt Universität, the Potsdam-Brandenburgisches Landeshauptarchiv; the Special Collections Library at the University of Michigan; the Massachusetts Historical Society; the Schlesinger Library; the Sophia Smith Collection at Smith College; Boston Medical Library in the Francis A. Countway Library of Medicine; the Archives and Special Collections on Women in Medicine and Homeopathy at Drexel University; and the Library of Congress. Jack Eckert at the Countway and Barbara Williams at Drexel University made it particularly easy to secure copyright permissions. My warmest thanks to Virginia Elwood, who is currently completing a biography of Caroline Severance and who photocopied and sent to me letters from and pertaining to Zakrzewska in Severance's correspondence. I am also grateful for all the help I have received from the staff in my department, especially from Vicki Swinehart and Brenda Hummel, neither of whom ever said no.

Parts of this book have been published in modified form in other venues. Thanks to *Isis* and to the *Journal of the History of Women* for allowing me to replicate some of that material here.

I have had many conversations over the years with colleagues whose comments have shaped this book in ways I can no longer recapture. Their insights have simply become part of the way I now think about gender and medicine. I have benefited greatly from conversations with Rima Apple, Charlotte Borst, Carla Bittel, Beth Conklin, Martha Gardner, Janet Golden, Margaret Humphreys, Katherine Crawford, Judith Walzer Leavitt, Susan Lederer, Regina Morantz-Sanchez, Ellen Singer More, Steven Peitzman, Rebecca Plant, Naomi Rogers, Susan L. Smith, Valerie Traub, and Russell Viner. I had the good fortune to participate in the National Library of Medicine's symposium "Women Physicians, Women's Politics, and Women's Health: Emerging Narratives" in March 2005, just as I was nearing the finish line on the final revisions of this manuscript. The feedback I received on my paper helped me to rethink my concluding chapter and to crystallize some ideas that were admittedly still vague. Thanks to the organizers of this conference, Elizabeth Fee, Ellen Singer More, and Manon Perry, and to all the participants for a wonderfully engaging two days. Thanks also to the members of the Medicine, Health, and Society group at Vanderbilt University, especially my colleague Matthew Ramsey, for their critical reading of my work. My department has provided a particularly nurturing and stimulating environment in which to work. I am grateful for the collegiality and friendship that define the culture of our department and for the lunchtime seminars, in which we read and critique each other's written work.

I owe a special debt to those individuals who read all or parts of this manuscript. These include Michael Bess, Katherine Crawford, Mona Frederick, Janet Golden, Judith Walzer Leavitt, Mary Lindemann, Rebecca Plant, Naomi Rogers, Helmut Smith, and David Zolensky. Their substantive and editorial suggestions forced me to rethink many of the assumptions I brought to this work, to tighten my argument, and to cut, cut, and cut some more. I am deeply grateful to the two previously anonymous readers for the University of North Carolina Press, Regina Morantz-Sanchez and Ellen Singer More. Not only did their suggestions for revisions make this book much better, but the ongoing conversations I have had with both of these scholars over the past decade have profoundly shaped my understanding of the history of gender and medicine and contributed immeasurably to my intellectual growth. Thanks to Allan Brandt and Larry Churchill, editors of Studies in Social Medicine at the University of North Carolina Press, for their support of my project and to Sian Hunter, senior editor at the press, for her intelligent suggestions and pleasant demeanor. It has been a true delight to work with her.

I have dedicated this book to my friends and family, who have done a masterful job keeping me sane throughout the many years I have spent on this project. I am grateful to Vivien Fryd, Brenda Hipsher, Susan Johnston, Sue Kay, and Hedy Weinberg for being there when I needed them. Janet Golden always knew how to turn a mountain back into a mole hill, and Mona Frederick had the uncanny knack of finding the humor in every situation. I am truly blessed to have such good friends.

My greatest debt is to my family. I wish to thank my sister, Shendl Tuchman, for never doubting that I would some day finish this book. My stepchildren, Rachel and Peter Zolensky, came into my life while I was in the middle of writing this biography. Their patience and good humor have sustained me in more ways than they can imagine. As interested as they have been periodically in this unusual woman whose story I have told, I know they are relieved to no longer have Zakrzewska's spirit at our dinner table. My son, Andrew, now five years old, was of course only vaguely aware of "mommy's work." Nevertheless, he was astute enough to extract the promise of a Scooby-Do sleep animal when "mommy sends off her manuscript." Finally, my deepest thanks go to my husband, David Zolensky, who has been looking forward to the completion of this book almost as much I have. He has read and reread drafts of this book until his eyes have glazed over. I am grateful for his love, his friendship, and his killer editorial skills.

Introduction

On 19 October 1942, radio listeners tuning in to the Du Pont radio series "The Cavalcade of America" would have heard the following introduction to that evening's broadcast:

> At a time in our history when women are doing the work of men in many fields—in science, industry and medicine—we recall another time when women had no equal place in the work of the world. Our story tonight is about a pioneer in medicine who fought to help achieve this equality. Her name is Marie Zakshefska (sic!), a courageous Polish girl who became one of the greatest woman physicians and a path-finder in American Medicine.[1]

Zakrzewska's name, which her contemporaries found unpronounceable and which the series' producers noticeably misspelled, has now been all but forgotten. As late as World War II, however, Zakrzewska (pronounced Zak-chef-ska) remained famous enough to be chosen to symbolize women who had successfully crossed traditional gender lines. She earned this reputation by establishing herself as a physician, educator, and hospital administrator at a time when most medical schools and institutions were closed to women.

The producers of "The Cavalcade of America" apparently chose this nineteenth-century woman as an example to inspire women physicians to serve the nation by joining the WAVES (Women Accepted for Volunteer Emergency Service) and WACS (Women's Army Corps). Focusing on her Polish ancestry rather than her German birth—hardly surprising during World War II—they fashioned her into the character they needed in order to promote a message that mixed patriotism with women's rights. Courageous, determined, and successful in the face of adversity, Zakrzewska became the Rosie the Riveter of the world of female physicians. This broadcast in 1942 was not the first time, nor would it be the last, that Zakrzewska's name and her work would be associated with various social and political agendas of the nineteenth, twentieth, and now twenty-first centuries.

Born in Berlin, Germany, on 6 September 1829, Marie Elizabeth Zakrzewska trained as a midwife at that city's famous Charité hospital and then spent six months working as the hospital's head midwife before immigrating to America to pursue an M.D. This she received in 1856 from Cleveland Medical College in Cleveland, Ohio, a traditionally all-male medical school that briefly opened its doors to women. Thereafter she helped Elizabeth and Emily Blackwell establish the New York Infirmary for Women and Children; she spent three years as director of a new clinical department at the New England Female College in Boston; and finally, in 1862, she founded the New England Hospital for Women and Children, one of a small number of all-female institutions that offered women an opportunity to study medicine and gain clinical experience. Zakrzewska directed the hospital for twenty-five years—some say with an iron hand—before handing over the reins. Unable, however, to let go of the institution she had created, she remained involved in hospital affairs until shortly before her death in 1902.[2]

Zakrzewska was known among her friends and students for her "magnetism" as well as her "fearless courage and persuasive tongue."[3] William Lloyd Garrison II, a close friend, once described her as "a woman of decided opinions and the frankest speech, a circumstance which gave zest and animation to any group in which she mingled."[4] Bold, outspoken, and often tactless, she forged a public persona that represented anything but the demure Victorian feminine ideal. She had a biting sense of humor, once ridiculing a physician who claimed women's small size, and thus small brains, rendered them unable to study medicine by asking him to lament with her "the death of the 600 pound man who died recently in New York and in whom we have certainly lost one of the greatest medical geniuses."[5] Many admired her for her forthrightness, others were intimidated, but most of her peers appreciated her willingness to fight for a woman's right to enter the medical field.

I first became interested in Zakrzewska more than a decade ago, when, in preparing to teach a new course on the history of women, health, and sexuality, I began reading about women physicians in the United States. My previous work had focused on nineteenth-century European medicine and science, but my teaching was more eclectic, drawing on material from countries outside Europe as well. The literature on women's battle to study medicine in the United States was particularly rich, offering a complex picture of the difficulties women faced and the diverse strategies they pursued as they sought to challenge cultural stereotypes of themselves as physiologically and mentally unfit for the study and practice of medicine.[6] Founding their own schools and hospitals at the same time that they sought to integrate all-male medical institutions, women set out to change the terms of the debate over whether they should study medicine. As Regina Morantz-Sanchez has demonstrated in her foundational study of women physicians in the United States, one of the most effective strategies women adopted was to counter men's claims that women's sympathetic natures rendered them unfit for the grueling practice of medicine. They did this by defining medicine itself as the caring profession par excellence. In this way they could argue that their possession of nurturing qualities placed them in a unique position to build a bridge between "sympathy" and "science," making sure that the knowledge gained by science would be applied in humane ways.[7]

Zakrzewska, along with Elizabeth Blackwell, who was eight years her senior, and Mary Putnam Jacobi, who was thirteen years younger, is always featured in studies of the first generation of women physicians in the United States. She has attracted attention not only because of the powerful influence she exerted as director of a teaching hospital over women who pursued medical careers in the second half of the nineteenth century but also because of her unusual stance on women's relationship to science. In marked contrast to the majority of her colleagues, who embraced the Victorian idea of unique feminine virtues, Zakrzewska insisted that all physicians, whether male or female, had first and foremost to develop their rational faculties and receive advanced training in the natural sciences. In her eyes, too much sympathy and compassion confused one's ability to reason, thus making it impossible to provide good medical care.[8] To be sure, what made Zakrzewska unusual was not her praise of science; the vast majority of her peers agreed that medical education and practice must be grounded in scientific knowledge. Where she stood out was in the iconic status to which she elevated science, coupled with her critique of sympathy, the very virtue her peers so revered.

Zakrzewska intrigued me immediately, and I found myself drawn more and more to a set of questions inspired by what I knew about her: Why, I wondered, did she so boldly claim science for women? Did others share her convictions? What, in fact, did terms like "science" and "sympathy" mean to her? Might they have meant something different to her because of her German background? Zakrzewska's writings on the place of science in medical practice resonated with the material I had read for my book on nineteenth-century German medical theories and practices. Here, then, was an opportunity to look anew at the differences and similarities between German and American medicine at a time when most American physicians remained skeptical of what they believed to be taking place in the German laboratories and hospitals.[9] Zakrzewska's story, it turned out, encompassed many intriguing twists: here was a German woman, trained in midwifery before she studied medicine, who was promoting European scientific medicine to a skeptical audience of American male physicians.

The story I tell begins with an exploration of Zakrzewska's German connections, something that historians have overlooked. Although Zakrzewska's career as a physician certainly took shape in the United States, her emphasis on the natural sciences makes little sense divorced from her German upbringing, training, and connections. She grew up in a nineteenth-century German bourgeois family that held rationality, secularism, and the natural sciences in high regard, associating them with all that was considered modern and progressive. Moreover, during her midwifery training, which took place at midcentury at one of the best midwifery schools in Europe, she became familiar with the demands of young, academically trained German physicians that medical education be grounded more firmly in the laboratory and clinical sciences. To these physicians, the call for what was alternately called "physiological medicine," "rational medicine," or "scientific medicine" served two ends. First, it sought to bring greater certainty to medicine by deriving therapeutic practices from a knowledge of the laws governing pathological processes. Second, it served as a democratizing tool, challenging elite professionals who claimed that the true physician possessed a certain talent or intuition that could not be taught. Drawing on revolutionary rhetoric, popular during the years leading up to the revolutions of 1848, these young physicians insisted that since the scientific method was something that anyone, regardless of class background, could learn, the doors to the elite profession should be opened to all.[10] Zakrzewska would draw on all these meanings in her promotion of the natural sciences. Although there was hardly an elite medical profession in the United States when she arrived in 1853, she found this rhetoric of egalitarianism useful in her battle to open the doors of the medical profession to women.

The German influence on Zakrzewska did not cease once she crossed the ocean. On the contrary, her appreciation of the political power of scientific knowledge only increased when she became deeply involved within a few years of her arrival in the United States with the community of radical German émigrés, most of whom had fled their homeland following the failed revolutions of 1848. For these radicals, science was more than a tool for acquiring information about the natural world; rather, it represented something akin to a worldview. Frequently describing society as a battleground between religion (especially the Catholic Church) and arbitrary authority, on the one hand, and reason and political democracy, on the other, they linked science, atheism, and materialism to humanitarian ends, convinced that the abolition of misery would not occur until individuals abandoned their belief in a higher being and acquired the skills to think for themselves.[11]

Zakrzewska, who embraced the views of the community of German radicals, thus grounded her moral values in a secular, materialist philosophy. This distinguished her from most other American women physicians, who, like Ann Preston, dean of the Woman's Medical College of Pennsylvania, derived their strength from "the inviolable authority of religion."[12] Indeed, it distinguished her from the vast majority of middle-class Americans, for whom religion, whether mainstream or unorthodox, provided the foundation from which they derived their sense of right and wrong. This was even true of such radicals as William Lloyd Garrison, Theodore Parker, Wendell Phillips, Angelina Grimké, and Sarah Grimké, many of whom became Zakrzewska's friends.[13] Zakrzewska may have joined with them in their fight to ensure justice for all, regardless of race, class, or sex, but her sense of justice did not stem from any belief in a divine being but rather from the conviction that the laws of nature, which science revealed, produced a world that was good in and of itself.

· · ·

As I learned more about the reasons for Zakrzewska's positive assessment of the sciences, I recognized the myriad ways in which her case complicated older assumptions about the relationship between gender and science. Certainly in the first wave of feminist work on women physicians, when scholars seemed particularly interested in Zakrzewska because of her germinal role in opening the medical profession to women, the dominant interpretive framework posited a fault line between femininity and morality, on the one hand, and masculinity and science, on the other.[14] Zakrzewska's conviction that science and morality were intimately connected, however, and that women needed to reclaim traits such as rationality for themselves fit poorly into this framework. As a result, the picture that emerged of Zakrzewska was highly confusing: we learned that she both promoted the idea of female uniqueness and "frowned on women who chose medicine out of female 'sympathy.'" She was cast as both a proponent of the "holistic, subjective quality of nineteenth-century medicine" and an advocate of microscopy, thermometry, and scientific medicine. Zakrzewska supposedly regretted that she never married and was exuberant that she never had to compromise her independence. Finally, she appeared as someone whose pragmatism usually led her to appreciate the importance of compromises, while being cast by others as unsympathetic, inflexible, and authoritarian.[15]

These conflicting pictures reflected in part Zakrzewska's complex personality and, as we will see, the way she changed as she aged. But they also stemmed from the difficulty of fitting her into a theoretical framework that pitted, in Regina Morantz-Sanchez's words, "'femininity,' 'feminism' and 'morality'" against "'masculinity,' 'professionalism' and 'science.'"[16] Subsequent feminist scholarship has, however, questioned whether such divisions were ever quite so entrenched as we had once thought. In recent years, intrigued by the multiple meanings of such terms as science and professionalism, historians have argued that many women physicians did not so much critique science and professionalism as define these terms differently than did the majority of their male colleagues.[17] They have also complicated the picture of men's professional practice, showing, for example, that male physicians who practiced in rural settings spent their days struggling to balance their public and private lives in a fashion once assumed to be peculiar to women.[18] And they have documented the lives of women physicians who publicly aligned themselves with new scientific techniques and the new professionalism, exploring in particular the gendered meanings of such an affiliation.[19]

The analysis I offer of Zakrzewska's life and work has been shaped by this revisionist approach to gender and medicine. It has also been informed by feminist scholarship on what is alternatively labeled "situatedness" or "positionality," which explicitly attacks the kind of binary oppositions that had shaped the older scholarship. Motivated by a desire to avoid the problems inherent in both cultural feminism's essentializing definition of "woman" and poststructuralism's tendency toward nominalism, many feminist theorists sought to destabilize the category "woman" while still retaining a loose definition of what it might mean to be a woman in any given situation. These theorists held that while essentialism offered them a clear picture of who and what they were fighting for, the price was a fixed definition of what it meant to be a woman, which both excluded those who did not fit this definition and ignored the changing nature of that category over time. Poststructuralism, on the other hand, provided a powerful apparatus for analyzing the discursive construction of gendered identities, but the category of "woman" threatened to disappear in this kind of analysis, along with the rationale not only for feminist analysis but also for political action.[20]

As a way out of this quandary, several theorists embraced a notion of gender as "situational" or "positional." Accordingly, a woman's subject identity, her actions, and her beliefs are all understood in relation to a specific and always changing context—a particular set of conditions, opportunities, and constraints —and not against an idealized notion of how women should behave.[21] This understanding of gender encourages exploration of the different kinds of personal and political negotiations that become necessary as contexts change. It also draws attention to the highly unstable nature of gender categories. Multiple understandings of masculinity and femininity have circulated at any given time, constantly threatening to subvert the rigid binary oppositions upon which power depends. Traditional boundaries must, as a result, constantly be reasserted or, in Judith Butler's terms, "performed."[22] In this sense, gender is neither a foundational category nor a meaningless category but rather a set of practices that individuals perform repeatedly and that aim to create the appearance of two and only two genders.

Focusing on Zakrzewska's "situatedness" led me to think of her as someone who, unlike many of her colleagues, rejected the option of empowering a set of allegedly feminine virtues as a way of justifying women's entry into the medical profession. Instead, recognizing the multiple and competing understandings of masculinity and femininity available to her, she tried, sometimes more successfully than others, to use these meanings to challenge the gender-based claims that functioned to keep women out of the public sphere. Zakrzewska, I realized, was engaged in her own struggle to dissociate science from gender by casting science and rationality as universal rather than masculine traits. The title of this book stems from a comment Zakrzewska made when offering a comparison of different nations' attitudes toward women physicians. "I am sorry," she wrote, "to be forced to say that it is not the Republic of America which has given the proof that 'science has no sex.' . . . But it is the Republic of Switzerland which has verified this maxim."[23] Zakrzewska was referring to the decision on the part of the University of Zurich to let women study medicine as early as 1864.[24] That only a republic could be the site of such momentous change Zakrzewska never doubted for the simple reason that only a nation committed to equal rights for all human beings would ever be capable of extending such rights to women.

. . .

Zakrzewska's battle to dissociate science from gender involved more than words. She also presented a different image of what it meant to be a woman. The few photographs we have indicate a woman who shunned traditional feminine markers such as ribbons and lace, preferring instead an unadorned and austere look. In addition, in stark opposition to the idealized construction of Victorian womanhood as pious, domestic, and dependent, Zakrzewska denounced religion, defended unwed mothers, and encouraged women to take on positions of authority. To be sure, few nineteenth-century women actually embodied this Victorian ideal, and certainly any woman who studied medicine at the time defied normative gender scripts.[25] Still, Zakrzewska stood out not only for the extent of the challenges she posed but also for the public nature of her challenges. Displaying her wit, using logic to ridicule opponents, even assuming the directorship of a hospital—these were all acts that highlighted her anomalous gender position and functioned (she hoped) to challenge assumptions about the true nature of woman. That she experienced such public displays as transgressive is evident in her comment that her father, who disapproved of her move to Boston, claimed she was "disgracing the family, and German womanhood in general, by accepting a position which caused my name to come prominently before the public."[26]

Zakrzewska challenged normative roles in her private life as well. Indeed, a kind of symbiosis existed between her public attack on the cultural stereotypes that functioned to constrain women's options and the alternative family she created for herself. Although Zakrzewska did not leave the volumes of personal material that biographers usually mine when they write their subject's life, enough has survived to paint a picture of a woman who flouted middle-class conventions by rejecting the institution of marriage and creating instead a family centered around two individuals: Karl Heinzen and Julia A. Sprague. Heinzen, a German radical émigré and political journalist, shared Zakrzewska's home for twenty years. Despite the controversy that later erupted over the nature of their relationship, this was not a romantic affair. Heinzen was considerably older, married, and a father, and when he moved into Zakrzewska's home, he brought his wife and child with him. The strength of their bond had rather more to do with their shared political convictions. As Zakrzewska once explained, she had been drawn to Heinzen because of his commitment to abolitionism and women's rights.[27]

Sprague, a women's rights reformer and founding member of the New England Women's Club, lived with Zakrzewska for forty years. Her name appears only a few times in the old but standard biography of Zakrzewska, published in 1924. Agnes Vietor, the author of *A Woman's Quest: The Life of Marie E. Zakrzewska, M.D.*, did, however, include the intriguing line that Sprague was Zakrzewska's "faithful friend and home companion for life."[28] Nevertheless, the nature of their relationship, like so many other same-sex relationships in the past, remained obscure until the recent discovery of roughly fifty letters of Sprague's, all written to the woman's rights reformer Caroline Severance, a close friend of both Sprague's and Zakrzewska's.[29]

These letters attest to the depth of the bond that developed between these two women over the forty-year period during which they shared their home and their lives. In exploring their relationship I have relied on the work of women's historians, who have radically altered our understanding of same-sex relationships. As they have shown, nineteenth-century women lived, worked, and traveled together at a time when emotional attachments between women did not evoke suspicion of a lesbian relationship. Some formed "Boston marriages," a label that, as early as the nineteenth century, came to describe two women, usually both middle-class professionals, who shared a household. While some formed Boston marriages as a way of sharing the many responsibilities and chores associated with running a household, for others, the decision to become partners for life grew out of their romantic love for each other.[30] The relationship between Zakrzewska and Sprague seems to have begun as a convenient arrangement, but it grew slowly over the years into a committed and caring partnership. Zakrzewska may never have married, but she created a rich life for herself in which she was never alone.

. . .

What follows, then, is the story of a woman who established a central place for herself in the nineteenth-century American medical community while also being active in radical political circles throughout her adult life. Zakrzewska arrived in the United States in 1853, a time of great turmoil: the Seneca Falls Convention in 1848 marked the formal beginning of a movement for women's rights; the passing of the Fugitive Slave Law in 1850 heightened tensions between the North and the South; and the growth of cities, coupled with the massive influx of immigrants from Ireland and Germany, was forcing Americans to confront expanding problems of urban poverty and disease. Within a few years of her arrival, Zakrzewska positioned herself on the radical fringe of those seeking reform; she did this not only through her German connections but also through her involvement in the radical wing of American political and social movements. Thus, Zakrzewska became an abolitionist and suffragist, serving briefly as a vice president of the Massachusetts Women's Suffrage Association. Her greatest contribution to social change came, however, through her founding of the New England Hospital for Women and Children, an institution she hoped would level the playing field for women in at least two ways: by providing poor, sick, and pregnant women with the same quality of care that wealthier women could purchase, thus offering them an alternative to the almshouse; and by creating a female-run teaching hospital, where women who aspired to the practice of medicine would have clinical opportunities otherwise denied to them.[31]

I first examine the New England Hospital as one of many social welfare institutions founded in the mid-nineteenth century to address the social problems linked to massive immigration and the resultant increase in urban poverty. Zakrzewska may not have ascribed to the mixture of Christian stewardship and Victorian moralism that inspired many of the founders of these institutions, but she still viewed her responsibilities as director of a new hospital to be a blend of medical care and moral education. Sharing with other founders a sense of obligation toward the poor and needy, combined with a reformist impulse that sought to discipline them, she too refused refuge to those she deemed unworthy.[32] Nevertheless, her political radicalism, particularly her concern for the plight of poor women, led her to draw such lines more loosely. At a time, for example, when some hospitals refused to establish lying-in wards for fear of the kind of women who would seek refuge and other maternity hospitals refused to admit unwed patients, Zakrzewska spoke out publicly in defense of unwed mothers, declaring it inhumane to limit care to those who possessed a marriage license.[33]

A closer look at the rhetoric and the practices of the New England Hospital thus offers an unusual glimpse at a mid-nineteenth-century social welfare institution created with the intention of fulfilling a radical agenda; at the same time, it allows us a deeper understanding of the difficulties and limitations that accompanied such a project, for the radicalism of the institution did not last. By 1872 the hospital had moved out to the suburbs and was trying to attract a "better" clientele; by the end of the century, its radical, even charitable, dimensions had all but disappeared. To be sure, hospitals throughout the nation were changing from largely charitable institutions to acute-care facilities, defined increasingly by new technological developments and surgical interventions, and catering more and more to the middle class and wealthy.[34] Yet since few had started out with as radical an agenda as the New England Hospital, few had been so utterly transformed.

Thus, national trends, as important as they may have been, cannot alone explain Zakrzewska's abandonment of her earlier radicalism; one must also take into consideration her personal limitations and aspirations. However committed she may have been to social justice for the poor, she came up against three obstacles that led her to redefine the hospital's mission: financial difficulties, a growing disillusionment with the increasingly Irish (Catholic) makeup of the patient population, and the realization that poor, chronically ill women did not best serve the needs of a modern teaching hospital. As with other middle-class reformers, Zakrzewska's actions revealed her class prejudices, coupled, in her case, with an extreme hatred of the Catholic Church. Given this, and given that her true passion had always been to open the doors of the medical profession to women, she had little incentive to continue a project that threatened to jeopardize that cause.

· · ·

As a result, Zakrzewska's hospital has not gone down in history as an example of an institution that provided justice to poor women; its claim to fame is rather through its role in opening the medical profession to women. Historian Mary Roth Walsh even dubbed the New England Hospital for Women and Children a "Feminist Showplace" because of its central role in demonstrating to the public women's ability to practice medicine, provide clinical instruction, and run their own hospital.[35] Like other all-women's institutions founded in the second half of the nineteenth century, whether clubs, colleges, or political organizations, the New England Hospital came into existence because of women's exclusion from the institutions that prepared men for work in the public sphere. Indeed, the founding and success of the institution depended, in Walsh's words, upon "the material and psychological support" Zakrzewska received from a network of women committed to advancing the cause of their own sex.[36]

The New England Hospital also relied upon the goodwill of a large number of men who were committed to advancing women's rights. Significantly, Zakrzewska's decision to found an all-women's hospital did not mark her embrace of a separate women's culture. On the contrary, her ultimate goal was full integration, and she hoped she was doing her part to convince society that women practiced medicine as effectively as, and certainly no differently than, men. She may have distinguished herself in this regard from some of the founders of all-women's clubs and colleges, who often used their culture's insistence on a separate woman's identity to expand their role in society, but Zakrzewska was not alone. Indeed, many of her peers who presided over all-women's medical institutions shared her preference for integration as well. Thus Elizabeth and Emily Blackwell, who founded the Women's Medical College of the New York Infirmary in 1868, did so only after they had failed repeatedly to open the doors of all-male institutions to women. For these women, the best way to advance the cause of their sex was to insist that, whatever differences might exist between men and women, they still needed to be trained in identical ways.[37]

Some of these pioneers also believed that training had to be in regular medicine. Thus Zakrzewska made sure to align herself and her institution with the elite medical community in Boston, joining other regular women physicians, such as Ann Preston and the Blackwells, in rejecting irregular practices.[38] Historians of medicine have argued convincingly that by midcentury the differences between orthodox and unorthodox approaches may have been as much rhetorical as substantive. Homeopathic physicians, who emphasized both the efficacy and painlessness of their infinitesimal doses, had often received training in regular institutions, whereas orthodox physicians, whose therapeutic practices consisted largely of bloodletting, purgatives, emetics, and tonics, had become more conservative in their approach.[39] Still, all differences had not disappeared, and by aligning the New England Hospital with regular medicine Zakrzewska was announcing her allegiance to the established medical profession and to traditional medical practices; at the same time, she sought to introduce some of the new scientific methods that were emerging from the German laboratories and clinics. Thus, not only did interns at her hospital learn standard medical practices, but they also charted their patients' temperature, pulse rate, and rate of respiration; they performed chemical and microscopic analyses of bodily fluids; and they witnessed the occasional autopsy. Although by modern standards this may seem unimpressive, few other hospitals—even those committed to regular medicine—did this much.[40] In this way, Zakrzewska gained the respect and the support of elite physicians, but she also distanced herself from the large number of women practitioners who received their degrees from irregular schools.

Some historians have judged Zakrzewska harshly for this, seeing her alliance with the orthodox profession as a failure on her part to show support for other women. Others have viewed her rejection of alternative medical practices, coupled with her attack on women's sympathetic natures, as predominantly strategic.[41] But these interpretations fail to acknowledge Zakrzewska's own perception of her move as radical, not strategic or conciliatory. Zakrzewska did not embrace orthodox medicine because she believed women would succeed only if they excelled in a man's world; she embraced it both because she rejected the gendering of that world and because it came closest to embodying the principles of science in which she believed. To be sure, Zakrzewska was not ignorant of the rhetorical power of laying claim to science and to orthodoxy, but when she set out to create a hospital that would best advance the cause of women physicians, she was also operating from a conviction that training in orthodox scientific medicine produced the best physicians: ones who could think for themselves, make their own deductions, and provide the truest and thus most humane care. In short, for Zakrzewska, science and orthodox medicine went hand in hand with moral actions and radical politics.

• • •

Zakrzewska's story thus draws our attention to the multiple meanings of science in the nineteenth century and to how one very public woman embraced a particular view of science as democratic and revolutionary in order to try to bring about radical change in gender relationships.[42] It is also a story that provides greater insight into the challenges women physicians faced as the century progressed and the practice of medicine underwent substantial changes. When Zakrzewska first began practicing medicine, medical care still took place largely in the home; the medical instruments available to physicians amounted to little more than forceps, microscopes, and thermometers; Louis Pasteur had not yet spoken of the germ theory; Joseph Lister had not yet developed antiseptic techniques; and no one had yet linked microbial agents with specific infectious diseases. By the time Zakrzewska began pulling back from hospital affairs in the early 1890s, shortly after she turned sixty years old, the world of medicine looked radically different. Bacteriology was a rapidly expanding field, the search for vaccines and antimicrobial agents was well under way, asepsis had already replaced antisepsis, new instruments were constantly being invented (the X-ray would soon be developed), and at least the larger hospitals were building laboratories and affiliating with elite medical schools.[43]

Scholars of women in medicine have long emphasized the difficulties that arose for women physicians as a result of these changes. In addition to the logistical problems of financing an ever longer and more expensive period of training, women had to struggle with the new image of a medical world that glorified everything exact and scientific while ignoring the caring, more human side of medicine.[44] This posed, of course, less of a problem for Zakrzewska, who had never embraced a notion of women as uniquely caring. Thus, she experienced little, if any, conflict between an image of herself as a woman and the emerging model of the physician-scientist. Indeed, given her lifelong advocacy of the natural sciences, one might very well have expected her to be among the loudest proponents of the changes taking place.

That was not, however, the case. Instead, by the 1880s Zakrzewska was voicing deep reservations, saving her harshest words for what seemed to her an obsession with bacteriology, gynecologic surgery, and the tendency to view disease as nothing more than the pathophysiological changes of the body. In their stead, she promoted prevention, hygiene, and moral education, thus embracing an older style of medical practice that many, in the last decades of the century, gendered female and contrasted with masculine practices located in the laboratory and the surgical theater.

It is tempting to see Zakrzewska's apparent change of heart as evidence of her move toward the notion of unique female traits, the sign of a mature woman who no longer needed to prove to men that she could function in their world. This is not the interpretation that I present in this book. Zakrzewska may have shortened the distance between herself and those who argued that women had a unique contribution to make to the reform of society, but she did so without couching her criticisms of modern medical practices in gendered terms. Most important, she did so without abandoning her staunch advocacy of science, rationality, or materialism. Central to her vision of good medical practice remained the scientifically trained physician, who had been taught how to dissect problems in order to best guide her or his patient toward recovery. At a time, however, when so many promoted the laboratory as the final arbiter in medical decision making, Zakrzewska's vision appeared to look backward rather than forward, no longer finding much resonance among the young physicians coming of age.

· · ·

In the end, Zakrzewska's life stands as a reminder of the problems inherent in reifying certain attributes as feminine or masculine, for inevitably one ends up with individuals who must be classified as "others" when they fail to fit the models being proposed. The story I tell is not, however, intended to raise doubts that the values associated with science—rationality, precision, objectivity—were gendered masculine at the time. They most definitely were. Over the past decades, feminist scholars have demonstrated convincingly that the *image* of the modern scientific method was and to a great extent remains masculine and that this gendering of science came about through a long historical process. They have also shown how the masculinization of science functioned to exclude women from professional scientific activity by setting up a contrast between the rigors of scientific thinking and appropriate feminine behavior.[45] But feminist scholars have also been emphasizing that as science became identified as a masculine activity, what it meant to be male and female was being redefined as well.[46] The huge amount of ink spilled in the nineteenth century proclaiming women's inability to engage in scientific activity testifies to the instability of these categories and the anxiety generated by the difficulty of fixing in place the boundaries of a moving target. But if the instability caused anxiety for some, it opened up possibilities for others, allowing individuals like Zakrzewska to embrace and perform alternative positions. This book is about Zakrzewska's twin battles against the gendering of science and the restrictive definitions of her gender; it is also about why those battles mattered in the past and continue to matter today.

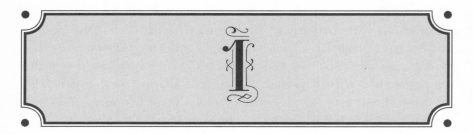

Aspiring Bourgeoisie

Marie Elizabeth Zakrzewska was born at home with the help of a midwife in 1829. At the time of her birth, her father, Martin Ludwig Zakrzewski, earned a modest salary as a quartermaster in the Prussian army; her mother, Caroline Fredericke née Urban, was a housewife. Over the next eighteen years, her mother would give birth to seven more children, one of them stillborn. Struggling to provide for their growing family, the Zakrzewskis decided that they could no longer manage on a single income. Caroline Fredericke thus entered the workforce when Marie was just six years old, first as a trader in porcelain and then, drawing on her own experiences with childbirth, as a midwife. Martin Ludwig's eventual move into a civilian position in the Prussian Ministry of Culture brought the family some financial relief, but only with the additional income Caroline Fredericke provided were they able to maintain a lifestyle that would count them among the newly emerging German bourgeoisie.[1]

And this was something to which they very much aspired. To belong to this class marked one as a member of the new elite.[2] Largely a product of legal, educational, and administrative reforms that were intensified following Germany's devastating defeat at the hands of Napoleon in 1806, the *Bildungsbürgertum* (urban educated elite) came to embody the values that would supposedly transform a rigid absolutist system based on estates into a civil society held together by a constitution. These values included, among others, hard work and industriousness, faith in rationality and the legal system, and the importance of education and economic security. For many men of Martin Ludwig's generation a position in the rapidly expanding Prussian civil service came to be seen as the most promising way to gain entry into this new social elite. As one contemporary later commented, by the 1820s "everyone looked to the state for his advancement."[3]

The Zakrzewskis struggled throughout their lives, however, to differentiate their lifestyle from that of a "wage laborer" and to secure for their family membership in the "middling" bourgeoisie.[4] Martin Ludwig's inability to achieve the economic security that would have guaranteed at least minimum standards of education for all his children posed one threat to their membership in this class; Caroline Fredericke's entry into the workplace posed another. The bourgeois lifestyle, in theory if not in practice, was predicated on a sharp separation between the female, reproductive, private sphere of the home and the male, productive, public sphere of employment. Like the bourgeoisie itself, this reconfiguring of social space was relatively new, developed as a means of excluding women from a political transformation designed to grant greater rights to men. The most vocal ideologues of the new bourgeois lifestyle coupled a theory of sexual difference grounded in nature with a redefinition of the family as the "natural" expression of such differences. Thus, according to one encyclopedia author in 1848, women's greater "dependence, uncertainty, sacrifice, [and] sympathy" led them "naturally" to confine their labors to the home, providing a moral education for their children and a safe haven for their husbands. Men, in contrast, were marked by "self-confidence, independence, power and energy, completeness, [and] antagonism," traits that sent them catapulting out into public spaces to engage in productive work.[5]

When Caroline Fredericke left the privacy of her home to enter the workforce, she thus broke with the ideal in a dramatic way. Other bourgeois women may have entered public spaces, extending their new position as moral guardians of their families by volunteering in religious or social welfare organizations, but it was another thing entirely to seek employment. Added to this, midwives traditionally came from the lower classes. For women of the middle classes who, in the early nineteenth century, needed to support themselves, the most respectable options were teaching or hiring oneself out as a governess, although these occupations were deemed appropriate for single women alone. Despite government efforts to make midwifery more attractive for "cultivated women," the Zakrzewskis struggled with the knowledge that Caroline Fredericke's status as a working woman threatened to collapse the distance separating them from the working and artisan classes.[6]

Many of the values and beliefs Marie Zakrzewska espoused as an adult reveal her deep roots in the bourgeois culture of mid-nineteenth-century Germany. These include everything from her work ethic to her embrace of rationality and secularism, her desire for independence and economic security, her high estimation of formal schooling, and her awareness of her social class. Yet Zakrzewska also broke sharply with this culture in significant ways, most directly by challenging the sexual division of labor. She would, for one, follow directly in her mother's footsteps by entering the workforce as a midwife and then—because she aspired to a position of greater esteem—as a physician and hospital director. She thus defined her life in and around public spaces, ensuring that she would have the economic security that always seemed to elude her parents. She would not, however, try to combine this with marriage and children. Instead, rejecting entirely the rigid structure of the bourgeois family, she would fashion for herself an alternative family structure made up of close friends and siblings. Finally, Zakrzewska would also claim for herself, as a woman, traits such as rationality and assertiveness, thus subverting the traditional gendering of mental and moral attributes and challenging those around her to rethink the categories that functioned to exclude women from public spaces. In all, Zakrzewska both drew on and rebelled against the environment in which she had been raised, and it is to her family background that we now turn.

· · ·

Zakrzewska's family history on her father's side is wrapped up as much in legend as in reality for the period prior to the early nineteenth century. The legend, first told in a memoir published one year after Zakrzewska's death, is attributed to one of her brothers—most likely Herman—who apparently traced the name Zakrzewski back to 911 to an aristocratic Polish family, which was counted among the "republican families of agitators." The family's fortunes, however, like those of all Polish nobility, changed in the late eighteenth century. In the aftermath of the territorial battles between Prussia, Russia, and Austria, which led to Poland's eventual disappearance from the European map, the Zakrzewskis lost their property to the Russians. Zakrzewska's great-grandfather fell on the battlefield defending his land, while her great-grandmother and several other family members died in the castle fire. Her grandparents, however, escaped to Prussia, where her grandfather, reputedly a liberal thinker, converted to Protestantism, leaving her grandmother alone in the family to defend the Catholic faith.[7]

One of the difficulties in verifying this story is the lack of documents from the Middle Ages that would allow one to trace the family name back to 911.[8] But whether the details of this story are accurate or not, what Herman Zakrzewski did was to link his family to two themes that assumed great importance in his sister's life: political radicalism and anti-Catholicism. By claiming that the Zakrzewskis were "republican . . . agitators," the brother was both positioning the family among the Polish nobility and highlighting the peculiar role the nobility played in Polish history—since at least the sixteenth century, it had ruled jointly with the monarch, promoting ideas of individual freedom, civil liberty, and, among a radical fringe, political anarchism. Thus in contrast to the absolutist systems that had started taking shape in Russia, Prussia, and France in the late seventeenth century, and even in comparison with England's consti-tutional monarchy, Poland enjoyed what one historian has termed a "monar-chical republic."[9] Emphasizing these Polish roots permitted Herman, more-over, to drive a wedge between his family and the imperialism and militarism that were flourishing in Germany at the time of his sister's death in 1902.

The story does not, however, simply foreground the Zakrzewskis' credentials as political radicals; it also links this radicalism to the grandfather's conver-sion to Protestantism, thus feeding upon anti-Catholic sentiments—powerful throughout the long nineteenth century—that cast members of this faith as backward, uneducated, superstitious, and intolerant while positioning Protes-tants as cultured, educated, and open-minded.[10] Zakrzewska, her brother knew, had early in life taken this one more step and turned her back on all religion, but she had always reserved her most caustic remarks for the practices of the Ro-man Catholic Church, which she had repeatedly cast as the absolute antithesis of all that was good and humane.

We may not be able to fully separate fact from embellishment in this legend, but since Marie was raised in the Protestant faith, there is a good chance that her grandfather did convert, joining many at the time who were inspired less by a sudden religious awakening than by a desire to embrace a growing secular culture more closely associated with Protestantism than with Catholicism. This would also fit with her grandfather's decision to become an elementary school teacher in 1807, immediately following a lengthy service in the Prussian army.[11] Although elementary schools remained denominational and teaching cannot, therefore, be seen as antireligious in any way, in the early nineteenth century the schools did come more squarely under the jurisdiction of the state, which sup-ported a secularizing trend.[12]

Zakrzewska's grandfather began his teaching career just as the government was implementing massive reforms designed to transform Prussian society following the army's humiliating defeat in 1806. Inspired largely by the Prussian minister of education and culture, Wilhelm von Humboldt, these reforms had as their goal the creation of a unified system of education that would awaken in each child an independent and creative spirit. Such changes necessitated more qualified teachers, and Zakrzewska's grandfather benefited as the government raised educational standards and transformed the position of schoolmaster into a public office, financed by the state.[13]

Enjoying greater economic security and social standing than their predecessors, the new schoolteachers were benefiting from their loose association with the newly emerging *Bildungsbürgertum*. Official acknowledgment of this social group's power can be linked to the creation of a new legal estate in the Prussian General Legal Code of 1794, which identified wealthy merchants, civil servants, academics, and industrialists as a new elite whose status derived from their advanced degrees. Entitled to such privileges as a reduction in or "exemption" from military duty, the so-called exempt persons (*Eximierte*) signaled the state's formal recognition that an individual who possessed an advanced education, or *Bildung*, deserved certain privileges and powers previously reserved for individuals of noble birth.[14] Elementary school teachers may not yet have belonged to this new elite—they neither possessed university degrees nor were counted among the *Eximierte*—but they had become civil servants with a public role that involved educating the nation's youth. If they were not yet considered members of the burgeoning *Bildungsbürgertum*, this did not mean that they could not aspire to belong one day or to pass on these aspirations to their children and grandchildren.

This is what Zakrzewska's grandfather seems to have done with his eldest son, who was born on St. Martin's Day, 11 November 1802. As a young man, Martin Ludwig set his sights on a civil service position, craving the security and opportunity for social mobility that such a position offered. Given Zakrzewska's later characterization of her father as a political liberal, he may also have been inspired by the rhetoric of the Prussian reformers, who had started out with a vision of a state government more responsive to the needs of the people. They may not have favored participatory politics, but many still encouraged legislation that promoted economic and social emancipation, religious toleration, and freedom of thought.[15]

The path to the civil service through the university being closed to him for economic reasons—schoolteachers may have been better off than their predecessors, but their salaries were still low[16]—Martin Ludwig pursued an alternative strategy for securing a government position: at the age of sixteen he began an unpaid four-year internship in the regional and municipal court system in the town of Mewe, with the intent, upon completion of his training, of entering the military and, ultimately, the civil service. That he could afford such an internship suggests that his parents, although perhaps too poor to send him to a good school, still had sufficient means to support a grown son for an extended period of time. It also suggests that the education he received was not of such a poor quality—indeed, he managed to learn some Latin—since the court system considered it sufficient to qualify him to study the legal and admin-istrative aspects of running a government.[17] With the skills he thus acquired, he entered military service in October 1822 as a hussar in the army's Second Cavalry Regiment, expecting after nine years of obligatory service to lay claim to a position in the civilian government.

Zakrzewski seems to have done well in the army, having advanced by 1830 to quartermaster with a yearly salary of 360 taler. At this point, he began inquiring about positions in the civilian sector, for his obligatory service was to end the following year. His requests, however, were initially turned down, presumably because no position was available.[18] In her autobiographical sketch, Marie would later claim that her father had been dismissed "from his position as military officer" because of his political views, but there is no evidence to sup-port this claim.[19] On the contrary, her father was even promoted to second lieutenant in 1836. He did, however, begin to suspect that it "takes, above all, effective protection" to secure a position in the civilian government.[20] Rhetoric to the contrary, Zakrzewski was beginning to realize that connections, rather than talent, determined who would end up in the service of the state.

By the mid-1830s, Zakrzewski had several pressing reasons for wishing to improve his situation. His health had begun to fail; indeed, he would be plagued by health problems throughout his career.[21] But the most important reason was that he had married in 1828, and he and his wife, Caroline Fredericke, were finding it increasingly difficult to support their ever growing family. Marie had been born in 1829, and in the ensuing five years, Caroline Fredericke had had four more pregnancies. One had ended in a stillbirth, but the other three, Sophie, Anna, and Herman, had all survived.[22] Three hundred and sixty taler a year was not an insignificant salary—it would have been the rare artisan who would have made this much in a year—but in addition to having a large family, the Zakrzewskis had certain expectations about the quality of life they wished to maintain, and this included above all ensuring that their children would attend good schools.[23] It was during Martin Ludwig's struggles to secure a position in the civilian government that Caroline Fredericke first entered the workforce. Although she would not pursue her training in midwifery until 1839, she was, if one accepts family lore, carrying on a family tradition when she finally chose that path.

As in Zakrzewska's paternal line, all we know about her mother's side of the family stems from the story Herman Zakrzewski told one year following his sister's death. However, where political radicalism had shaped his account of his father's family, medicine was now the central theme; and where he had used his father's Polish roots to erase any connection to Germany, he now focused on his mother's Gypsy heritage. Accordingly, his great-great grandfather, a member of the Gypsy tribe of the Lombardi family, had joined Frederick the Great's army as a surgeon during the Seven Years' War. From this moment on through to Marie's decision to become a physician, someone in each generation had practiced a healing art. Her great-grandmother and namesake, Marie Elizabeth Sauer, "a Gypsy Queen of the Lombardi family," had learned surgery from her father and worked as his assistant during the war. She was said to have saved the life of another member of their Gypsy tribe, a Captain Urban, by removing a bullet that had lodged in his chest. They eventually fell in love and married, bringing nine children into the world, all of whom were "of unusual size, the daughters almost six feet tall, with hair flowing down to their feet, the sons seven feet tall, of perfect stature."[24] The middle child, Zakrzewska's grandmother, became a veterinary surgeon and married another Urban, most likely a distant relative. They had three daughters, one of whom was Caroline Fredericke.

Even more than the story about the Zakrzewskis, this one seems apocryphal, especially with its six- and seven-foot Gypsy ancestors. Gypsies, who had first migrated from northwest India at the beginning of the previous millennium, were so feared and despised in eighteenth-century Germany that it is doubtful Zakrzewska's ancestors, even if they had stemmed from Gypsies, would have been allowed to join the Prussian army had their membership in this group been self-evident.[25] In Herman's story, however, the emphasis on a people known for their nomadic culture, alternative lifestyle, and persecuted status functioned not only to erase his family's Germanness (as had his focus on his paternal Polish roots) but also to provide a context for understanding his sister's unusual life choices, the most important of which was her refusal to embrace a traditional family structure. According to this story, moreover, Zakrzewska stood at the head of a long line of women who lived their lives challenging gender norms, whether through their physical stature, their activities as surgeons, or their preference for travel and adventure over the home. Finally, both Zakrzewska's and her mother's decisions to practice a healing art seem almost predetermined, driven by a family history of women (and some men) entering the world of medicine.

Unfortunately, we know next to nothing about Caroline Fredericke's childhood other than the likelihood that she grew up in Prenzlau, about a hundred miles north of Berlin, where her father worked as a superintendent of an almshouse.[26] It is certainly possible that this setting stimulated her interest in midwifery, but whether she felt drawn to this line of work or not, it is highly unlikely that she relished the idea of pursuing this career in the mid-1830s. With four small children at home the thought of becoming a midwife must have felt overwhelming. Not only did the training course require time and money, but the work was also arduous. Added to this, as we have already mentioned, midwives were usually of lower-class origin. Their work, moreover, necessarily took them out into the streets, often at night and frequently unchaperoned. This must have produced anxieties, particularly as the ideology of separate spheres gained force and women who went out in public alone risked being viewed as prostitutes.[27]

Thus Caroline Fredericke's first attempt at earning money led her to try her hand at trading porcelain, hoping, most likely, to sidestep some of these problems by working out of her home. But the business did not pan out, and the Zakrzewskis ended up in debt. Only at this point did Caroline Fredericke apply to the school of midwifery at the Berlin Charité hospital, but as Martin Ludwig later commented, "here, too, we were not blessed with luck."[28] Four years in a row she applied, and four times she was turned down. In the midst of all this, she also gave birth to their fifth child, a daughter they named Wilhelmine (Minna), and the Zakrzewskis' financial situation worsened.[29] Perhaps they should not have been surprised by the stiff competition for the midwifery school: it accepted only two pupils each year from the city of Berlin (another twenty-eight came from the larger regional district of Potsdam). But what troubled the Zakrzewskis most was that here, once again, connections seemed to be necessary. Indeed, when Martin Ludwig finally succeeded in securing a civilian position in 1837, it was because of the interventions of Adalbert von Ladenberg, an adviser in the Ministry of Culture and soon to become director of educational affairs. This connection may very well have been responsible for Caroline Fredericke's acceptance to the school of midwifery two years later.[30] Obviously, the Zakrzewskis were not above using protection when they could.

The Zakrzewskis thus went into debt to hire a servant to help out at home, and in the fall of 1839 Caroline Fredericke began her training. Most of the women in her class signed up for a sixteen-week course, lasting from mid-October until mid-March, at which time they took their licensing examinations. The two women from Berlin, however, had a more rigorous course to follow. Believing that city midwives required more extensive training than those who practiced in rural areas, government officials had stipulated that the Berlin pupils had to attend the midwifery course two years in a row, acting as assistants to the instructor during the second year. They were also required to spend the intervening summer in the hospital, helping out in the obstetrics wards. Thus, from October 1839 until March 1841, Caroline Fredericke spent her days—and some nights—at the Charité, acquiring the skills that would allow her to become a licensed midwife.[31]

In the spring of 1841, Caroline Fredericke passed her examinations and was licensed by the state to practice midwifery.[32] She had pursued this path to help with the family's finances, especially the expense of the children's education, but in the first few years following her graduation the Zakrzewskis' situation did not improve.[33] Caroline Fredericke and her husband had gone further into debt to pay for her books, instruments, examinations, and license as well as for the servant to watch their children. To make matters worse, the government had assigned her to the "bleakest and poorest" section of the city, where most individuals had difficulty paying a midwife for her services. Midwives, like physicians, surgeons, and apothecaries, had little choice in these matters. Government officials had long ago exerted control over the distribution of health care practitioners, trying to prevent their concentration in the wealthier sections of the city. As it turned out, the Zakrzewskis were surprised by Caroline Fredericke's assignment. They had already moved to a better part of town in anticipation of an assignment to that district and had even signed a new lease (on Stralauer Street). Why they would have expected this is unclear, but when Caroline Fredericke was told that she would be practicing instead near the Hamburg gate, the family had to move again, and the Zakrzewskis were caught paying rent on two apartments. It seemed that no matter how hard they tried to improve their financial standing, things just kept spiraling out of control.[34]

Caroline Fredericke was not, however, someone who accepted her situation without a fight. She may not have been able to alter her assignment, but when she realized that some of her financial woes stemmed from the fact that swaddling women (*Wickelfrauen*) were taking away business by illegally attending women in labor, she became involved in a turf battle that pitted the city's midwives against practicing obstetricians, medical students, and even the professor of obstetrics at the University of Berlin. The problem was that swaddling women, who trained as physicians' assistants in the university's obstetrics clinic, were neither permitted nor licensed by the state to handle deliveries themselves. Indeed, state law stipulated that obstetricians, when called to a laboring woman, had to perform the delivery themselves or entrust it to a licensed midwife. What annoyed Caroline Fredericke and other midwives was that physicians frequently ignored this ruling and left the delivery to a swaddling woman while they visited other patients. Even worse, medical students, who themselves were not yet qualified to perform deliveries, frequently engaged swaddling women when, as part of their university training, they went to the homes of the poor to offer medical assistance and practice their skills. Most aggrieved by this practice, Caroline Fredericke and her cohorts directed their complaints at the practices of Dietrich Wilhelm Heinrich Busch, professor of obstetrics at the University of Berlin. They insisted that medical students be required to follow the law and take along either an obstetrician or a licensed midwife when they attended women in childbirth. Their demands did not go unheeded. The police passed on a warning to Professor Busch that he cease such practices immediately. Although it took years before this problem was fully resolved, Caroline Fredericke did pick up some cases as a result.[35]

Caroline Fredericke's willingness to fight for her rights, even to challenge a university professor, must have had an enormous impact on Zakrzewska, who would fight her own battles with government officials when she assumed the position of head midwife at the Charité later in the decade. Zakrzewska does not, however, discuss this specific incident in her autobiography, other than to write approvingly of the steps the government took in the nineteenth century to regulate, and thus to improve, the training and status of the midwife.[36] However critical she may have been of the Prussian state, she must have recognized that her mother had benefited from the protection the government provided through the law, protection that worked in two directions by staving off competition both from above and from below. Indeed, Zakrzewska inherited from her mother not only a willingness to challenge authority but also an arrogance toward those who acquired their knowledge through unofficial channels and thus lacked the imprimatur of the state (or whatever body had the authority to grant such privileges). Throughout her life, she would look favorably upon the official signs and symbols that distinguished the so-called qualified from the so-called unqualified, whether they came in the form of university degrees, government licensing, or membership in exclusive organizations. Her own battle against unorthodox physicians, which she waged with great determination in the 1870s and 1880s, must be understood in this light.[37]

Caroline Fredericke's victory against Professor Busch may have brought her satisfaction, but her family's financial situation did not improve, and in some ways it worsened. The civilian position her husband had finally landed in 1837 had actually come with a reduction in salary from thirty to twenty-five taler a month. The only reason the Zakrzewskis had been able to survive this cut in pay was that Martin Ludwig had been receiving a small disability pension from the military of eight taler per month. But one year after his promotion the military informed him that he would need to give up his pension, since its official policy was to terminate a veteran's pension six months after he began earning a fixed income.[38] Although Zakrzewski requested repeatedly that an exception be made, the War Ministry not only refused but also insisted that he refund the money he had drawn in the interim. Small wonder that Caroline Fredericke's assignment to one of the poorest neighborhoods in Berlin made the Zakrzewskis feel desperate. By the summer of 1841, Martin Ludwig was writing impassioned letters to the state minister, pleading for any help at all—a raise, a loan, or a gift—just anything to help him gain control over his skyrocketing debts. Drawing as much attention as he could to the threat these financial burdens posed to his lifestyle, he complained bitterly that his living standard could no longer be considered even that of a "modest bourgeois [Bürger] but rather of a wage laborer."[39]

There is no reason to doubt the sincerity of Zakrzewski's laments, but we also need to bear in mind that he was rehearsing a script that he suspected would fall on sympathetic ears. Government ministers were themselves interested in ensuring that members of the civil service maintain a certain image, for it reflected well on the government as a whole. Martin Ludwig was speaking the correct language, emphasizing their shared values and deploring his inability to create a life for himself and his family that would bestow honor on the government as well. Thus, throughout the years he received small gifts of twenty-five to thirty taler or advances on his salary. Moreover, the combination of his connections and his complaints landed him a promotion in August 1841 to secretary in the Privy Chancellery of the Ministry of Culture at an annual salary of five hundred taler. This marked a turning point in the Zakrzewski household, and for at least a few years the family was able to breathe more easily. By the fall of 1842, Martin

Ludwig was thanking the state minister for his "current contentedness, health, honor and domestic happiness."[40]

It is significant that this promotion did not result in Caroline Fredericke's remaining at home with her children, not even following the birth of their sixth child, Rosalia, in 1844 or the birth of their seventh (a boy, who does not seem to have survived) in 1847. Although we do not know for certain why she continued to work, chances are once again that this was not by choice. Following her last pregnancy, Caroline Fredericke had become ill, apparently suffering from dropsy (a condition similar to edema), but she had been able to remain at home only three weeks before the family's financial situation required that she return to her midwifery practice. The Zakrzewskis seemed, in fact, to be trapped between two incompatible desires for their family. While they yearned to maintain a bourgeois lifestyle, they showed no inclination to limit their family size, as other members of this social group had begun to do. Forced to choose between maintaining separate spheres, which would mean a decline in their standard of living, and blurring the separation between public and private, which would allow them to pay for a decent apartment and a good education for their children, the Zakrzewskis chose the latter.[41]

Indeed, much of the reason Caroline Fredericke worked was to allow the Zakrzewskis to send their children to better schools.[42] Had they been willing for their children to receive a basic education, their expenses would have been considerably lower. But the reformed Prussian school system, despite its goal of providing a universal national system of education, was not classless, and the Zakrzewskis did not wish to see their children follow the path of the vast majority, who attended the elementary schools until only the age of thirteen or fourteen. After this they either entered the workforce, sought an apprenticeship, or pursued some form of technical training. Girls from a more privileged background tended to leave the *Volkschule* after three or four years (around the age of eight) in order to attend private ladies' seminaries, which were designed primarily to prepare girls for running a household. This is where the Zakrzewskis sent their daughters, starting with Marie.[43]

For their son, Herman, the Zakrzewskis had other options. He could either go to one of the reformed classical secondary schools, where he would follow a curriculum that emphasized Latin, Greek, and the classics, or he could attend one of the newly founded nonclassical secondary schools (*höhere Bürgerschulen* or *Realschulen*), which focused on the so-called *Realwissenschaften*—subjects such as mathematics, natural science, history, and the modern languages, which, in certain German educational circles, had come to count as "modern."[44] They chose the latter and in doing so positioned themselves, whether intentionally or not, on one side of a fierce pedagogical battle that was waging at the time between defenders of a classical education and those who believed Latin and Greek were becoming increasingly anachronistic in a world slowly dominated by railroads, steamships, and power-driven mills. The Zakrzewskis' choice thus signaled their attraction to a particular vision of progress, and it was one that embraced rather than feared the social and economic changes that had been slowly transforming the German landscape over the previous few decades.[45] Zakrzewska would later announce her own embrace of this vision by declaring "history, geography and arithmetic" to be her "favorite studies," even though it is doubtful that she received much introduction to any of these subjects in the all-girls' seminary she attended.[46]

With five school-age children at home in the mid-1840s, the Zakrzewskis' decision to give their children a more privileged education was costing them about seventy-five taler per year.[47] Marie and Anna had, moreover, reached the age at which they needed to be confirmed in the church, and their father estimated that between the purchase of clothing, the fee to the priest, and other expenses, this would run one hundred taler. (Marie would later claim that her parents were "Rationalists" and did not belong to any church, but at the very least her parents understood the need to keep up appearances.)[48] By 1847, whatever relief the family had felt five years earlier was no longer palpable. "I'm a poor man," Zakrzewski wrote the state minister; "I am in debt to the grocer, the baker, the doctor and the midwife."[49] In addition, that spring Marie began to suffer from rheumatism, an illness that worsened as the year progressed and was expensive to treat. All of this must have been particularly frightening to Martin Ludwig, whose own health was fragile enough that he frequently missed work. Indeed, ever since his dismissal from the military he had suffered from terrible "catarrhs" and "nerve fevers" that kept him home for weeks and some-times months at a time.[50]

Zakrzewski's fears and frustrations appear to have found a brief outlet, how-ever, for in the early months of 1848 political protests began taking place all over Europe, and he ended up getting involved. The protesters, a mixed group that included peasant farmers, artisans, factory workers, professors, lawyers, and civil servants, sported a diverse array of grievances: some were cold and hungry; others wished to limit the power of the nobility and the king through the establishment of a constitutional monarchy; yet others wanted nothing less than the creation of a democratic republic. These differences would eventually render the reform movement ineffectual, but in the early months of the revolution this was not yet evident.[51] It certainly was not clear on 18 March, when Berliners put flowers in their hats and took to the streets to celebrate King Frederick William IV's stated willingness to work with reformers to draft a constitution for the state of Prussia. Events soon took a tragic turn, however, when the troops who were guarding the king's palace reacted nervously to the ever growing crowd and fired some shots, killing a number of civilians. The street battles that ensued were not subdued until the king agreed to put a liberal ministry in place. For the next six months it seemed to many that true change was going to take place.[52]

Given Zakrzewska's later insistence that her father had been persecuted by the Prussian government, his involvement in the revolutionary events of 1848 is worthy of note. Nevertheless, the exact nature of his participation is difficult to pin down. The government later investigated whether he had participated in the events on 18 March, but it was unable to come to any conclusion. In contrast, there is no question that he joined, at least briefly, the people's militia, which was founded in the aftermath of the shootings to assume many of the responsibilities previously held by the military troops. Moreover, in mid-May, Martin Ludwig's name was put forth as the democratic party's candidate in elections for a platoon commander in the militia.[53] He lost the election, but this indicates a certain level of engagement on his part with left-wing politics. The democratic unions that were cropping up all over Germany in the late spring of 1848 were taking form because of a growing disillusionment among their members with the moderate course of political reform. They feared a loss of their dream to create a radical democracy based on a constitution that would guarantee rights and representation to all (at least, to all men).[54]

The democrats' wishes, however, were not heeded. Indeed, by the fall of 1848, the king was already able to reinstate a decidedly conservative ministry. Although he accepted a constitution in December, he managed by the following spring to disregard any efforts at universal suffrage. Instead, he instituted the famous Three Class suffrage system, which all but guaranteed that power would remain unevenly distributed, with the lion's share resting in the hands of the top 5 percent of the electorate.[55] Then, in the early spring of 1850, the government began its investigations into the political activities of its subjects. Zakrzewski did not escape scrutiny. An "extract" submitted to the ministry and placed in his personnel file cited three events that linked him to the democratic party: he was the party's candidate during the elections for a local militia; he attended a ball in February 1850 put on by the democratic party; and he was present on the streets of Berlin on 18 March "with a flower in his hat," a charge, as previously noted, that was eventually dropped.[56]

At first, Zakrzewski denied everything, but he ultimately chose a different strategy that emphasized both his ignorance and his loyalty. He claimed, for example, that he had been unaware of the political nature of the ball he had attended. As for the elections, he contended that he had been so taken by surprise when his name had been put forth as the democratic party's delegate to the elections for a people's militia that he had not thought to recuse himself. But he insisted that although he had expressed his pleasure at being nominated and had acknowledged that he was "a friend of the people," he had added: "But I obey, honor and love the King just as much, and only in this sense will I cast my vote."[57]

Zakrzewski's entire response reads like a prepared script, as well it may have been. The fact that he had begun the day by denying everything only to recant later on and confess his mistakes suggests that he may have received some coaching. If so, odds are that the advice came from von Ladenberg, who had been "protecting" Zakrzewski for more than a decade and who had assumed the position of minister of culture in 1848.[58] Why Zakrzewski changed his tune is not, however, entirely clear. More than likely, he had grown fearful that he might lose his position in the civil service, but he may also have become critical of the revolutionary uprisings as they became increasingly radical. If it was the latter, he would not have been alone. A significant number of dissatisfied civil servants had taken to the streets in the early days of the revolution, but as the revolution came to be marked by more popular and spontaneous expressions of violence, and as the focus of these violent outbreaks came to rest more on eradicating social and economic misery than on establishing a constitutional democracy, many among the middle class pulled back.[59] Whether this describes Zakrzewski is unknown, but whatever his motivations, it turned out to be a smart move to cast his actions as mistakes. One day after submitting his confession, he was reprimanded and forgiven. The government official who presided over the case seemed to be following his own script when he opened his report by accepting Zakrzewski's "pronounced assurances of [his] true and patriotic sentiments." Still, he held Zakrzewski responsible for the unfortunate events that followed, expressing his disbelief that anyone could have been fully ignorant of the political nature of the events that occurred in the city in the

spring of 1848 and, consequently, blaming Zakrzewski for giving "the appearance of being in agreement with the views of [the democratic] party." Appearances, in other words, mattered, although certainly not as much as actions.
For his transgressions, Zakrzewski was required to approve and sign the report,
which included a promise that in the future "he would everywhere, including
outside of his office, prove himself to be a true servant of his King."[60]

In her autobiographical sketch, Zakrzewska did not directly address her
father's interrogation by the police in June 1850. Her comments were of a more
general nature and simply characterized him as someone who "would not
consent to endure wrong and imposition."[61] She also claimed that he, "who
held liberal opinions and was of an impetuous temperament, manifested some
revolutionary tendencies, which drew upon him the displeasure of the government; and caused his dismissal, with a very small pension, from his position as
military officer. This involved us in great pecuniary difficulties; for our family
was large, and my father's income too small to supply the most necessary wants;
while to obtain other occupation was for the time out of the question."[62]

In this passage Zakrzewska appears to be drawing on several different events,
collapsing them into one story as though they had occurred at the same time
and creating, as a result, an inaccurate picture. We have, for example, already
seen that her father was never dismissed from the military; nor was he ever
unemployed. Instead, he had remained in the military until he had been guaranteed a civilian position. Indeed, a military attest, placed in his file at the time
of his departure, stated that he had "conducted himself in an exemplary fashion" throughout his service.[63] It is true that he lost his military pension, but that
was because of a government ruling that canceled the pension once a person's
salary exceeded a specified amount, not because of any political persecution.
Only in the aftermath of the revolutionary events of 1848 was he subjected to
any harassment, but even here, disturbing and frightening as this experience
may have been, it was resolved without any concrete consequences for the
family. Zakrzewski was forced to confess and repent, an action that allowed the
government to save face and Zakrzewski to keep his job. Whatever political
views he may have shared with his daughter within the confines of their own
home, there is very little evidence that he ever suffered professionally because
of them.

This is not to say that personal alliances and petty intrigues did not affect
Zakrzewski's career. He may very well have enjoyed more protection under
certain ministries than others. This is also not to deny his democratic sympa-

thies. Later in life, Zakrzewska claimed her father had introduced her to the writings of Karl Heinzen, a radical republican and political journalist who would be forced to flee Germany in 1850 as a consequence of the failed uprisings and who would eventually become part of her alternative family in America.[64] Still, whatever Zakrzewski's political sympathies may have been, for most of his career he showed himself to be anything but radical. Instead, he worked hard to succeed within the Prussian civil service system, and in public and in his official letters he consistently presented himself as an obedient servant of the state. Not only did he declare himself to be a member of the Protestant Church when he was sworn into his new position in the Privy Chancellery in 1841, and not only did he make sure his daughters were confirmed in the church, but he repeatedly assured his superiors that he was raising his children to be of value to the "King, the State and the Magistracy [König, Staat und Obrigkeit]."[65] Even if we consider that Zakrzewski may have done this solely for the purpose of appearances, the point is that he performed according to expectations, aware that movement up through the ranks of the Prussian civil service provided him with perhaps his only chance of improving his own situation and, by extension, that of his family.

Zakrzewska's misrepresentation of her father in her autobiographical sketch cannot easily be ascribed to the usual tricks of memory, which often lead one to recall events in a distorted fashion. True, she may have been only eight years old when her father lost his military pension, but she was twenty-one when he was interrogated by the police. Moreover, she penned the autobiographical sketch just nine years later. As I argue later in this book, there can be no question that Zakrzewska's autobiography was a highly constructed text, designed more as a vehicle for creating a certain image of herself at a critical point in her career than as an accurate account of her childhood. In the case of her father, by portraying him as both a radical and a victim of persecution, she accomplished several things: she grounded her own radicalism in her family history; she strengthened her diatribe against the authoritarian Prussian government; and she may very well have given her father the life he wished he could have led had he not had a large family to support. She may also have given herself the father she wished she had had.[66]

Unfortunately, the only document Zakrzewska left that describes her experiences during the first twenty years of her life is this autobiographical sketch, and it must be used with great caution. The story surrounding her father's persecution is just one case in point. In other examples, the problem is less one of distortion than of selectivity. Zakrzewska tells us, for example, that she spent the summer of 1840 with her mother at the Charité, which may very well have been the case. But most of what we learn about this prolonged stay is that she was, at one point, accidentally locked up in the dead house, having gone to examine the corpse of a young man who had turned green from the poison that had killed him.[67] Whether this ever really happened is not clear, but for Zakrzewska the story seemed to matter more for the opportunity it gave her to emphasize her bravery (when she realized she could not get out, she simply lay down on the floor and went to sleep), her interest in dissection (considered improper for girls), and her early attraction to medicine (she was only ten years old). Indeed, as Susan Wells has argued, this story follows a narrative structure that captures symbolically the obstacles faced and overcome by nineteenth-century women who wished to study medicine, a profession that was, for them, as forbidden as the dead house.[68] We learn little else about Zakrzewska's extended stay in the hospital.

Another time, Zakrzewska tells her readers that she quit school in defiance at the age of thirteen, furious at the school officials for refusing to let her miss a morning of lessons in order to visit a close friend, a teacher of history, geography, and arithmetic, who was on his deathbed. When he died that very morning, she "left the schoolroom, . . . and never entered it again."[69] What Zakrzewska failed to mention is that it was not unusual for German children, especially girls, to end their schooling at this age. Indeed, with a working mother and five younger siblings, she was probably under considerable pressure to leave school and help out at home. But by portraying this solely as an act of defiance instead of also as an act of necessity, Zakrzewska could cast herself as intolerant of arbitrary and unfair rulings and in control of her life.[70] The fact that her close friend taught history, geography, and arithmetic rather than religion, reading, and sewing is also not coincidental. As we have already mentioned, Zakrzewska could thus present herself as a proponent of those subjects her brother had studied in the nonclassical secondary schools and that she had come to view as symbols of modernity.

The stories Zakrzewska shared in her autobiographical sketch are thus not entirely reliable sources for gaining insight into the actual events and experiences that marked her youth. Nevertheless, since they are probably less fabrications than embellishments, and since in some cases we find corroboration in the letters her father wrote to his superiors, we may be able to draw some conclusions about her experiences growing up. By all accounts, Zakrzewska did assume considerable responsibility for running the household, raising her siblings, and even assisting her mother in the practice of midwifery. She once claimed to have "become a regular appendage to my mother; going with her in the winter nights from place to place, and visiting those whom she could not visit during the day."[71] As the oldest daughter of seven children (in 1849, her parents adopted her mother's half brother, who was orphaned upon his father's death), a significant level of responsibility would not have been unusual.[72] How she felt about it is another matter. In her autobiographical sketch, she described the years she spent caring for her family and assisting her mother as "among the happiest of my life"; yet she also expressed resentment that she "should be forced to do housework when I wanted to read, while my brother, who wished to work, was compelled to study."[73] Chances are that she both enjoyed the power that came with responsibility and felt burdened by the endless household duties that were preventing her from engaging in more satisfying work. We do not know what language Zakrzewska might have used at the age of fourteen to describe her disapproval of the traditional sexual division of labor, but her experiences in her family certainly contributed to her eventual decision to flout gender norms. It must have been difficult enough to accept that her brother's formal education mattered more than her own and that she was expected to limit her activities to the domestic sphere, but watching her mother struggle to reconcile "production" and "reproduction" may very well have had the greatest impact of all.

Zakrzewska seems to have decided relatively early in life that she would not follow in her mother's footsteps and try to combine work with marriage. She also seems to have been clear about which of the two she would prefer. Several sarcastic comments about marriage in her autobiographical sketch suggest that, at least by the time she had turned thirty, she had developed a distaste for the institution. She referred to it, for example, as "an institution to relieve parents from embarrassment. When troubled about the future of a son," she elaborated, "parents are ready to give him to the army; when in fears of the destiny of a daughter, they induce her to become the slave of the marriage bond."[74] It is possible, of course, that Zakrzewska was not yet so cynical when she was still in her early twenties and living at home, but she certainly would have had ample opportunity to observe her mother's difficulties trying to sustain a midwifery practice while still being in her own childbearing years. Not until Zakrzewska turned sixty did she lament that she had "no young life, which belongs to me."[75] For most of her life, in contrast, she seemed clear that if she had to choose between work and marriage, there was only one choice to be made.

Thus, at the age of eighteen, when many girls were either contemplating marriage or already wed, Zakrzewska applied to the same school of midwifery from which her mother had graduated. Clearly in this regard she was modeling her life on that of her mother, not turning away. Zakrzewska once claimed that the summer she had spent in the Charité marked the point at which she had decided to pursue a medical career.[76] But whether she made this decision at the age of ten or not, chances are that her more formative experiences occurred during the years she accompanied her mother to the homes of laboring women. During these visits, Zakrzewska later remarked, she had the opportunity both to observe her mother in the practice of midwifery and to learn firsthand about the consequences of social inequality.[77] One can easily imagine the young Zakrzewska beginning to draw connections between the political theories she was learning from her father and the people before her who seemed trapped by their illnesses, poverty, and lack of education and political power. Zakrzewska would eventually build on these experiences when she founded her own hospital and became a champion of the poor. She may not have been without her own class prejudices, but her views would nevertheless place her on the far left of the political spectrum in nineteenth-century America.

Midwifery thus marked a site where Zakrzewska's political upbringing, her interest in medicine, and her desire for economic independence could all come together. Of course, the pursuit of a medical degree might have had more appeal, but German universities, as embodiments of bourgeois culture and the separation of the sexes, excluded women until the end of the century.[78] Zakrzewska's experience in the school of midwifery would prove, however, to be the next best thing, for midwifery, like medicine, was experiencing as much turmoil around midcentury as was politics, and Joseph Hermann Schmidt, the man who became her mentor, advocate, and friend, was at the center of Prussian medical reform.

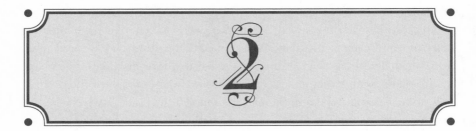

Master Midwife

In the fall of 1847 Zakrzewska applied to the city magistrates for admission to the Charité's school of midwifery. She had just turned eighteen, the minimum age for anyone wishing to attend the school. She did not, however, submit her application without first seeking the support of Joseph Hermann Schmidt, associate professor of obstetrics at the university, director of the obstetrics ward at the Charité, and one of the most important medical personalities in Berlin at the time. At an early age—most likely because of her parents' experiences—Zakrzewska seemed only too aware of the need to establish relationships with powerful individuals in order to accomplish her goals. Fortunately for her, this contact soon blossomed into a deep and lasting friendship.[1]

Schmidt's support did not, however, prove sufficient in 1847, and Zakrzewska repeated her mother's initial experiences as she, too, received several rejections from the city magistrates. She later blamed this on her youth and unmarried status, but this would not have been consistent with the government's official policy, which stated explicitly that anyone between the ages of eighteen and thirty, whether married, widowed, or single, could apply to a school of midwifery.[2] Undaunted, Zakrzewska waited one year and tried again, but again she was turned down. "During this time," she later explained, "Dr. Schmidt became more and more interested in me personally." Determined to apply again and encouraged by Schmidt's support, she spent the following year reading midwifery texts and assisting her mother in her practice. When, in 1849, she received her third rejection, Schmidt intervened more directly. According to Zakrzewska, he took his request straight to the king, arguing "that he saw no reason why Germany as well as France should not have and be proud of a La Chapelle."[3]

The reference was to Madame Marie Louise Lachapelle (1768–1821), chief midwife of one of Paris's lying-in hospitals and the renowned author of an important midwifery text, *Pratique des Accouchemens*, the first volume of which had been translated into German in 1825.[4] If Schmidt did in fact make this argument to the king, it was because he saw in Zakrzewska a young woman who could assist him in his efforts to improve the training and thus the status of midwives. By emphasizing the science of midwifery, the importance of training pupils in the use of instruments, and the need to bridge theory and practice, Schmidt was linking his proposed changes not only to the general educational reforms in which the Prussian government had been investing since the beginning of the century but also more specifically to recent reforms in medical education and licensing. Historians of medicine have explored in considerable detail the various curricular and legislative changes instituted by German governments around midcentury that strengthened the elite medical profession; less attention has been paid to the effect of these reforms on the training and practices of midwives. Yet Schmidt, who drafted the plan that informed the revamping of Prussia's medical system in 1852, was committed to making changes in midwifery as well.[5]

Whether it was because of Schmidt's alleged audience with the king or his promotion to director of the Charité's midwifery institution, Zakrzewska was formally accepted as a pupil in the fall of 1849, ten years after her mother had begun her studies. She would spend the next three and a half years at the hospital, gradually working her way up to the position of head midwife. During these years, she acquired greater knowledge of the natural sciences and excellent skills in delivering babies. She also learned, by observing the continued battles between midwives and physicians, how professional hierarchies were formed around claims to expert knowledge that were then sanctioned by law. Zakrzewska would take this understanding with her when she left for the United States in 1853, a land where licensing was virtually nonexistent and medical practitioners of all ilks were vying with one another for patients and prestige.

• • •

Certainly no one had a greater impact on Zakrzewska's early appreciation of the natural sciences than Joseph Hermann Schmidt (1804–52), the central architect of the rules and regulations that helped create a powerful medical profession in Prussia.[6] Born in Paderborn, Schmidt specialized in obstetrics during his medical studies. An ambitious man, he wrote the prizewinning *Lehrbuch der Geburtskunde für die Hebammen in den königlichen Preussischen Staaten* (Textbook of

Obstetrics for Midwives in the Royal Prussian States) in 1839, while he was teaching midwifery in his hometown, directing the city hospital, and serving as head physician of the city's poor commission. According to the government-appointed prize committee, its advantages over the previous textbook included its greater attention to science, its increased focus on understanding rather than memorization, and its more careful delineation of the midwife's rights and responsibilities.[7]

Educational reform coupled with greater regulation would mark the twin sides of the government's increased legislation with respect to medical personnel over the course of the century. Schmidt's deep appreciation of the intimate relationship between the two attracted the attention of Prussia's minister of culture, Johann Albrecht Friedrich Eichhorn, who was looking for someone to help revamp the state's medical system. Schmidt came to Berlin in 1843 to assist with the task. Two years later, after being promoted to privy medical councillor in the Ministry of Culture, associate professor of obstetrics at the university, and director of the obstetrics ward in the Charité hospital, he completed his massive work, *Die Reform der Medizinalverfassung Preußens* (The Reform of the Prussian Medical System), which became law in 1852.[8]

Schmidt's recommendations for restructuring the Prussian medical system echoed those of a large group of academically trained physicians throughout Germany who had been trying since the early 1840s to convince their state governments to institute both curricular and licensing reforms. Their campaign for an extension of the term of study from three to four years, greater time spent in laboratory and clinical courses, and a graded curriculum was coupled with a push to establish a more powerful and elite profession by eliminating several categories of medical practitioners still licensed at that time by the state. Thus, in Prussia, before Schmidt's reforms were enacted, degree-holding medical practitioners were divided into physicians, surgeons of the first class, and surgeons of the second class.[9] Next in line were obstetricians, eye doctors, and dentists, followed by midwives. As a result of Schmidt's reforms, the first three groups were collapsed into a single category, "physician," and aspirants for this title had to pass examinations in internal medicine, surgery, and obstetrics. Historians have paid most attention to the merging of medicine and surgery, which dissolved the centuries-old division of physicians into those more knowledgeable of theory and those who engaged in manual labor. But of equal significance, as Schmidt himself remarked, was that obstetricians, who had "been cut off from . . . physicians, and placed together with opticians and dentists," were now included among the elite.[10]

Zakrzewska's later decision to immigrate to the United States to study medicine probably reflected her desire to stand at the pinnacle of the medical hierarchy and not in the subordinate category retained for midwives. Once in the United States, she would even speak out against midwifery schools, insisting that women who wished to practice obstetrics should instead become physicians.[11] But while in Germany, Zakrzewska saw herself as a central player in Schmidt's campaign to raise the status of the midwife. Coupling educational reform with legal protections, he instituted curricular changes designed to increase the knowledge base of midwives and battled successfully to prevent the elimination of midwives from the list of licensed medical personnel. Zakrzewska may have eventually rejected Schmidt's commitment to midwifery, but her knowledge of the battles he fought and won taught her about the power both of the law and of claims to certain forms of knowledge in defining and protecting professional identity.[12]

Schmidt's struggles to protect midwives is a story unto itself and must be dealt with only briefly here.[13] Suffice it to say that they lasted approximately five years and harkened back to the dispute in which Zakrzewska's mother had participated over swaddling women. Schmidt, who sided with the midwives, insisted that obstetricians refrain from using swaddling women as their assistants. In staking out this position, he was pitting himself against the Berlin Society of Obstetricians, which he had helped found and which wished to see the position of midwife abolished. Schmidt was not, it should be emphasized, trying to elevate the position of midwife to one even remotely on a par with that of physicians; still, he insisted that she had rights and responsibilities, which he was determined to protect. These rested upon a division of duties such that "the obstetrician is assigned chiefly to the irregular (unusual) cases, the midwives, on the other hand, chiefly to the regular (usual) cases."[14] No ruling, he insisted, ever described a situation in which a case was supposed to be assigned to swaddling women.

Schmidt eventually won this battle. In February 1852, as part of the government's implementation of his plan for a total revamping of the medical hierarchy, it also forbade obstetricians from having a swaddling woman represent them at a delivery. Convinced, however, that physicians required assistants, the government agreed to increase the number of midwives in Berlin from fifty to one hundred. In the long run, the additional midwives were to come out of the Charité's official training program, but in the short run, the government took the fifty most talented swaddling women and put them through a two-month course in the Charité. This instruction, as we will see, fell to Zakrzewska, who had by that time advanced to the position of head midwife.[15]

There is no direct evidence that Zakrzewska followed this battle in detail, but between her mother's experiences trying to ban swaddling women, her close relationship with Schmidt, and her own role as instructor of the swaddling women in 1852, the general issues must have been familiar to her. For this reason, at least some aspects deserve attention. The first is the way each side used science to bolster its position. Carl Mayer, president of the Berlin Society of Obstetricians, insisted, for one, that only men had played a role in raising obstetrics to its current state as a medical science because only they "possess the scientific acuity and impartiality of the . . . senses." What troubled Mayer was that by assigning all normal births to midwives, the state had created a situation in which the "material" (by which he meant the laboring women's bodies) was "almost without exception lost to science."[16] Schmidt, in his rejoinder, turned to science as well, but he did so to distinguish not between physicians and midwives but between midwives and swaddling women. The former, he explained, were taught "small science [kleine Wissenschaft]," which helped them to recognize the boundary between natural and artificial assistance. "One calls this small science with its particular rules," he emphasized, " '*the art of midwifery*'; the state does not yet recognize '*the art of swaddling*.' "[17] Thus both men used science rhetorically to justify the unequal distribution of power, but whereas Mayer wished to exclude women altogether from scientific activity, Schmidt claimed science for his midwives, albeit in a diminutive form. In this way, he too was inscribing gender distinctions: only physicians learned "big" science, and only men (by law) were physicians. Small wonder Zakrzewska would eventually speak out against midwifery schools in the United States. Her goal was to ensure that women received the same education as men, not that they be taught "small" science.[18]

The other aspect of this battle that deserves attention is what it reveals about the power of the law and its role in shaping a professional identity. The 1852 legislation both raised the status of obstetrics by including it as one of the three examination areas for all physicians and strengthened the position of midwives by removing a formidable competitor. True, the government also grew more invested in impressing upon midwives their place as physicians' *assistants*, but one need only think of the country that would later become Zakrzewska's home to understand the significance of this legislation. The weakness of any licensing laws in the United States meant that when tensions mounted between midwives and physicians in the nineteenth century, American midwives had no recourse to state regulatory bodies that might have offered them some protection. Although not the only reason for their eventual decline, the lack of any effective legislative protection certainly contributed to the American midwife's gradual disappearance from the birthing room.[19]

The midwives who benefited from the Prussian legislation formed an elite group. The decision to protect midwives had nothing to do with an appreciation of the knowledge of lay practitioners, who usually acquired their expertise through oral traditions and experience. The winners of this battle were midwives who attended a formal course of instruction at a state-run institution, followed by examinations that, if they passed, licensed them to handle normal births on their own and to assist physicians in the case of any abnormalities. This was the group of midwives to which Zakrzewska belonged as long as she remained in Germany. One can only wonder whether much of her own sense of professionalism—which she would later carry with her to the United States and which would shape her views on women's medical education, training, and behavior—might not have had its roots in this formally trained community of midwives.[20] Zakrzewska may have eventually turned her back on this community, but she had learned a valuable lesson about the role of the law, knowledge claims, and a common educational experience in shaping and solidifying a group's identity.

• • •

Schmidt's efforts on behalf of midwives did not focus entirely on protecting their legal rights. He also set out to improve their knowledge base. For Schmidt, as we mentioned briefly, this meant greater attention to *Wissenschaft*, a difficult term to define but one that, by the 1840s, had come to refer to the pursuit of new knowledge through in-depth scholarly work. Schmidt's choice of the term "*Wissenschaft*" must be seen as an intentional move on his part to link his own curricular reforms to the pedagogical revolution taking place in the German universities. Friedrich Wilhelm III's decision to create a new Prussian university in Berlin in 1810 to "replace intellectually what [the state] has lost physically" to the French, coupled with Wilhelm von Humboldt's emphasis on *Wissenschaft*, had fostered an educational environment that emphasized independence of thought and, perhaps even more important, independence of spirit.[21] Schmidt did not, it should be emphasized, expect midwives to produce new knowledge (hence the qualifier "small"), but he did seek to deepen their understanding of the theoretical underpinnings of their subject and to integrate this knowledge with their practical skills.

It is possible to reconstruct in considerable detail the instruction Zakrzewska received from Schmidt during her years of study. Not only did his textbook form the basis of midwifery education throughout Prussia, but he submitted yearly reports to the government as well as publishing a lengthy article in the first issue of the *Annalen des Charité-Krankenhauses* in which he elaborated on both his pedagogical intentions and his style of teaching. As Schmidt made clear, one of his primary goals was to integrate both theory and practice in the training of midwives.[22]

In promoting an intimate connection between theory and practice, Schmidt was echoing one of the rallying cries of physicians who were fighting for medical reform at midcentury. But where physicians were trying to counter an over-emphasis on "theory" in university education by insisting that students be re-quired to attend both laboratory and clinical courses, Schmidt was trying to raise the status of the midwife by more fully developing her theoretical under-standing of her field, albeit while linking it intimately to practical exercises.[23] He thus developed a program that combined lectures with both visual demonstra-tions and hands-on experience examining and attending women in labor.

Midwifery pupils attended lectures six days a week for one hour a day. Schmidt followed the content of his textbook closely, beginning with the anat-omy and physiology of the female pelvis and reproductive organs before moving on to pregnancy, birth, and confinement under normal conditions. Here he covered conception, the signs of pregnancy, the ways of noting when the time of delivery was approaching, the midwife's responsibilities during the birthing process, the birth, and finally the care of mother and newborn in the first weeks following the birth. He then turned to abnormal conditions, discussing the problems that could arise from an irregular pelvis or reproductive organs, from the positions of the fetus, and from a premature or prolonged delivery. He followed this with a discussion of the accidents and illnesses that could occur during the birthing process, ending with a clear statement of the therapeutic measures midwives were permitted to provide and those that were strictly for-bidden to them.[24]

Throughout this instruction Schmidt made extensive use of visual aids, in-cluding skeletons of both the female body and the newborn, wax forms, organs soaked in preservatives, manikins, dolls, and birthing chairs—in short, any aids that would help his students grasp more concretely the scientific underpinnings of midwifery. He even permitted at least some of his pupils to attend dissections of the mothers and infants who died during birth.[25]

The core of Schmidt's pedagogical program was, however, the coordination of these lectures with instruction in clinical practice. He organized the latter into two parts, which he named casuistic and systematic. The former he defined as the observation and management of the birth, and his goal was to ensure that each midwife received as much experience as possible.[26] As he proudly wrote in his yearly reports to the government, he consistently exceeded the state-mandated requirement of two births for every midwife. In his clinic, each pupil had sole responsibility for at least four and often five births over the course of her training; she assisted in another eighteen cases, which included giving a full examination to the mother; and she observed as many as one hundred more deliveries. In the event of an abnormal delivery, Schmidt or one of the other physicians always took over, but the pupils were allowed to remain in the room. This afforded them the opportunity to observe the conditions under which forceps needed to be used or the fetus turned. One could well imagine Carl Mayer and other obstetricians worrying that midwives might as a result believe that they had learned enough to handle such difficult deliveries themselves. In fact, Schmidt did once permit a student to handle a breech birth on her own. He was thus skating on thin ice. Still, he insisted that his goal was both to help midwives discern when it was necessary to send for a physician and to provide them with the skills to assist the obstetrician when he arrived.[27]

It bears mention that Schmidt may also have discussed with his midwives the need to take special precautions to avoid spreading puerperal fever (otherwise known as childbed fever). This postpartum septicemic infection posed one of the most serious threats to both European and American maternity wards before the introduction of antiseptic techniques in the last decades of the century.[28] Schmidt was well aware of the work of the physician Ignaz Semmelweis, who in the 1840s had attributed the high rates of puerperal fever at the Vienna General Hospital to the practice of leading medical students straight from the dissection room to the examination of parturient women. Schmidt, like most professors of midwifery at the time, did not subscribe fully to the notion that puerperal fever was being spread by the direct introduction of putrefying matter into the women's bodies. He preferred the more commonly held view that "the hospital atmosphere of the maternity rooms" was principally responsible, but he considered the charge serious enough to warrant consideration. Of course, he would not have worried about his midwifery pupils spreading puerperal fever—even those who observed dissections were not performing them—but more than likely he would have discussed with them his reasons for recommending, even if he did not require, that his medical students take the precaution of washing their hands in a solution of chloric acid before examining the parturient women.[29] This may, in fact, explain why Zakrzewska instituted similar procedures when she opened her own hospital in 1862 and, as a result, had a comparatively low incidence of puerperal fever in her wards.[30]

In addition to these "casuistic" lessons, which took place whenever a woman went into labor, Schmidt provided scheduled "systematic" clinical instruction. This occurred at least twice a week for an hour at a time and focused on how to examine the parturient women. Here, Schmidt was most concerned with helping midwives to develop their sense of touch. They needed, he explained, to learn how "to have their eyes on the tips of their fingers."[31] But other senses were also important, as was the use of instruments and techniques that could supplement the knowledge a midwife acquired through her own hands. Thus Schmidt introduced midwives both to the speculum, which relied on their sense of sight, and to the techniques of percussion and auscultation, which required a developed sense of sound. Throughout, moreover, he tried his best to develop his pupils' powers of discernment by providing as many comparisons as possible, presenting, for example, women who were pregnant for the first time together with those who had given birth before, women who had pelvises of different sizes, or those who had fetuses in different positions. As Schmidt once explained, "Nothing is easier than to distinguish between a *uterus descendens* and a *uterus ascendens* when both are right next to one another."[32]

Schmidt recognized that such comparisons were possible because the midwifery school was housed in a large urban hospital that could provide adequate clinical material. But the quantity of material was not the only advantage a hospital conferred. Although Schmidt never stated this explicitly, it was also evident that only in a large hospital would midwives have the opportunity to practice the various techniques that allowed them to perfect their skills. Schmidt may have started his pupils on manikins, but he soon took them over to the station for syphilitics, where the women, mostly prostitutes, could raise few objections to having their bodies probed and prodded. During these visits, his pupils could practice how to percuss, use the speculum, insert catheters, apply leeches, and give injections.[33] For all of Schmidt's insistence that he saw "something more than a living phantom even in people who have sunk as low as they can go," his conduct resembled that of most nineteenth-century hospital physicians who viewed their patients, almost all of whom came from the poorest segments of society, as clinical material on which to practice their craft.[34]

Zakrzewska would eventually develop a greater concern for the dignity of the poor and try her best to guard against the abuse of the patients who frequented her hospital. This sensitivity may very well have stemmed both from her experiences assisting her mother in practice and from her observations of the way poor women were frequently treated at the Charité. Zakrzewska never said as much; yet when she described her experiences at the hospital, she emphasized the respect she tried to show the prostitutes, refusing to treat them as totally lost souls. Still, Zakrzewska's class upbringing comes through in a story she told about one of the prostitutes at the Charité, whom she engaged as a "servant" and to whom she "trusted every thing [*sic*]."[35] To Zakrzewska what was important was the trust she placed in a woman whom others dismissed as beyond redemption. That she showed her respect by placing this woman in a position of servitude remained fully unproblematic for her. Much like other middle-class reformers who were committed to building a just society, Zakrzewska frequently mixed compassion for those in need with a sense of her own superiority.[36]

The education in midwifery Zakrzewska received at the Charité was outstanding by any measure of the day. One need only consider that at that time most American medical students sought out clinical instruction, if they did so at all, on their own time. Few medical schools offered bedside training, let alone formal instruction in auscultation, percussion, or the use of the speculum.[37] Perhaps even more impressive is the fact that Zakrzewska's obstetric training, at least the practical end, differed little from what medical students at the University of Berlin were being taught. Schmidt, who was responsible for instructing both groups, saw no reason, in fact, to distinguish between the two in his detailed descriptions of his pedagogical methods, since he considered "the foundations of the one to repeat themselves, with the necessary changes, in that of the other."[38]

If this was true in general of the instruction Schmidt provided his midwifery pupils, then the education Zakrzewska received as one of the Berlin students may even have surpassed in some ways that of the university students. Not only did she sit through the course twice, but she also spent several months living in the Charité when the midwifery institute was not in session, taking responsibility for the deliveries for which a medical student was not available. As a result, during her midwifery studies, Zakrzewska delivered about thirty babies a year, not to mention the large number of deliveries in which she assisted or that she simply observed. In addition, she functioned both as a tutor and as a "house mother" to the midwifery pupils during her second year of instruction, helping them to master the information required of them while she kept "peace and order" among them as well.[39] Small wonder Zakrzewska would later claim that the education she received at the Charité was every bit as good as that of any medical student. She may not have learned as much "big science," but she certainly made up for that in the practical experience she acquired and the responsibilities she assumed vis-à-vis the other pupils.

· · ·

Schmidt may have granted Zakrzewska more responsibilities than was usual for a second-year pupil because he was preparing her to become the next head midwife, a position he once referred to as the "right hand not only of the leading physician but of the midwifery instructor as well."[40] This was a state-level position, usually reserved for an experienced midwife who lived in the Charité and helped to take care of the women in the obstetrics wards. In her auto-biographical account, Zakrzewska stated that Schmidt had even higher goals, wishing "to reform the school of midwives by giving to it a professor of its own sex." She even claimed that he wished "to surrender into my hands his position as professor in the School for Midwives, so that I might have the entire charge of the midwives' education."[41] But this could not have been true. Anyone familiar with the German system of higher education would know that someone with Zakrzewska's educational background—she had not attended the *Gymnasium* let alone the university—could never assume a professorship. Indeed, one could hardly imagine that Schmidt, who had a deep commitment to raising the standards of midwifery, would have fought to bestow a professorship upon anyone who lacked a formal education. Nevertheless, he did show a commit-ment to redefining the status, responsibilities, and even power of the head midwife. As early as the spring of 1850, when this position became vacant, Schmidt decided he had an opportunity to articulate and push through his reforms, and he chose Zakrzewska to help him execute his plans.

Schmidt disliked the arrangement he had inherited from his predecessors by which the midwifery pupils were trained and supervised. To begin, his assistants were young physicians who were themselves in training, rotating every month or two through the hospital's various wards. As a result, the midwifery pupils had several different instructors during their five-month course. He was also critical of what he believed to be a "peculiarity" of the Charité, whereby the pupils were under the supervision not only of a "house *mother*" but also of a "house '*father*.' " As he wrote to the hospital's directors in the spring of 1850: "In all the other lying-in institutes of the world the head midwife, when she is capable, is the virtual female soul of the institute."[42] Schmidt, who disliked the decentralized nature of this arrangement, recommended that the instructional and supervisory responsibilities of the assistant physicians and the house father be transferred to the head midwife. In fighting for these reforms, he clearly sought to empower the position of head midwife, yet in shifting responsibilities in this way he was also enhancing his own control of the institute. The head midwife would be answerable only to him, whereas the assistant physicians and house father enjoyed a certain level of independence. Schmidt, who had no interest in a "co-director," set out in the spring of 1850 to make the appropriate changes.[43]

Schmidt realized that his success depended upon finding not an "ordinary midwife" but a "master midwife" to fill the vacant position. For him, this meant a person with endurance, humanity, good clinical skills, and "a brilliant understanding." He had received a list of midwives to consider for the position but had rejected each and every one in turn. One he found incapable of helping with either the theoretical lessons or the practical instruction; another he rejected because her fingers were "drawn together and crooked"; a third he turned down because she had a husband and children "and because of the former has prospects of increasing the latter." A fourth candidate he considered seriously because she had the right kind of experience, having trained in the obstetrics clinic at the University of Bonn and in the lying-in institute in Petersburg. Yet he showed some concern because she was Catholic while most of the women in the obstetrics ward were Protestant.[44]

Having thus cleared the slate, Schmidt moved on to recommend Zakrzewska, who had not appeared on the government's recommended list. In a previous communication with the hospital directors he had already made clear his conviction that the surest way of getting a master midwife was "to train a young talented single woman or widow with long fingers and of evident morality from the very beginning."[45] Now, two weeks later, he asked them to consider

the unmarried woman, Marie Elisabeth Zakrzewska, who is listed by the local magistrate as a midwife of the city of Berlin and who already made it to a short list in the previous year because she was without question the most qualified of thirteen applicants sent to me. Of course, she has not applied, and could not, because she has not yet completed her studies. But that does not seem important to me when one is searching for people to fill positions. She has an unusual ability to comprehend things, and a hand which one could not find more fitting for a midwife. . . . Notwithstanding her one failing, which grows smaller every day, and that is her youth, . . . she would be a much more successful choice than the first four women.[46]

Since Zakrzewska had, at the time, completed only the first year of her two-year course, Schmidt knew she could not yet assume the position of head midwife, but he wished to avoid the appointment of an accomplished midwife who would preclude his hiring Zakrzewska the following year. He recommended, therefore, that a midwife by the name of Franz be hired temporarily. Widowed and poor, Franz would, Schmidt believed, be helped by the temporary arrangement, but she would also be in no position to expect to remain longer.

The directors of the Charité were less than enamored of this plan, but they did eventually agree to hire Franz. However, what must have been a direct blow to Schmidt was the directors' dismissal of Zakrzewska—they refused to consider his recommendation until she completed her studies—at the same time that they informed him of their decision to hire a deaconess by the name of Catherine Stahl as an assistant to the head midwife. Stahl, a graduate of Theodor Fliedner's deaconess institute in Kaiserswerth, had acquired experience as a nurse during a serious typhus epidemic in Silesia, but she had no particular skills in midwifery. In fact, she, like Zakrzewska, had only just begun her studies. The directors' plan was to hire Stahl as a nurse and to promote her to the position of second house midwife when she completed her training.[47]

This was not the first time Zakrzewska and Stahl had come into competition with each other. According to Zakrzewska, her application to the school of midwifery had been rejected the previous fall because of the preference for a deaconess among a religious faction in the government.[48] The snub Schmidt received in March 1850 may very well have stemmed from a similar source. But paralleling these religious concerns were more than likely political ones, for it was exactly at this time that the government began its investigations into the political activities of Zakrzewska's father, suspicious that he had long been supporting the democratic party. Although Martin Zakrzewski was, as we have seen, eventually exonerated, the head physician at the Charité, Ernst Horn, was a well-known reactionary, and he may have wished to have nothing to do with the daughter of a Prussian civil servant who had generated cause for concern.

Nothing, however, prevented Schmidt from singling out his favorite pupil in order to groom her for the position of head midwife, which is exactly what he did. For example, as his health began to fail (Schmidt was suffering from tuberculosis),[49] he let Zakrzewska take over much of the instruction of the pupils, an experience that surely proved valuable when she began teaching in the United States six years later. It may also have contributed to her superb performance at her final examination. As Zakrzewska described that event, Schmidt had "invited some of the most prominent medical men" to come and observe his star pupil, for he wished to prove to them that she could " 'do better than half of the young men at *their* examination.' " She continued:

> The excitement of this day I can hardly describe. I had not only to appear
> before a body of strangers, of whose manner of questioning I had no idea,
> but also before half a dozen authorities in the profession, assembled especially for criticism. Picture to yourself my position: standing before the table
> at which were seated the three physicians composing the examining committee, questioning me all the while in the most perplexing manner, with
> four more of the highest standing on each side,—making eleven in all; Dr.
> Schmidt a little way off, anxious that I should prove true all that he had
> said in praise of me. . . . It was terrible.[50]

Zakrzewska passed with flying colors, having answered every single question asked of her as well as demonstrating to everyone's satisfaction her practical skills on a manikin. She was awarded a diploma "of the first degree."[51]

Schmidt must now have felt ready to proceed with his plans, for he took the first opportunity to mention Zakrzewska again to the hospital directors. The immediate occasion was the latter's decision to promote Stahl, who had received her midwifery license in December of the previous year, to the position of second house midwife. Schmidt did not voice any objection to this move, but he followed up one month later with his own request that Zakrzewska be promised the position of head midwife when Franz left in May.[52]

While Schmidt waited for the directors' response, Zakrzewska was informed that she needed to report to the district medical officer in order to be assigned to the section of the city she would service. Anxious not to lose Zakrzewska, Schmidt pressured the Charité directors to make a decision. In response, Horn sent him a list of concerns about Zakrzewska, beginning with his belief that the

Charité needed someone with more practical experience. He also felt that because of her youth, she had not yet had the chance to provide a "guarantee of the strength and seriousness of her moral deportment," without which, he feared, she might "succumb to the many temptations" that would arise through the contact the head midwife had with the young medical students. Finally, and one cannot help but wonder whether this was also more to the point, he complained that "during her stay in the Charité as a midwifery pupil, Zakrzewska had at times shown a hint of a snappish nature, impudence, and a lack of control."[53]

Horn may have intended this exchange to be in friendship and confidence, but Schmidt, angered by the insults both to his own judgment and to his protégée and perhaps convinced that he had little to lose, told Zakrzewska what Horn had said. Zakrzewska's response was immediate: she withdrew her application and wrote a long, indignant letter addressed to Schmidt but with the expectation that it would be forwarded to the hospital directors (which it was). Zakrzewska remarked pointedly that although she coveted the position and also believed she deserved it, she did not *need* the job. She also insisted that it had been Schmidt's idea, not hers, to apply for the position of head midwife. Clearly, though, what angered her most was Horn's insinuation that she had acted improperly when she had been a pupil in the Charité. Zakrzewska believed she knew the incident to which Horn was referring, and it was one, she claimed, in which she had done no more than stand up for what she believed to be her right. Apparently, as she wrote to Schmidt, several weeks after she had assumed her role as supervisor of the other midwifery pupils, she was told that she could no longer leave the house, for any reason, without first requesting a signed pass from the director. Not only had Zakrzewska found this demeaning, but she had believed that the privilege of leaving the hospital at will was crucial in order to strengthen her position in regard to the other midwifery pupils, who needed to view her with respect. The bottom line though, as she explained, was that after voicing her objections she had accepted the ruling and requested the passes as required. That she would nevertheless be considered disrespectful disturbed her not because she might have jeopardized her chances of attaining the position of head midwife but rather because one "would have found any reason at all for reproach."[54]

Zakrzewska demonstrated in this letter none of the feminine traits so revered in her day. On the contrary, she wrote with anger and indignation, denying

Horn's charge of wrongdoing and accusing him instead of improper actions. She was, in other words, taking the high moral ground, much as her mother had done in the battle over swaddling women, and she was doing so by displaying self-confidence and forthrightness rather than uncertainty and passivity. Already at twenty-two years of age, Zakrzewska was developing a public persona that flouted gender norms and claimed attributes most commonly associated with men.

That this performance did not end Zakrzewska's tenure at the Charité right then and there had to do with the intervention of the undersecretary of state, Hermann Lehnert. Having learned from Schmidt's wife that her husband's health had been so affected by this turn of events that she now feared for his life, Lehnert had pressured the hospital directors to reverse their decision. Nevertheless, he also cared little for Zakrzewska's style and assured the hospital directors that should she get uppity they "had sufficient means for disabusing Zakrzewska of the loathsome qualities which have become noticeable in her, and to breed into her the qualities of subordination and modesty."[55] She could, in other words, be forced into a different gender performance, one more compatible with the expectations of her sex. Events would not, however, take that turn. Indeed, when relations between Zakrzewska and her superiors turned sour less than six months later, rather than submit to their will, she quit.

That conflict had not yet surfaced when, on 10 May 1852, Horn and Esse granted Schmidt permission to hire Zakrzewska with the understanding that Schmidt would "be at Zakrzewska's side."[56] Five days later, however, Schmidt succumbed to his illness. Zakrzewska did not hear of his death until the following day when she arrived at the Charité to begin her new job. The shock of the news left her shaken and trembling, but her grief was also mixed with fear as she realized that she was now "without friendly encouragement and support." For the next few days, until Schmidt's funeral, she "moved about mechanically as an automaton," confused and yet acutely aware of the extreme vulnerability of her position. Having been appointed not because she "was wanted by the directors of the hospital, but because they had been commanded by the government," she recognized that she had to build new alliances quickly. Acting shrewdly, she decided to try to placate Stahl, who had resented being placed in a position subordinate to someone with so little experience and who was eight years her junior. Zakrzewska hoped thereby also to please the directors, who seemed all along to favor Stahl. Her proposal was to eliminate any difference of power between the two positions by dividing the responsibilities of the head midwife equally between them. For the time being, she at least hoped, peace would thus be made.[57]

Zakrzewska felt now that she could focus on carrying out the responsibilities associated with her position as head midwife. This basically entailed performing whatever duties the director of the midwifery institute delegated to her. In Zakrzewska's case, these seem to have been quite extensive, perhaps a reflection of the uncertainty that reigned while the government sought a replacement for Schmidt. Zakrzewska claims to have provided both the theoretical and the practical instruction to the midwifery pupils; to have offered practical instruction to the medical students as well; to have supervised the care of the newborns with medical problems; and to have basically taken on the general management of the maternity ward.[58] It has not been possible to find independent corroboration of these claims, although guidelines spelling out the various expectations of the head midwife do mention that the practical instruction of both the medical and midwifery pupils may fall under her purview, depending upon the wishes of the institute's director.[59] (No mention is made of theoretical instruction.) Thus, it is reasonable to assume that Zakrzewska did not exaggerate the extent of her responsibilities.

Zakrzewska did not, however, remain long at the Charité. Whatever peace she may have believed she had secured did not last. The incident that brought everything to a head stemmed from the government's decision in 1852 to enlist fifty swaddling women in a two-month course at the Charité in order to increase the number of assistants available to the city's obstetricians. Although this instruction was assigned formally to two physicians at the Charité, they both immediately turned around and handed it over to Zakrzewska. Stahl, who resented this obvious favoritism, turned on Zakrzewska and complained to the directors that she had behaved inappropriately, accepting presents from her pupils, despite this being forbidden. Zakrzewska was summoned before Horn, who most likely welcomed this opportunity to take the young midwife down a peg. Unfortunately, the only account we have of their meeting is the one Zakrzewska provided in her autobiographical sketch. According to her, she admitted that she had kept the presents but had done so because to have returned them would have hurt her pupils' feelings. She had, though, put them away, realizing that any other action would have been improper. Zakrzewska claims that Horn showed some embarrassment at the assumptions he had made about her motives but that he refused to back down. This made her so angry, she added, that

"I soon ceased to be the humble woman and spoke boldly what I thought, in defiance of his authority. . . . The end was, that I declared my readiness to leave the hospital."[60]

Horn would probably have described the encounter differently, presenting Zakrzewska as the upstart that he believed her to be. It turns out that the acceptance of presents was a highly regulated affair; the government's instructions for the head midwife dictated exactly the conditions under which they were allowed. Most important, presents, whether from her pupils or from the parturient women and their families, had to be offered without any coercion and had to be shared with the wards' attendants. By accepting and then storing the presents, Zakrzewska had clearly broken the rules. Her reasons may have been noble, but Horn, who must have viewed this as yet another example of Zakrzewska's unwillingness to submit to the regulations governing her position, saw this as the opportunity he needed to encourage termination of her appointment. Zakrzewska must have realized this was coming when she took matters into her own hands and quit.[61]

By 15 November, six months after she had assumed the position of head midwife, Zakrzewska was contemplating what to do with her life. She possessed an outstanding education in midwifery, had held a position of considerable responsibility, and had become acutely aware of the need for protection if one was to survive as a government employee. Schmidt's wife, who had retained a friendship with Zakrzewska following her husband's death, suggested to Marie that she remain in Berlin and establish her own private hospital. Zakrzewska contemplated this option seriously, but ultimately she decided against it. Instead, like so many other Germans at the time, she began thinking about immigrating to the United States. Restless and ambitious, she set her sights on studying medicine abroad, the United States being the only country at the time where women could earn the M.D. Earlier in the year, her mentor had told her about the Female Medical College in Philadelphia, which had opened in 1850 and was granting women medical degrees. "In America," she claims Schmidt told her, "women will now become physicians, like the men; this shows that only in a republic can it be proved that science has no sex."[62]

Zakrzewska would soon learn that many of the same prejudices against women that she had had to endure in Germany existed in the United States. But early in 1853, as she was contemplating this move, she shared the excitement of millions of individuals who had been looking across the ocean for almost a decade with great hope and high expectations. Between 1844 and

1854, the United States opened its doors to three million immigrants. As far as Germans were concerned, many left for economic reasons, preferring emigration over starvation. In the years following the revolutionary events of 1848, a smaller group of political refugees joined those who continued to leave for economic reasons. Some emigrated because they feared persecution, others because they found Germany increasingly intolerant and believed America offered better soil for building a true democracy.[63] Zakrzewska, who probably came closer to the latter, had of course the added hope that she would be able to do what remained forbidden to women in her own country: pursue a medical degree.

Zakrzewska claims her mother "consented with heart and soul" when she heard of her plans.[64] Her father also gave his approval, although he made it a condition that she take along her younger sister, Anna. Presumably he did not want Marie to travel alone, but perhaps he also suspected that all his children would eventually follow their oldest sister, forming part of the transatlantic crossing that so altered the face of American society. Of all her siblings, Marie would leave the greatest mark on the land that would soon become her home; within a decade of her arrival she would become the director of one of the few hospitals at which women interested in studying medicine could receive clinical training. What she later remembered about her departure, though, was less her excitement than her sadness at leaving her mother. "Upon my memory," she wrote, "is for ever imprinted the street, the house, the window behind which my mother stood waving her handkerchief. Not a tear did I suffer to mount to my eyes, in order to make her believe that the departure was an easy one; but a heart beating convulsively within punished me for the restraint."[65] Zakrzewska, who was all of twenty-three years old, was about to cross the ocean to a land she had read about only in books.

This Land of Liberty, Equality, and Fraternity

In April 1853, Marie and Anna Zakrzewska set sail for New York on board the *Deutschland*. It was a clipper ship, with room for eighteen people in the first cabin and scores of others down below in steerage. The two sisters, who were among the more privileged, kept to themselves, finding their fellow travelers to be "not sufficiently attractive to induce us to make their acquaintance."[1] They may have been going to the new world of freedom and democracy, but like other middle-class travelers they carried their old "baggage" of class with them. For forty-seven days they struggled, sometimes with stormy and inclement weather but mostly with boredom, anxious to reach their destination and begin their new lives. On 22 May they finally sighted land, surprised by the greenness of the landscape that met them as they pulled into the quarantine at Staten Island. "I was at once riveted by the beautiful scene that was spread before my eyes," Zakrzewska later remembered, ". . . and a feeling rose in my heart that I can call nothing else than devotional; for it bowed my knees beneath me, and forced sounds from my lips that I could not translate into words, for they were mysterious to myself."[2]

Zakrzewska's sense of awe grew as the ship continued its journey toward its final destination, the island of Manhattan, where it docked at Pier 13 on the Hudson River. Pastoral scenery now gave way to an urban environment as the *Deutschland* pulled into a busy commercial port, filled with people and abuzz with the activity and sense of purpose so characteristic of city life. Zakrzewska viewed this sudden transition not with dismay but with excitement. To her, this city, which would be her home off and on over the next six years, was "beautiful," and whatever joy she had felt as she gazed upon Staten Island's bucolic setting was now "mastered by another feeling—a feeling of activity that had become my ideal."[3]

Zakrzewska thrived on city life. There was something about the pace of life and the intensity of experience that inspired her, making her hopeful that she would be able to fulfill her dream. Of course, all cities were not equal. She had left one because "a despotic government and its servile agents" had not allowed her to continue her study of medicine, but now she had found another urban setting, which she believed would present fewer obstacles to a young woman intent on pursuing a medical career. Zakrzewska had come to New York, believing that "in this land of liberty, equality and fraternity" things would be different.[4]

· · ·

Zakrzewska may have left Germany behind her, but she still landed in a city with the third largest population of German-speakers in the world. By 1855, just two years following her arrival, roughly 154,000 Germans lived in New York City, a significant number but still just a small part of the almost 1.5 million Germans who came to the United States between 1843 and the Civil War.[5] Most immigrants chose their final destination based on where they had immediate family, distant relatives, or even close friends. Marie and Anna lacked such intimate ties, but they did arrive with letters of introduction, some to physicians who Marie hoped would help her pursue her medical career, others to friends of her family and even distant acquaintances who had crossed the ocean years before. The two sisters did not, however, expect to be met at the dock and were thus all the more surprised and even a bit shocked when they heard their names being called. An old acquaintance of theirs, a "Mrs. G," had heard from her family in Berlin that the two young women would be arriving alone, and she and her husband had decided to extend a helping hand. In this way, Marie and Anna were pulled immediately into New York's "Little Germany," or *Kleindeutschland*, a community located on the lower east side of Manhattan where the vast majority of the city's German-speaking population resided and worked.[6]

Language may have held this community together, but beyond that differences abounded. Whether in terms of class, religion, politics, or occupation, the residents made up a markedly heterogeneous group. Still, it would be fair to say that the community tended to be more secular than religious, more Democratic than Republican, more artisanal and skilled in employment than unskilled. Indeed, the largest occupational group in *Kleindeutschland* consisted of those involved in some capacity with the tailoring business, and it was to this group that Zakrzewska's hosts belonged. As a manufacturer of fringes and tassels, Mr. G managed to make a modest living, although by no means a comfortable one. His dwelling consisted of no more than his shop, a small kitchen, and two additional rooms, one that they used as a sitting room, the other as a bedroom. Nevertheless, he and his wife did not hesitate to offer their sitting room to the two sisters, something that touched Zakrzewska deeply but that also increased her resolve to find accommodations as soon as possible. She succeeded by the end of the week in finding what she referred to as "a suite of rooms," which, given that she paid only $5.50 a month in rent, probably consisted of little more than a parlor, a single bedroom, and a kitchen. But Marie and Anna were pleased, and having moved in the furniture they had brought with them from Germany, they settled in quickly and turned their attention to the more important business of figuring out how to support themselves.[7]

Most female immigrants who arrived in New York City around midcentury found employment either as a domestic or in tailoring or needlework. The first, although providing better compensation than the others, subjected the women to the scrutiny of their mistresses, who frequently moved beyond supervision of the work routine to the regulation of personal habits and behaviors. The latter trades, whether carried out in small shops or through outwork, allowed greater personal freedom, but the work was poorly paid and unreliable, subject as it was to the whims of the business owner and the seasonal demand for goods. By one estimate, a woman who managed to sew full-time could earn about ninety dollars a year, just barely enough to support herself. But such constant employment was rare, not to mention the impossibility of surviving on such a low wage should there be any dependents. Seamstresses and needlewomen thus lived on the edge of poverty, occasionally engaging in casual prostitution to supplement their income when other forms of work proved inadequate.[8]

The latter was not an option for either sister, whose bourgeois upbringing made it impossible for them to think of casual prostitution as an economic choice, part and parcel of a system of sexual bartering that had, by midcentury, come to mark urban working-class culture.[9] Nor, however, was it even remotely a threat, since they always had the option of writing home for additional funds should their situation deteriorate too far. The two sisters had thus a buffer around them, distinguishing them from most other immigrants who came off the boat penniless and therefore dependent upon an exploitative labor market to make ends meet.

How they ended up supporting themselves their first year in New York highlights the ambiguity of their situation. For a while their only income came from
piecework Anna was doing as a sewer for a dressmaker. Working eleven hours a
day, six days a week, she would have made $2.75 a week had she received her
wages regularly. But Anna, like other pieceworkers, was not always paid for her
work, and she and Marie watched their savings dwindle rapidly. The anxiety
they experienced stemmed in part from their concern that they might have to
seek additional support from their parents, but in some ways the shrinking of
any economic separation between themselves and the poor seemed to matter
less than the indications that socially the line was blurring as well. Thus when
Anna had initially sought the piecework, she had done so, she explained to
Marie, only because "no one here knows me." And when Marie decided to
pawn a watch chain in order to get some additional money, she did so "by giving
a fictitious name," reasoning that it was tolerable to borrow money in this way
because "[n]o one knows us."[10] Much like their parents, they seemed most
concerned with the appearance of impropriety, especially any behaviors that
would suggest their abandonment of bourgeois values.

Marie is the one who finally secured the family's finances, and she did so by
engaging in outwork as well. However, rather than seek piecework, as Anna was
doing, she set up a small business knitting worsted into fancy wares. To do so
had been risky; she had had to take the last few dollars out of the family's funds.
But Marie had neither the personality to work for others nor much fear that she
would fail. Indeed, she turned out to be a shrewd businesswoman—much better
than her mother had been—and at one point had thirty women in her employ.
That she had basically become an exploiter in this labor market never occurred
to her. Instead, she viewed herself as a savior to many women who would
otherwise have been unemployed. Whether she was indeed a compassionate
employer or not, the truth is that her business did so well that she and Anna
were able, by the fall of 1853, to move into more comfortable quarters in a better
neighborhood, renting part of a house on Monroe Street for two hundred
dollars a year.[11]

Zakrzewska had not, though, come to the United States to run a business but
rather to pursue a medical career. In fact, her original plan had been to go
directly to Philadelphia to try to gain entry to the Female Medical College, but
she had realized quickly that she lacked the language skills to do so. Still, even
before she had turned to the worsted business, she had called on a Dr. Reisig, a
physician who had worked with her mother back in Berlin. Her hope was that

he would consent to be her preceptor, a standard arrangement at the time that paralleled the artisanal relationship between master and apprentice. Accordingly, an established physician took a young physician-to-be under his wing, introducing him (rarely her) to basic medical theories and practices while the young protégé worked as his assistant. For many physicians, four to seven years of such an apprenticeship was all the education they received before setting up their own practice; others began their studies this way, entering medical school after a few years of such training. Zakrzewska had hoped that with her midwifery skills a physician might be willing to take her on, but much to her disappointment the reception she received differed little from what she had experienced in her native land. Her visit to Dr. Reisig ended in his offer of a nursing position, and Zakrzewska, refusing to be patronized in this way, decided she would be better off trying to establish a midwifery practice on her own. It was only when this failed to bring in sufficient income that Zakrzewska had turned to the worsted business; but now, in the spring of 1854, with the household finances fairly stable, she decided that it was time to return to her original plans.[12]

Zakrzewska was beginning to recognize that American society had its own obstacles in place, making it hard for women to pursue a medical career. Finding a preceptor had proved difficult. Gaining acceptance to medical school did not promise to be much easier. In the early 1850s, few medical schools accepted women, although since most schools relied upon student fees to finance their operating budget (in contrast to Germany, where medical schools were financed and operated by the state), every once in a while opportunities did present themselves. Thus, Elizabeth Blackwell, the first woman in the United States to receive a degree from a regular medical college, had gained admission in 1847 to Geneva Medical College in upstate New York because of a misunderstanding. The dean of the college had given the students, whom he had no wish to antagonize, the final word as to whether Blackwell should be allowed to attend, fully convinced that they would say no. The students, however, believing the entire affair to be a joke, voted to accept her application. Two weeks later, Blackwell turned up to begin her studies, and although the students stayed true to their word, she spent the two years it took her to earn her M.D. in relative isolation. Upon her graduation, Geneva closed its doors once again to women. "Miss Blackwell's admission was an *experiment*, not intended as a *precedent*," the dean firmly told another female applicant in 1849.[13]

Slowly, however, the number of women who gained acceptance to medical school did grow, so Zakrzewska had reason to have some hope. Progress was slowest among orthodox medical schools, but even here some changes took place. Most important was the opening of the Female Medical College in Philadelphia in 1850; two years later Cleveland Medical College began accepting a small number of female students each year (although it, too, ended its "experiment" after four years); and in 1856 the New England Female Medical College gained the right to confer the medical degree. Women who applied to unorthodox medical schools had somewhat greater success, although they, too, encountered resistance. Still, their acceptance rate was higher than at regular institutions. Whether this reflected unorthodox physicians' greater tolerance of female practitioners or the pecuniary needs of the medical institutions is unclear. But the outcome was that, of the roughly 250 women who received a medical degree from a chartered medical school by 1862, more than half had attended an unorthodox institution.[14]

Zakrzewska never considered applying to an unorthodox medical school. To understand this one must recognize that for women the decision whether to pursue an orthodox or unorthodox education carried particular meaning because they struggled with questions of legitimacy on two counts: accused of being incapable of practicing medicine because of their sex, they risked being further discredited, at least by regular physicians, should they pursue an unorthodox path.[15] Indeed, the fledgling American Medical Association (AMA) had, at its creation in 1847, established a code of ethics forbidding regular physicians from consulting with all other practitioners. According to the AMA's founders, unorthodox practices were "based on an exclusive dogma." Whether homeopaths were prescribing infinitesimally small doses of medicines, hydropaths were recommending water cures for most ailments, or Thomsonians were promoting botanical cures, all were allegedly endangering the lives of their patients by discarding therapeutic measures that had stood the test of science and had been part of the profession's medical arsenal for centuries.[16] Unorthodox physicians, in response, went straight to the regular profession's Achilles' heel—the high mortality rates, especially during outbreaks of epidemic diseases—and they held the harsh practices of the regular profession, foremost the excessive bleeding, purging, and puking, responsible for such poor outcomes. As for the charge that their practices lacked any scientific foundation, unorthodox physicians begged to differ. Homeopaths in particular insisted that the laws upon which they based their practices (the laws of "like cures like" and of infinitesimal doses) had more scientific legitimation than the "heroic" measures so beloved by regular practitioners.[17]

Many of the battles fought among nineteenth-century medical practitioners centered on competing understandings of science, but one also cannot ignore the sheer power of the claim that one's group alone was proceeding scientifically. Much of the tension between orthodox and unorthodox physicians at midcentury should, in fact, be seen as largely rhetorical in nature, fueled by competition and turf battles. This is not to say that there were few differences between the various medical philosophies. Regular medicine relied largely on depletive measures, such as bloodletting, cathartics, and purgatives, to restore the sick body to health; homeopathy, in contrast, may have sought the same goal, but it did so by administering small doses of medicines that were found to mimic the symptoms brought on by the disease; hydropathy went even further, promoting a therapeutic regimen that consisted largely of applications of cold water. To the patient certainly it mattered whether one was prescribed small pills and drops whose action on the body remained invisible or whether one was given violent purgatives and emetics.[18] Still, a closer look at actual practices indicates that at the time the AMA forbade consultation with unorthodox practitioners, a number of so-called homeopathic physicians used some traditional therapeutic regimens. Conversely, regular physicians sometimes prescribed homeopathic remedies. Indeed, despite the acrimony of their rhetoric, regular physicians and homeopaths often socialized together, attending the same parties and meetings and even, on occasion, referring family members to one another. The members of the AMA had, in other words, made a strategic choice to highlight the differences between regular medicine and homeopathy rather than focus on the similarities. Accusations of being "unscientific" drew attention to this chosen rift.[19]

It is against this background that we must understand Zakrzewska's decision to pursue a regular medical education. There can be no question that she questioned the therapeutic efficacy of irregular practices, but she was also acting on her ambition to be accepted by the elite of the medical profession.[20] Nor was she alone. Elizabeth Blackwell, Emily Blackwell, Ann Preston, and Mary Putnam Jacobi, among others, also believed that an orthodox education would render women better practitioners and that it would confer the desired cultural legitimacy on practitioners of their sex.[21] Indeed, some women, like the gynecologic surgeon Mary Dixon-Jones, who received her first degree from New

York's Hygeio-Therapeutic Medical College in 1862, even sought a second degree later in life from an orthodox school because of the greater prestige bestowed on a regular education. And Sarah Adamson Dolley, who graduated from an eclectic school in 1851, later turned her back on her own unorthodox education when she helped found a medical society restricted to regular women physicians in Rochester, New York.[22]

Zakrzewska was thus among those women who cast their lot with the regular medical profession. As good fortune had it, a contact she had made earlier with the matron of a homeless shelter led her to Elizabeth Blackwell, a woman whose commitment to orthodoxy paralleled her own. The two women liked each other right away. Perhaps this stemmed from their shared European background; Blackwell was born in England and had moved with her family to the United States when she was twelve years old.[23] But certainly what drew them together most was their shared determination to challenge the medical profession's discrimination against women. Describing their first meeting in May 1854, Zakrzewska later commented that "from this call . . . I date my new life in America."[24] As Blackwell explained to her sister, Emily, just after this meeting: "I have at last found a student in whom I can take a great deal of interest— Marie Zackrzewska [sic], a German, about twenty-six. Dr. Schmidt, the head of the Berlin midwifery department, discovered her talent, advised her to study, and finally appointed her as chief midwife in the hospital under him; there she taught classes of about 150 women and 50 young men, and proved herself most capable. . . . There is the true stuff in her, and I shall do my best to bring it out. She must obtain a medical degree."[25]

Blackwell, who also dreamed of founding a hospital for the medical care and training of women, had already opened a small dispensary in 1853.[26] Located in *Kleindeutschland*, the dispensary catered primarily to poor German immigrants who had not yet lived long enough in the United States to have mastered the English language. Blackwell's excitement at meeting Zakrzewska thus also reflected her realization that the young German could help her in caring for this population. She suggested that Zakrzewska begin immediately to assist her at the dispensary. She also offered to tutor her young protégée twice a week in English. In the meantime, she promised to try to secure a place for Zakrzewska in a medical school. Zakrzewska, who could not "comprehend how Blackwell could ever have taken so deep an interest in me as she manifested that morning," left Blackwell's home secure that she had found a good and powerful friend.[27]

During the summer and fall of 1854, a number of things came together. Most important, Blackwell succeeded in getting Zakrzewska enrolled at Cleveland Medical College for the winter term. Blackwell's sister, Emily, had just graduated from that institution; she was the second woman to receive her degree there since 1852. (All in all, six women graduated from Cleveland Medical College before it closed its doors to women in 1856.)[28] The timing was good for Zakrzewska because although her family had grown during the year—her sister Sophie had arrived the previous autumn, and before the year was out both Herman and her half brother had come to New York as well—one by one they were settling in. Anna was engaged to Albert Crouze, the son of a family the Zakrzewskis had known in Berlin; Sophie had set up her own millinery business; and Herman had found a position as a mechanical engineer.[29] Besides, Zakrzewska's business had taken a turn for the worse. As the demand for worsted goods had declined, she had taken up the production of silk coiffures and then the embroidering of caps, but she had not been as successful in this line of work. Indeed, her finances had dwindled to the point that had Blackwell not arranged for the subsidy of some of her school fees she would not have been able to afford her medical education.[30] For Zakrzewska, the winter term could not start quickly enough.

· · ·

Zakrzewska left for Cleveland almost seventeen months after her arrival in New York. She had spent that entire period living among family members in the well-marked ethnic community of *Kleindeutschland*. Surrounded by other Germans, speaking her native tongue at home and on the streets, and providing medical care to German immigrants whose knowledge of English was markedly worse than her own, Zakrzewska must have wondered at times whether she had ever really left home. She would not have such doubts once she arrived in Cleveland, despite the city's well-developed German-speaking population.[31] Indeed, her first experiences there were a painful reminder of her poor language skills and how little progress she had actually made during the past year and a half. Having arrived earlier than expected, she felt reluctant to trouble the family that had agreed to be her host, and she ended up spending the first night in a hotel. Her knowledge of English was not, however, good enough to allow her to request that dinner be brought to her room, and she ended up going to bed hungry. Nor, apparently, did she know a word as simple as "breakfast," for she tells an amusing story of how, in desperation, she barked out an order for a "Beefsteak" the following morning when she awoke, famished from the long hours she had gone without food. To Zakrzewska, the English language was still "like chaos." It took another three months before she felt comfortable with the language and another full year before she approached anything remotely like mastery. "I am not," she once claimed in a classic understatement, "a linguist by nature."[32] Indeed, like many people who learn a new language as an adult, Zakrzewska never fully lost signs of her native tongue.

Zakrzewska finally met her host, Caroline M. Severance, the following afternoon. This marked the beginning of a friendship between the two women—Severance, who was born in 1820, was nine years older than Zakrzewska—that lasted almost fifty years.[33] It also signaled Zakrzewska's introduction to the world of American politics, for it was through the Severances that she first met many of the leaders of the antislavery and women's rights movements, providing her with a political education that matched the medical education she received during her stay in Cleveland. Zakrzewska later described this period as the beginning of her political awakening. A "new world," she wrote, appeared before her eyes as she made the acquaintance of such individuals as William Lloyd Garrison, Wendell Phillips, Theodore Parker, Ralph Waldo Emerson, Frederick Douglass, Sarah and Angelina Grimké, Harriot Hunt, and Caroline Dall.[34]

Zakrzewska had arrived in Cleveland in the midst of battles that were already threatening to divide the country. The Fugitive Slave Law was four years old, the Kansas-Nebraska Act barely five months old, and the Republican Party had only just started taking shape. "Discussions pro and con on all kinds of subjects agitated the people," Zakrzewska remembered, "and more than once did I hear the 'Boston Trio'—William Lloyd Garrison, Wendell Phillips and Theodore Parker—denounced as disturbers of Law and Order."[35] Zakrzewska would eventually find the radical views of the "Boston Trio" most to her liking, but during the years she spent in Cleveland, she moved comfortably among a wide variety of political groups. This was especially the case at the Independent Christian Church, a Unitarian-Universalist church that the Severances had helped establish and where Zakrzewska spent a considerable amount of time during her two years in Cleveland. "The congregation," Zakrzewska later wrote, "was the most heterogeneous imaginable. Most of the people were in a transition stage from the darkest orthodoxy to atheism, neither of these extremes satisfying their ideals. There were also reformers in other directions dissatisfied with all existing codes of religion and law who sought refuge in the companionship of malcontents. Thus, we had not only Unitarians and Universalists to meet, but also Spiritualists, Magnetists, Fourierists, Freelovers, Women's Rights advocates, Abolitionists—in fact, followers of all kinds of *isms* then existing."[36]

Zakrzewska's attraction to this group had much to do with its roots in a liberal religious movement dating from the eighteenth century. Universalist and Unitarian churches in particular had long rejected religious orthodoxy (particularly the Trinity), as well as religious enthusiasm, church hierarchies, and the harsh and judgmental God of New England Calvinism. Their emphases were, instead, on reason in religious affairs and free and independent inquiry; moreover, they held firmly to a belief in a benevolent deity who endowed individuals with an innate moral sense meant to guide them in their actions and help them to create a humane and just society.[37] It had been exactly this innate moral sense that had directed the Severances to leave the Presbyterian Church in the early 1840s and help form a church organized largely around the antislavery movement. Thus when Zakrzewska joined the Severances' household in October 1854, she entered the heart of this small community of social and political reformers. Her ties to this group were strengthened when she moved in with the family of the church's new pastor, Amory Dwight Mayo, in April 1855. Zakrzewska never mentioned whether she temporarily embraced Unitarian doctrine, but there can be no doubt that she felt comfortable with the philosophy, if not the theology, of this religious community. Although she would eventually become an avowed atheist, she maintained close relations throughout her life with several of the more radical Unitarian ministers, predominantly Theodore Parker and James Freeman Clarke.[38]

The members of this congregation also publicly supported the movement for women's rights. Among them, Caroline Severance may very well have been the most directly involved. As early as 1851, at the second statewide convention for women's rights in Ohio, she had been a commanding figure. The following year she was elected to the vice presidency of the newly formed Ohio Woman's Rights Association and a year later to the vice presidency of the National Woman's Rights Convention; by 1854, the year Zakrzewska moved into her home, she was addressing the state legislature on behalf of "suffrage and such amendments to the state laws of Ohio, as should place woman on a civil equality with man."[39] Like other members of the more radical wing, Severance was throwing her weight not only behind the struggle for married women's rights to own property, have joint guardianship of their children, and control their own earnings but also behind the more controversial demand for suffrage.

Severance thus introduced Zakrzewska both to antislavery issues and to the battle for women's rights. Zakrzewska later claimed that she initially had had a more difficult time understanding the need for the latter. "I was shocked," she wrote, "that Mrs. Wright and others had demanded the emancipation of women. That a Woman's Rights Convention was held in New York State seemed to me so ridiculous."[40] This may seem a surprising comment for someone who had been fighting for her own rights for years, but Zakrzewska does not appear to have appreciated at first the broader context of the battles in which she was engaged. Perhaps this is because in Berlin she had not fought to enter a male domain; rather, she had aspired to the position of head midwife, which had always gone to a woman. It is true that Schmidt had wished to increase the power of the head midwife, but the resistance he encountered, and Zakrzewska experienced, may not have been strong enough to push her toward a deeper analysis of her problems. Besides, an experience of discrimination does not always lead one to an understanding of how power operates.[41]

However "shocked" Zakrzewska may have felt when she first heard about the women's rights movement, she soon came to a deeper understanding of the politics of discrimination. No one seems to have been more influential here than Harriot Kezia Hunt, whom Zakrzewska met at the Severances shortly after she arrived in Cleveland.[42] One of the best-known women's physicians in Boston at the time, Hunt had been practicing medicine since 1835, although she had never been formally trained. She, like Blackwell, had tried to gain acceptance to an orthodox medical school in the late 1840s, but her decision to apply only to Harvard (which did not admit women until 1945) suggests that she was most interested in making a political statement.

Hunt, like Severance (and many other women's rights advocates at the time), had strong ties to both the antislavery and women's rights movements. In attendance at an antislavery meeting in Boston in 1850, she had been one of ten women who had called for, planned, and then spoken at the first National Woman's Rights Convention later the same year. Hunt's engagement with these issues also led her to issue a formal protest to the Boston city authorities in 1852, and to continue registering this complaint year after year, against "taxation without representation." She resented, as she explained to the treasurer of the city, "the injustice and inequality of levying taxes upon women, and at the same time refusing them any voice or vote in the imposition and expenditure of the same." Yet, she went on, "[e]ven drunkards, felons, idiots, or lunatics of *men*, may still enjoy that right of voting, to which no woman—however large the amount of taxes she pays, however respectable her character or useful her life—can ever attain. Wherein, your remonstrant would inquire, is the justice, equality, or wisdom of this?"[43]

When the forty-nine-year-old Hunt was introduced to Zakrzewska in the fall of 1854, she felt as though she had met a kindred spirit. She had heard of the young German woman studying in Cleveland but had known little more about Zakrzewska. "[W]hen I met her," Hunt later remarked, "an electric communication was instantly established between us. I felt that here was a combination of head and heart, which was as uncommon as it was beautiful."[44] Zakrzewska must have felt the same way, for a warm friendship developed between the two women over the years. Through Hunt Zakrzewska began to understand the connection between her own struggles to pursue a medical career and the battles of women's rights advocates both to gain legal rights for women and to alter not only the way men thought about women but also how women thought about themselves. This education continued when Zakrzewska visited Hunt in Boston in the fall of 1855, right around the time of a New England Woman's Rights Convention over which Hunt presided and that met to review the legal status of women in the various states. Whether Zakrzewska attended this convention is unknown, but she did spend her days meeting and socializing with Sarah Grimké, Angelina Grimké, Theodore Parker, William Lloyd Garrison, and Wendell Phillips. She also met Walter Channing, one of Boston's elite physicians, who would later become one of her staunchest supporters. Indeed, many of the people she met during this stay would provide critical support to her when she returned to Boston at the end of the decade to found her own hospital.[45]

By the time Zakrzewska visited Hunt in Boston, she was well aware of how much she was personally benefiting from the social and political goals of this circle of reformers. In fact, it was Hunt who had informed her of the female support network that had made her study of medicine possible. Zakrzewska had, of course, appreciated the generosity of the Severances, but she had been unaware that more was going on than the willingness of some good people to open their home to a young medical student. What she learned was that Severance had joined together with a group of prominent Cleveland women in November 1852 to form the Ohio Female Medical Education Society, which had been established explicitly for the purpose of promoting women's entry into the medical field by helping them to defray much of the expense of acquiring an education. Severance was elected secretary of the group, and a board of managers was established, whose task it was to screen applicants and ascertain who would be most likely to succeed.[46] This is the group Blackwell had contacted when she sought to help Zakrzewska defray some of the expenses of a medical school education.

The Ohio Female Medical Education Society was clearly modeled after early nineteenth-century women's benevolent associations, but rather than assist the poor and hungry, it was helping middle-class women enter an area of public life traditionally restricted to men. As Zakrzewska soon learned, many individuals who were otherwise committed to social reform nevertheless found this goal threatening. During her second year in Cleveland, she boarded with the Vaughan family, former southern slaveholders who had moved to Ohio in the 1840s and freed their slaves but who had avoided the more radical wing of the abolitionist movement. Among their friends, even among those who claimed to be supportive of women's rights, Zakrzewska found "the same prejudice . . . against all women who attempted to step out of the domestic sphere."[47] She found it puzzling that the same women who would join in political discussions and articulate their views intelligently, even in opposition to their husbands or fathers, would speak disapprovingly of her decision to study medicine. "I was often," Zakrzewska later remembered, "taken by surprise when, on the brink of forgetting that these manifestations of independence could exist side by side with the most ludicrous prejudice against me and my medical companions, I would be seriously questioned, 'Do you want to turn women into men?' "[48]

These are words Zakrzewska penned later in the century, as she was looking back on her days in Cleveland. Chances are she would not at the time have phrased things in this way, addressing directly the way her actions subverted traditional gender roles. Only over time did she come to understand the deeply gendered meanings ascribed not only to specific behaviors but also to mental and moral attributes. She would eventually challenge such gendered meanings, believing that only in this way would women ever gain the freedom to pursue their own interests. But such insights took time to develop. More than likely in the years Zakrzewska spent in Cleveland she did not yet fully understand why her study of medicine posed such a threat to men and women who were otherwise committed to reform.

Fortunately for Zakrzewska, though, whatever resistance she may have encountered from the Vaughans and their circle of friends was offset by the support she received from the Severances, Hunt, and other advocates for women's rights. How different her experience must have been from the one Elizabeth

Blackwell had had to endure in Geneva, where she had spent two years living and studying in relative isolation. How different as well from her own ordeal in Berlin, where, once Joseph Hermann Schmidt died, she had lost all protection. During her two years in Cleveland, Zakrzewska came to understand that she might never have even gotten into medical school without the support of others who were fighting not simply for the education of a handful of women physicians but for radical changes in gender relations. She recognized that the roots of what she had once viewed as her own personal battle went far deeper than she had imagined and that her own personal success would mean little if legal, social, and gender barriers remained largely intact, just opening a crack to let her through. Thus Zakrzewska's initial resistance to a Woman's Rights Convention gradually dissolved, and she came to see that despite her earlier view of these women as "hens which want to crow," she "had tried to crow as hard as any of these women without realizing it."[49]

Zakrzewska's greatest support came from the community of women's rights advocates, a fact she well appreciated, but others encouraged her as well. As previously mentioned, she felt welcome at the Independent Christian Church, where she found a community of like-minded individuals most of whom supported her efforts. She also felt particular gratitude toward the Reverend Mayo. Zakrzewska once wrote that there was no one in Cleveland among her "many dear and valued friends" to whom she owed more, for although he had little, he had given willingly when she was in need. Finally, she also received much encouragement from John J. Delamater, dean of Cleveland Medical College, professor of midwifery and diseases of women and children, and a committed abolitionist. In short, Zakrzewska's support network during the two years she spent in Cleveland, and indeed during the rest of her life, consisted of men and women who both shared and helped shape the political goals she came to value most highly.[50]

• • •

John J. Delamater became Zakrzewska's mentor almost as soon as she arrived in Cleveland. It was, as one historian has suggested, as though she had re-created the same kind of relationship she had had with Schmidt, one based on fondness and mutual respect, from which she received substantial protection. Zakrzewska remembered Delamater receiving her "like a father," taking her under his wing, and helping her to feel "perfectly at home."[51] It is easy to understand why she would have been drawn to her new mentor. Active in the temperance and abolitionist movements most of his adult life, Delamater had been a member of the college since its establishment in 1843 and was the leading force behind Cleveland Medical College's decision to open its doors to women. As a result, in the six years Cleveland experimented with coeducation nine women matriculated, of whom six received the M.D.[52] Delamater had thus succeeded in putting the college on the map, albeit briefly. The year Zakrzewska graduated the school changed its policy. Not until 1880 did it grant another woman an M.D.[53]

In trying to understand Cleveland's decision to end its experiment with coeducation, one must separate the question of why it opened its doors in 1850 from why it closed them six years later. Linda Lehmann Goldstein has argued persuasively that the willingness to experiment had come about because of the presence on the faculty of several powerful individuals, none more important than Delamater, whose general commitment to social and political reform translated as well into a specific interest in promoting the higher education of women. At various times Delamater had received important backing from Jared Potter Kirtland, professor of the theory and practice of medicine and a committed abolitionist as well. The two men had known each other from the early 1840s when both had taught at Willoughby Medical College in Chagrin, Ohio, twenty miles east of Cleveland. Both had left that school in 1843, along with two other faculty members, to found Cleveland Medical College, the medical arm of Western Reserve University, still located at that time in Hudson. As Goldstein demonstrates, these two men were primarily responsible for convincing the other members of their department to accept female students. Still, as she also shows, Cleveland's openness to women never became official policy; rather, it always depended upon the presence of particular individuals willing to persuade their colleagues, quietly and from behind the scenes, of the importance of this cause. "It was," she wrote, "as if an equal medical education is what happened to six talented women while the faculty debated the Woman Question."[54] The greatest support for this claim was Cleveland's decision to close its doors to women in 1856, just about the time that Delamater and Kirtland were nearing retirement and no longer able to exert as great an influence on their colleagues.[55]

But more may have contributed to Cleveland's decision to reverse its policy. Indeed, what remains puzzling in this account is Kirtland's ambivalence toward the "Woman Question," for one year after recommending that women be accepted as students he turned around and suggested that it might be inadvisable to admit any more women. A resolution that he submitted to the faculty to this effect passed unanimously. Then, two years later, in 1853, he submitted another resolution recommending that the dean be given ultimate authority to admit women on a case-by-case basis.[56] Kirtland's behavior may, however, be explainable if we take into account the opening of the Western College of Homeopathic Medicine in Cleveland in 1850. Since unorthodox medical schools, as we have already noted, sometimes demonstrated a greater openness to female students than regular institutions, coeducation and unorthodoxy were perceived by some to go hand in hand. Thus when Cleveland Medical College accepted two women in 1850, it risked blurring the boundary separating its institution from the newly founded Western College of Homeopathic Medicine. The fact that Cleveland's medical faculty explicitly distanced itself from homeopathic institutions in 1851, the same year Kirtland judged it unwise to admit any more women students, suggests how strongly these two issues were linked in the minds of the faculty.[57]

Thus, the reversal in 1856 of Cleveland Medical College's policy toward women may not have rested solely on Delamater's and Kirtland's declining power within the medical faculty. After all, Delamater continued teaching until 1861, Kirtland until 1864. What may also have changed was their perception of the threat posed by the neighboring homeopathic institution. In fact, during the six-year period in which women studied at Cleveland, total enrollments dropped from a high of two hundred to a low of seventy-two.[58] Although this decline cannot be, and apparently was not, ascribed directly to the presence of women, the medical faculty, including Delamater and Kirtland, reacted by trying to distinguish its institution more definitively from homeopathic schools. If that meant abandoning coeducation in order to rid itself of the taint of unorthodoxy, so be it.

The reaction of male regular physicians to female physicians cannot thus be understood without paying attention as well to contemporary concerns about the professionalization of medicine.[59] For at least some men, perhaps even for many, the question was not so much whether women were capable of practicing medicine as what effect their inclusion, both in institutions of medical learning and afterward in medical practice, would have on physicians' professional image. Even those men who favored the advancement of women never attributed as much importance to that goal as they did to the advancement of their profession. There is a noticeable parallel to the situation Susan B. Anthony and Elizabeth Cady Stanton encountered as their fellow abolitionists pressured them to table their fight for women's suffrage until the civil rights of the black man could be secured. Women physicians, too, were being given the message that their battles had to be subordinate to those aimed at establishing a respectable and powerful medical profession.

· · ·

Zakrzewska was lucky, however, and in the fall of 1854, two years before Cleveland closed its doors to women, she began her training in regular medicine. Such training, whether at Cleveland or at any of the other mid-nineteenth-century American medical schools, was, as we have already mentioned, sorely lacking. Until the postbellum period, admission requirements at most medical schools in the United States, at least if one was white and male, often amounted to little more than the ability to pay tuition fees. The standard course of instruction typically involved two four-month terms, with the second session often being no more than a repeat of the classes one had attended the previous year.[60] With the exception of exercises in dissection, there was next to no laboratory instruction, and even dissection was not taught at every school. In addition, clinical instruction could be quite erratic. While some schools offered weekly clinics, it is not at all clear whether the students actually examined patients or whether the instructor merely lectured to the students from the bedside. Indeed, as late as 1878, one medical student complained that "at the clinics the patient is simply exhibited to the students."[61] In general, most schools expected their students to acquire clinical experience on their own, often by working under their preceptors' tutelage during the summer months or by attending private courses or studying abroad. Still, as Kenneth Ludmerer has pointed out, students could graduate "without having attended a delivery, without having witnessed an operation, and often without having examined a patient."[62]

Cleveland's course of instruction followed this general pattern, although the apparent regularity with which it held dissection classes, its insistence that every student write a medical thesis, and the weekly clinical courses it held may have made it one of the better schools. Even though Zakrzewska later claimed that the subjects were "well known" to her, she felt as though she had benefited from the time she spent there.[63] Her only complaint was that clinical experience there, as elsewhere, depended upon the willingness of the instructors to take their students along when they attended the sick, and for female students that spelled disaster. "[E]ven our kind and beloved Dr. Delamater," she explained, "could not often venture upon such an innovation as to take a female student with him, even when visiting the poorest patients."[64]

During the first few weeks of the term, Zakrzewska lived with the Severances and was the only female student in the school. But in November both of these situations changed. Another woman, Sarah Ann Chadwick, joined her at Cleveland Medical College, and the Severances, who had decided to move to Boston at the end of the year, helped the two students find different lodgings. This turned out to be more difficult than expected, for not everyone was willing to take in female medical students, but Caroline Severance eventually found a boardinghouse for both Zakrzewska and Chadwick, and the two women roomed together for the rest of the term.[65]

Once the regular term began, Zakrzewska spent six hours every day listening to lectures in anatomy and physiology, materia medica and botany, chemistry, surgery, the theory and practice of physic, and the diseases of women and children. She then went back to her room and studied another six hours before returning to the college in the evening to practice dissection. By the second week of the semester she had so impressed her teachers that they proposed to let her graduate at the end of the term provided she passed examinations in surgery and chemistry and wrote a thesis in English.[66] Their confidence in her speaks to the strength and sophistication of the knowledge she had acquired while in Berlin. Not only had she worked as an apprentice to her mother, but she had also received ten months of instruction at the Charité in medical topics related to midwifery; she had tutored younger students during her second year of instruction; she had delivered at least one hundred babies; and she had been the chief midwife of Berlin's major city hospital for a six-month period. Few American medical students at the time brought such knowledge and skills with them to their studies.

That Zakrzewska did not graduate at the end of her first term rested most likely with her inability to master the English language quickly enough. Indeed, she claimed that during the fall when she lived in the boardinghouse, her language skills were so poor that she "never conversed with any one . . . , nor even asked for any thing at the table; but was supplied like a mute."[67] Preparing for examinations was not much better: at first she had to surround herself with four dictionaries when she studied, trying to figure out the English equivalents of the medical terms she had learned in German. Knowing she would need to return for a second year of study, Zakrzewska decided to spend the summer months in Cleveland. This was when she moved in with the Mayos, and, as we have seen, she found this experience to be extremely rewarding.

The summer of 1855 ended, however, with a personal tragedy for her. In July she heard that her mother had decided to come to the United States with the two youngest children to visit the rest of her family and to figure out whether there would be any opportunities for her husband should she wish to remain. Zakrzewska later wrote to a friend of the great happiness she had felt "at the prospect of beholding again the mother whom I loved beyond all expression, and who was my friend besides." But on 18 September, the Mayos received a telegram from Zakrzewska's siblings with the message that they should "[t]ell Zakrzewska that she must calmly and quietly receive the news that our good mother sleeps at the bottom of the ocean, which serves as her monument and her grave." Caroline Zakrzewski had died at sea three weeks earlier, apparently from a violent hemorrhage, and the two daughters traveling with her (Minna and Rosalia) had chosen to have her lowered to the bottom of the ocean rather than, as Zakrzewska later explained, "bring to us a corpse instead of the living." When Zakrzewska received this news, she set out immediately for New York, feeling very much the need to be with her siblings during this time of mourning.[68] She remained there several weeks, returning once again in December, ostensibly to deliver her sister Anna of a baby boy but perhaps also to seek the comfort of her family circle.[69]

Unfortunately we lack letters from this time of Zakrzewska's life that would provide more insight into her response to her mother's death. All we have is her autobiographical sketch, written four years later, in which she tells her friend Mary (to whom she is "relaying" her life's story) that "this is the most trying passage that I have to write in this sketch of my life." "[Y]ou must not think me weak," she went on, "that tears blot the words as I write."[70] She tells us, however, little more, although that in itself may be significant. Zakrzewska was and remained an extraordinarily private individual, viewing public displays of emotion as highly distasteful. The autobiographical sketch, which was intended for publication, would consequently have been an unlikely site for expressing the depth of her distress. Besides, one of her goals in writing this "letter" to Mary was to paint a picture of women as anything but sentimental. Tears were thus allowed but, as she took pains to emphasize, no signs of weakness.

Thus it should come as no surprise that she turned immediately in her autobiographical sketch from her account of her mother's death to the time she devoted while on the East Coast to expanding her professional network. Perhaps she sought solace in her work, or perhaps she wished to communicate to her readers that women should choose work over self-indulgence and self-pity. Whatever her intent, she did meet frequently with Elizabeth Blackwell while she was in New York in order to plan an infirmary they hoped to establish when Zakrzewska returned from Cleveland. The small dispensary Blackwell had earlier operated was no longer in existence; she had not had the time to attend the clinics on a regular basis herself. But she now planned together with Zakrzewska the establishment of a larger institution, which Elizabeth's sister, Emily, would also help run. Not wasting any time, the two women invited a few wealthy friends to Blackwell's home, and they organized right then and there an association whose task it was to raise, through the holding of fairs, the ten thousand dollars they calculated they would need in order to purchase a house for their new infirmary.[71]

Before beginning her journey back to medical school, Zakrzewska took the brief excursion to Boston referred to earlier. When she returned to Cleveland, she moved in with the Vaughans, the Mayos no longer needing her help, and she set herself the task of fulfilling the obligations for the M.D.[72] This included attending a second term of classes, studying for her examinations, and writing a thesis in English. Although Zakrzewska scarcely mentions her thesis in her autobiographical sketch, Cleveland's medical theses are extant, and it has been possible to get a copy of her work. Interestingly, although perhaps not surprisingly given her background in midwifery, Zakrzewska chose to write on "the organ of parturition." She decided, however, not simply to describe the physiology of this organ but also to challenge prevailing views on the centrality of the uterus for understanding women's nature. One can just imagine Zakrzewska returning to Cleveland from her visit with Harriot Hunt, Sarah Grimké, Angelina Grimké, and other radical reformers, fired up over issues of women's rights and determined to begin establishing links between her medical and scientific studies and the social reform causes to which she had become committed.

• • •

The first evidence of this commitment was a fourteen-page study that, on the surface, dealt with the similarities and differences between the organs of parturition in the various classes of the vegetable and animal kingdoms. Without question, though, Zakrzewska's goal was to challenge the biological "facts" upon which physicians based their argument for fundamental differences between the sexes and thus for a division of labor between men and women. One can easily imagine Zakrzewska viewing this as an opportunity to dismantle the claims of someone like Carl Meyer, president of the Berlin Society of Obstetricians, who had denied women's ability to think scientifically.[73] Her barbs were, moreover, directed specifically toward those who attributed women's alleged limited mental abilities to their possession of a womb.[74]

Understanding fully the rhetorical power of a claim to science, Zakrzewska began by placing her work within a European tradition that had long been concerned with a "science of obstetrics." This she contrasted with the approach of the American medical community, which still treated the subject "too much as a mere mechanical process," ignoring the use of comparative physiology and embryology to understand better the developmental history of specific structures and their functions.[75] Zakrzewska, whose central goal was to understand the organs of parturition in "the genus man," nevertheless insisted that "a correct knowledge of the human uterus, with its functions, qualities and different relations . . . [can be] obtained only by a strict and critical comparison with creatures below the human species."[76] Through such a study, she explained, one learns that there are three basic types of organs of parturition: the one found most commonly in plants, where the organ in which the ovum develops is lost when the ovum is expelled; the type more common among the lower animal forms, where the organ is retained for "future procreation"; and the one, typical of higher animal forms, in which a separate organ, the uterus, functions as a separate repository for the fertilized ovum.

Zakrzewska believed (mistakenly) that this comparative approach demonstrated that the uterus was nothing more than a highly developed differentiation of the intestines. She defended this by insisting that a rudimentary uterus in the lower animals was little more than "a mere enlargement of the oviduct" and that the oviduct itself was "connected with the intestinal canal," even retaining a "structural analogy with the intestines" higher up the scale. Thus, although "in the mammalia this organ [the uterus] is very distinct and conspicuous and seems to have lost its affinity with the oviducts and intestines," what the comparative approach demonstrates is that the pattern has just been obscured.[77] "It therefore cannot," Zakrzewska went on,

> be a matter of surprize [sic] that during pregnancy the uterus not only assumes an intestinal appearance, but also through different sympathetic disturbances, producing an effect upon the whole system, reminds us of its derivation. The shortning [sic] of the cervix and the development of the muscular tissue, which is enlarged to produce the peristaltic motions at the time of labor—prove that pregnancy is the return of the uterine sys-

tem, to the type of the intestinal system. And in this fact is concealed the secret of the opening of the os uterii and labor pains, which result from the peristaltic motions thus established. But labor . . . is not only the process of transformation to the intestinal but appraoches [sic] also the type of the egg, for the pyriform shape is entirely changed to the form of an egg, the two extremities becoming more and more oval until they have assumed a similar form. At the time when the return to this type is completed, parturition takes place.[78]

It bears mention that Zakrzewska was not suggesting an evolutionary connection between the three different uterine forms she described. Rather, in the years before Darwin published *On the Origin of Species*, most embryologists believed that such similarities revealed instead the particular plan, idea, or "type" that defined the parameters according to which development occurred. The "type" established connections or relations between different classes of organisms not because they shared a common ancestor but rather because the members of a particular group shared a fundamental structural pattern unique to the members of the group. This pattern, Zakrzewska believed, was more evident among the "simpler" organisms, growing ever more obscure as one climbed the ladder of complexity. Thus her justification for taking a comparative approach was that by studying "a similar organ or its equivalent in the lower organism . . . we find the functions and other qualities comparatively simple and distinct."[79]

As may be evident from the passage cited above, Zakrzewska drew not only on a comparative tradition but also on arguments of analogy frequently associated more closely with German nature philosophy. Indeed, in other sections of her thesis she wrote about sensibility and irritability as "the two poles of life" and wondered whether the organization of higher forms could best be characterized as one of "Unity or Duality."[80] At still other times she cited Alexander von Humboldt or drew upon her knowledge of the therapeutic effects of certain drugs. In short, this was a highly eclectic piece, and while the level of scientific knowledge may have been modest, what Zakrzewska demonstrated was her ability to cull information from a variety of sources in order to drive home her point, to wit, that the uterus was little more than an outgrowth of the intestines.

Two aspects of Zakrzewska's thesis deserve note. First, unlike the two other female graduates of Cleveland Medical College who had also practiced medicine before beginning their studies, Zakrzewska chose to write on a scientific rather than a clinical topic.[81] More than likely this decision stemmed from her strong identification with the scientific tradition that had developed in Germany in the 1840s, a tradition she had embraced during her studies with Schmidt. But Zakrzewska's thesis was more than an advertisement for European approaches to the "science of obstetrics." She also seemed determined to demonstrate, by example, women's ability to employ scientific reasoning.[82] As Zakrzewska explained in her introduction, she could have written on any number of topics, all of which would have fallen under the rubric of obstetrics. That she chose to focus on "the organ of parturition" marked her first attack on the biological arguments used to justify women's confinement to the home. Thus, in contrast to those who claimed that women's mental and physical abilities were dictated by their possession of a womb, Zakrzewska denied that any meaningful sexual differences existed at all. Instead, she insisted that the womb be understood as part of the intestinal tract; that labor be compared to the peristaltic motions of the intestinal system; and that the relation between the uterus and the ovaries be seen as "somewhat similar to that of the bladder to the kidneys."[83] Clearly, Zakrzewska's decision to dethrone the quintessential female organ—to challenge, in her words, one physician's mystification of "this portion of the human frame" as the "Wonder of Nature"[84]—indicates that by 1855 she had already come to understand that her scientific and medical studies could be turned to political ends.

Zakrzewska submitted her thesis in the winter of 1855. It was, she later wrote, "considered exceptionally good, and was the cause of my not failing as a candidate for a diploma, because I received only mediocre marks in all the branches of study, even falling below the passing mark in one branch."[85] Such mediocre grades may very well have reflected her difficulty with the English language, but Zakrzewska chose instead to attribute them to her own rebelliousness. As she later claimed, parroting the rhetoric of Prussian educational reformers like Wilhelm von Humboldt as she did so, she found most "pernicious" the insistence on memorizing "isolated facts and filling the brain to its fullest capacity with the names of authors and their opinions," leaving no room "for individual reasoning or for the power of making original deductions and applications."[86] As we will see, Zakrzewska would make the link between independent thinking and scientific reasoning one of her central leitmotifs; she would also challenge the gender stereotypes in circulation at the time by insisting on women's ability to engage in this form of reasoning as well.

Zakrzewska graduated from Cleveland Medical College in March 1856. She was one of four women who received the M.D. that day out of a class of forty-two students. The room, as Zakrzewska described it, was packed not only with friends and family but also with "a goodly number of the curious of the city who had come to get a look at the women doctors."[87] To be a woman and a doctor, especially one who graduated from an orthodox medical institution, was still a novelty. Cleveland Medical College, as we have already mentioned, would not continue the experiment. Indeed, all-male orthodox institutions would not open their doors to women on a regular basis until the 1870s. As a result, until that time the vast majority of women who received an orthodox education in the third quarter of the century did so at one of four all-female medical institutions: Female Medical College of Pennsylvania (1850; in 1867 the school changed its name to the Woman's Medical College of Pennsylvania), Boston's New England Female Medical College (1856), Woman's Medical College of the New York Infirmary (1865), and Chicago's Woman's Hospital Medical College (1870). (A fifth institution was founded in Baltimore in 1882.) Zakrzewska was thus not only unusual among women for having studied medicine; as a graduate of a coeducational regular institution, she stood out among female doctors as well.

Immediately following graduation, Zakrzewska headed back to New York City. She wished to be with her family again, but, perhaps more important, she could not wait to join Emily and Elizabeth Blackwell and finally set in motion their plans for a hospital for women and children. Highly skilled, thoroughly committed to regular medicine, and acutely aware of the ground they were breaking as female doctors, Zakrzewska was anxious to start the next phase of her life.

The First Hospital for
Women and Children

A return to New York City meant, for Zakrzewska, a return to her family. By this time, all her siblings had immigrated to America, and while her two brothers had decided to travel west to seek their fortunes, her sisters had remained together, moving to Hoboken, New Jersey, the seat of a large German-language community. Her family circle now included her sister Anna, her brother-in-law, Albert Crouze, and their three-month-old baby; her sister Sophie, who was managing a flourishing millinery establishment; Minna, who remained at home to run the household; and Rosalia, who was still young enough to be in school. They were, moreover, looking forward to a visit from their father, who had remarried after their mother's death and wished to come to America to assure himself that his children were all well and comfortably settled.[1] Much, however, as Zakrzewska may have wished to re-create the living arrangement she had enjoyed before she left for Cleveland, she decided that she had to set up her medical practice in New York rather than in New Jersey. Thus almost immediately upon arrival, she began looking for rooms to let, only to find that the prejudice against women physicians made this an impossible task. Her one encouraging conversation led nowhere when the woman's husband refused to have his home tainted by association with a female doctor. Zakrzewska's response was to point out the irony of placing obstacles in the path of women whose ultimate goal was to be of service to others.[2]

Unable to find her own accommodations, Zakrzewska accepted Elizabeth Blackwell's offer that she move in with her family, letting the back parlor for medical practice. In this way, Zakrzewska was drawn into the Blackwell family, repeating her experience in Cleveland as she once again became part of a reform-minded household. Elizabeth's father, Samuel Blackwell, was an abolitionist; her brothers, Henry and Samuel, supported both the antislavery and women's rights movements. Henry married Lucy Stone, one of the nation's leading women's rights advocates, and Samuel married Antoinette Brown, the first woman to be ordained as a minister in the United States. Elizabeth's sisters, Anna and Sara Ellen, became painters, and Emily, like Elizabeth, studied medicine. "We were," Zakrzewska later recalled, "a delightful family, suffering more or less from social ostracism but happy in spirit, and feeling far above the ordinary run of mankind in the belief of our superiority in thought and aim."[3] Zakrzewska would remain in New York City three years. In that time she would have her first experience planning, establishing, and then helping to run a hospital by and for women. It was the first such hospital in the United States.

• • •

Once Zakrzewska settled into the Blackwell household, she and Elizabeth turned their attention to finalizing their plans for an all-women's hospital. Emily, who was at that time in England, did what she could from abroad. One of the first tasks they embarked upon was the writing of a small pamphlet, spelling out in detail the exact nature of the enterprise they sought to establish. *An Appeal in Behalf of the Medical Education of Women* built on two central premises: that women physicians had to be "thoroughly qualified" in order to keep the practice of medicine out of "ignorant or unworthy hands" and that a good education meant combining theoretical instruction with practical training.[4] The reference to the "ignorant" and "unworthy" may have been a veiled criticism of unorthodox physicians. All three founders had been educated in regular schools and intended to offer clinical training in orthodox medical practices.[5] However, they may also have been attacking female abortionists. Although they do not develop this point in their pamphlet, at other times Zakrzewska described abortionists, like the infamous Madame Restell, as the greatest threat to the reputation of women physicians. Advertising their services, often under the title of "Doctress," they confused the public, Zakrzewska believed, blurring the boundary between competent female physicians and those who "disgrace decency and undertake abhorred practice."[6] Zakrzewska's condemnation of abortionists was, it should be emphasized, typical of women's rights advocates at the time, who argued that such practices allowed men to avoid responsibility for their sexual behavior, assured that any pregnancy that occurred could be terminated for a fee.[7]

Both Zakrzewska and Blackwell were determined to undo any such confusion. Their hospital, they insisted, would train the best physicians possible, complementing the more theoretical education women received in medical school with an education at the bedside. "[T]he mere attendances on courses of scientific lectures, even if fully illustrated by cases, &c., is altogether insufficient," Zakrzewska and Blackwell argued. "[Students] cannot learn from words the characteristics of disease, which must be appreciated by all the senses. The physician deals with physical symptoms, and those can only be studied by the bedside; and not in a few scattered cases, but by the examination of hundreds and thousands of individuals, before varieties can be distinguished, and delicate but important shades of difference thoroughly known."[8]

Male students, we have already noted, had the opportunity to gain practical experience by attending patients with their preceptors or by walking hospital wards with their professors. Female students, on the contrary, had to rely on the goodwill of a hospital physician who, even if he himself harbored no objections to instructing women, often found it difficult to withstand the disapprobation of his colleagues. This, as we have seen, had been Zakrzewska's experience with Delamater. Blackwell and Zakrzewska thus insisted that women must have their own hospitals; it was the only place where they could become "really acquainted with disease."[9]

In emphasizing the importance of practical training Blackwell and Zakrzewska were by no means alone. Indeed, the desire for clinical training is what sent thousands of American medical students to the European cities of Paris, London, and Edinburgh during the antebellum period.[10] Attempts, however, to create similar opportunities in the United States rarely succeeded: poorly endowed medical schools could not afford to construct their own hospitals, and hospital trustees generally refused to grant neighboring medical schools the authority they needed to conduct proper clinical classes.[11] Aware of this problem, Blackwell and Zakrzewska were seeking to create a teaching hospital, unaffiliated with any medical school but one nevertheless whose central purpose would be to train physicians. They saw this as a radically new departure in the American system, for it made the hospital "the foundation of a medical education." They were, they stated simply but emphatically, promoting "a very different method of education *from anything yet attempted*."[12]

Their model was not, however, the European clinics visited by male medical students who went abroad to further their clinical training but, significantly, the training programs for midwives. In Europe, they proclaimed, even common midwives received an education that was largely practical.

> [T]hey reside in a hospital for one or two years, having all the ordinary cases of their specialty in their own hands, under the supervision of superiors; they assist in the medical and surgical treatment of extraordinary cases; their powers of observation are cultivated by detailed records of cases, which they are required to make, day by day, at the bedside; their hand is carefully trained to the delicacy of touch, indispensable in this department of medicine, and through the whole period of instruction they go from the lecture-room to the bedside, receiving at every hour of the day practical illustration of the subject discussed by their professors. If such thorough training is considered necessary for a class of practitioners whose position in medicine, is a limited and subordinate one, how much more is it necessary to the wider duties and higher responsibilities of the physician.[13]

Historians of medicine who have studied European influences on American medical education have focused on the sites where male physicians trained when they went abroad, that is, on the medical clinics and hospital wards of Paris, London, and Edinburgh (and later in the century on the German laboratories).[14] But both the New York Infirmary and the New England Hospital for Women and Children, two of the earliest and most successful teaching hospitals in the United States, took their inspiration from schools of midwifery. This is, of course, hardly surprising. Zakrzewska was the product of one of the best midwifery programs in Europe. Elizabeth Blackwell, too, had spent several years following her graduation from Geneva Medical School at the Paris La Maternité, honing her clinical skills and observing a similar training program. Still, it must have rankled many physicians to have the system of medical education in the United States compared unfavorably to the training of midwives, a group most physicians considered beneath them.

Blackwell's and Zakrzewska's focus on the "Hospital" (which they capitalized) did not preclude an appreciation of laboratory exercises. On the contrary, they asserted that "[a]s soon as possible a laboratory and good anatomical rooms will be added to the hospital, which shall afford thorough practical facilities to students."[15] Thus under "practical," which they believed to be the "most important part of medicine," they placed both clinical training and exercises in the laboratory and dissection rooms (although there can be no question that they placed greater importance on the former). In doing so they were parroting the demands of German physicians, who had been pressuring their governments for almost a decade to make such "practical" exercises a required part of the medical curriculum. We have already noted that Zakrzewska was still in Berlin when Prussia and several other German states began to reform their medical schools in accordance with these demands. In the United States such requests for reform could be heard as well, although in contrast to Germany they appealed only to a small elite until much later in the century.[16] Blackwell and Zakrzewska counted themselves among this elite.

Armed with this message, the two women began to try to raise money for their hospital. Most of their financial backing ended up coming from the community of social reformers who saw this as an opportunity to provide quality care to poor women while also advancing the cause of women physicians. The Quakers, to whom Blackwell had particularly strong connections, provided critical support. Zakrzewska also reached out to more radical groups, although she claimed Blackwell was "often repelled by the theories advanced by them." Exactly which groups troubled Blackwell is unclear, but Zakrzewska described attending the salon of the literary sisters Alice and Phoebe Cary; joining Alpha, an association for the advancement of women; and meeting with Free Lovers, "the admirers of the socialist Fourier," and Spiritualists. She became, she explained, "acquainted with the leading minds who agitated the public, and who helped to advance our plans for the establishment of a hospital."[17]

"We were the happiest," she once reminisced, thinking of the women who gave their support to the hospital, "even if materially the poorest, of a group of women which included friends engaged in different lines of work, such as journalism, art and music. Of these, none identified herself so closely with us as Mary L. Booth . . . who spent every Sunday with us."[18] Booth (1831–89), who was a reporter at the *New York Times*, covered issues related to women and education. Upon request, she received her editor's permission to run announcements for the hospital in the newspaper, soliciting funds for the cause and helping to raise considerable sums. An active member of the Anti-Slavery Society of New York and a founding member of Alpha, she shared many of Zakrzewska's political passions, and the two women gradually became extremely close. Booth went on to earn a national reputation as both the editor of *Harper's Bazaar*, a literary-fashion magazine founded in 1867, and a translator of French works, being responsible for the translation of roughly forty volumes in her lifetime. In addition to producing English editions of literary works, she translated the writings of European sympathizers with the Union's cause. As we will see shortly, she and Zakrzewska also pursued a number of political projects together, including an aborted attempt to found a women's journal during the early years of the Civil War. Their friendship lasted until Booth's untimely death in 1889 at the age of fifty-eight.[19]

In her fund-raising attempts, Zakrzewska also received substantial backing from the Boston community of social reformers. Walter Channing, a Boston physician with a deep and abiding interest in the promotion of women physicians, had convinced her to visit his city to seek funds. She made her first trip in early July 1856. Although she traveled to other cities over the next few months, she returned to no city as often as to Boston; nor did she find anywhere else the same level of enthusiasm for a women's hospital. Zakrzewska was able to take advantage of her connections to Harriot Hunt and Caroline Severance, but it was primarily through Channing that she met Lucy Goddard, Mary Jane Parkman, Abby May, and Ednah D. Cheney, all of whom would become her most ardent supporters when she decided to found her own hospital in Boston several years later. Her circle of friends also soon extended to William Lloyd Garrison II, with whom she stayed during one of her Boston trips. As he wrote his brother, Wendell Phillips Garrison, he found her "a charming woman, and a splendid scholar. She is the easiest person in conversation that I ever saw, & interests everyone whom she converses with."[20]

Zakrzewska returned from Boston with the promise of half the rent for three years. This, in addition to the other funds she and Blackwell raised, allowed them to open the first all-female teaching hospital in the country in 1857. The New York Infirmary for Women and Children was located at 64 Bleeker Street, right on the outskirts of the neighborhood known as Five Points. Zakrzewska and Blackwell had scheduled the official opening for 12 May, which coincided with the twenty-fourth meeting of the American Anti-Slavery Society. Whether this was intentional is unclear; it may be that they hoped to draw a larger crowd to their opening. Unfortunately, in some cases it backfired. Zakrzewska, who had hoped that William Lloyd Garrison II would attend, learned with disappointment that he had other obligations to fulfill. Nevertheless, they did manage to get together during his stay.[21]

Garrison's absence could not, however, quell Zakrzewska's excitement for long. Two days after the opening, she wrote Harriot Hunt, who had by this time become a close friend. "Will you not come to New York this spring? I am homesick for you, I wish to see you & also Mrs. Severance. I feel the first time

myself since my life in New York, I wish to embrace the whole world for gratitude of this feeling, as if they had bestowed it upon me, & all this together makes
me thanking God, that I live, lived & will live to be useful to my contemporaries
& perhaps even to posterity."[22]

This is one of the few letters I have come across that captures the combination of youthful enthusiasm, verve, and sense of purpose that seems to have
made Zakrzewska attractive to so many individuals when they first met her. It
allows us to understand more easily Elizabeth Blackwell's comment to her sister,
shortly after meeting Zakrzewska, that "[t]here is the true stuff in her" or Hunt's
remark that "when I met her, an electric communication was instantly established between us."[23] Zakrzewska seems to have made friends easily, quickly,
and intensely. This was certainly true of her friendships with Mary Booth and
Karl Heinzen in New York. It would also characterize her first encounters with
Lucy Sewall, Caroline Healey Dall, and Julia Sprague once she moved to
Boston. Zakrzewska's spiritedness may, moreover, have inspired many of her
donors, both in New York and later in Boston, who sensed in Zakrzewska a
young woman of conviction and passion.

Zakrzewska now applied this energy to her work at the New York Infirmary.
She was, she later claimed without any sign of modesty, "really the soul of that
establishment."[24] She and the Blackwell sisters (Emily had since returned from
England) agreed that Zakrzewska would assume the role of resident physician,
living in the hospital while managing its day-to-day affairs. The infirmary had a
total of twenty-four beds: two general wards each with six beds; a maternity
ward; and sleeping quarters that could accommodate four students, three servants, and the resident physician. Zakrzewska shared with Elizabeth and Emily
the care of the patients and the instruction of the students; they also all took
turns running the dispensary, which they kept open six days a week from nine
until noon. In addition, Emily handled most of the surgical cases while Zakrzewska mixed medicines in the apothecary, a skill she had acquired while studying medicine in Cleveland. In no time at all they had filled all the beds in
the hospital and were often seeing thirty people a day through the dispensary.
Emily later estimated that by the end of their first year, thirty-seven hundred
women and children had benefited from the New York Infirmary's outpatient
practice.[25]

The novelty of the New York Infirmary was not, it should be emphasized, in
providing care for women and children. Other hospitals in America already
offered that service. What was new was that the hospital was run by an entirely

female staff; in addition, this staff provided clinical training to women interested in pursuing a medical career. In its first year, four medical students lived in the hospital, paying three dollars a week for board and receiving in exchange instruction "at the bedside," both in the wards and at the dispensary. The level of supervision they received may very well have been higher than at most other hospitals that permitted clinical instruction, a reflection of the high standards Zakrzewska and the Blackwells set out to impose. With three physicians and four students, the New York Infirmary avoided what had become a central criticism of many other hospital arrangements both at home and abroad: that with so many students following their instructors on their rounds, only the most aggressive ever got to see anything, let alone practice their own skills.[26] Indeed, Zakrzewska and Blackwell had made it a goal to avoid "the rush of students . . . , crowding and elbowing one another for the best place, peering over each other's shoulders in the effort to see as well as hear what is going on." They did this by keeping the classes small; in fact, at any given time, only two students were in the dispensary and two in the wards. As they explained, this was done "so as to keep them completely under the supervision of the professor, to enable him to acquire a full acquaintance with the ability and needs of each individual student, and to allow the latter to obtain that special aid of which the want is so much felt by those who have been members of a large hospital class."[27]

The arrangement Zakrzewska had made with the Blackwells was that she would work for two years in exchange for room and board. Whatever earnings she made had to come from her private practice, which she continued to pursue in the late afternoons and early evenings. "In truth," she later remembered, "often I had to earn by outside practice, the money to buy a holiday or Sunday dinner, as the Institution was too poor to afford a decent table."[28]

During the first year of the infirmary's existence, all three women worked together, but in the second year Elizabeth went to England to help advance women's entry into the medical profession in her native land. The work, Zakrzewska later remembered, grew more difficult—she and Emily often saw sixty patients a day in the dispensary—but she continued to find it extremely rewarding. What she also deeply appreciated was the constant support they received from some of the city's more established physicians, such as Richard Kissam, a well-known obstetrician; Willard Parker, professor of surgery in the College of Physicians and Surgeons; and Valentine Mott, another well-respected surgeon. Some of these physicians came to the hospital to consult on a case or provide clinical instruction; others invited the female students to visit their dispensaries;

yet others joined the hospital's board of consulting physicians. Thus what the female students must have learned, in addition to the medical knowledge they acquired, was something that Zakrzewska had long ago appreciated, and that was the value and importance of the support that prominent men could offer their cause.[29]

. . .

By the end of the decade Zakrzewska had come to realize that "their cause" extended far beyond simply breaking down the barriers keeping women out of the medical profession. She even came to believe that linking their cause to the movement for women's rights, however important that may be, was not enough; it had also become necessary to fight for sweeping social, political, and moral reforms. In this regard, no one influenced her more than Karl Heinzen, a German "Forty-Eighter," whom she met sometime after returning to New York. Zakrzewska would end up sharing her home with Heinzen and his wife for twenty years.

The "Forty-Eighters" were Old World democrats who left their homeland for political reasons following the failed revolutions of 1848. Frustrated in their inability to establish a constitutional democracy in Germany and put an end to the monarchical system that denied the majority of the population any part in the political process, many turned to America as the "promised land," hopeful that they could more easily work toward creating a truly democratic society here. Although they never constituted more than a small minority of the German immigrant population in the United States, their visibility and impact on American political and social life surpassed their numbers. Not surprisingly, they became defenders of individual freedoms, outspoken and sometimes militant in their attack on slavery and in their battles for freedom of the press and religion and voting rights.[30]

Heinzen had made a name for himself in Germany as a radical republican and political journalist. He had first been forced to flee his homeland in 1844 after publishing several scathing critiques of the Prussian bureaucracy. Following a long sojourn in Switzerland and a much briefer stay in the United States, he returned to Europe in March 1848 to join the revolutionary forces in Baden, the German state where the possibility of establishing a true democracy seemed most promising. When the revolution failed, he once again had to flee. Heinzen returned to the United States in the fall of 1850, this time to make it his new home. Although he would make several trips to Europe later in life, he never again set foot on his native soil.[31]

Zakrzewska had heard of Heinzen through her father, who had read the journalist's banned publications on the sly.[32] She may thus have actively sought him out after he moved to New York in 1855. More than likely, though, she came across his name through his editorship of a politically radical German-language weekly he had founded two years earlier, *Der Pionier*, a paper William Lloyd Garrison once described as "the ablest, most independent and outspoken, and most uncompromising in its opposition to slavery, of all the German newspapers in this country."[33] "Uncompromising" was surely the best way to describe not only Heinzen's newspaper but the man himself. As Horace Greeley once commented, no other European exile wielded "so trenchant, merciless and independent a pen as Mr. Charles Heinzen." "A radical democrat," he continued, "avowing his opinions on religion, literature, politics or individuals, with perfect coolness and indifference to the opinions of the majority, he necessarily often shocks the feelings of his readers and makes foes where he might make friends, but he also often tells the truth."[34] Heinzen's biographer, Carl Wittke, writing almost a century later, agreed with this assessment. Heinzen, he wrote, rather unpoetically, "never pricked with a needle when he could hit over the head with a hammer."[35]

In the next chapter we turn to Heinzen's writings in greater detail; for now I wish to mention only that he was as committed to promoting materialism, atheism, and the dangers of the Roman Catholic Church as he was to the abolition of slavery and the fight for equal rights for all people, regardless of sex or race. All these political concerns eventually became Zakrzewska's as well. When they first met is unclear, but by the fall of 1858 they were contemplating a move to Boston together. Their friendship, as Zakrzewska once described it, was "based not simply on affinity, by nature, but also on principle, making the object for which we spoke, our real life's cause, and we pledged ourselves to devote our strength and means to further our convictions & realizations."[36]

In October 1858 two events came together. Heinzen decided to take *Der Pionier* to Boston, where he believed the community of radical German émigrés had a stronger following than in New York. He had his paper up and running in his new hometown by the beginning of the new year. By that time, he may already have known that Zakrzewska would eventually follow, since she had received a letter from the trustees of Boston's New England Female Medical College in early October asking that she consider the directorship of a teaching hospital that they were planning to found in connection with their school. Zakrzewska did not, however, move as quickly as Heinzen. First, she visited

Boston in February to give a lecture and speak in person with the trustees of the school. Only after receiving a formal offer later that month did she decide to accept the position of professor of obstetrics and diseases of women and children and resident physician in the hospital-to-be. Even then, she remained in New York a while longer, tying up loose ends. Not until early June did she finally move.[37]

In the intervening months she stayed in close touch with Heinzen, even penning two articles on women and medicine for his paper. Zakrzewska would never again be so prolific. Aside from her autobiographical sketch, which she published in 1860, she wrote only a handful of articles, three of which appeared in German in *Der Pionier*. She leaves us no clue as to why she published so little. Perhaps she lost interest in writing for a German audience but lacked the confidence to communicate her ideas in English. Perhaps she simply lacked the time. Certainly, the founding of the New England Hospital for Women and Children in 1862 changed her life radically, leaving her precious little time to do much else other than care for her institution. But perhaps the question should not be why she did not continue writing but rather why she ever wrote at all. The few months in the spring of 1859, when Zakrzewska was "between jobs," may simply have been an anomaly, a time, like no other, when she had the luxury to spend her days collecting her thoughts for publication. It is also possible that Heinzen had suggested that this would be a good way for her to make a name for herself in the community of radical German émigrés she would soon be joining in Boston.

· · ·

In the spring of 1859 Zakrzewska published two articles in *Der Pionier*, "Weibliche Aerzte" (Female Physicians), which appeared on 19 March, and "Sind Hebammenschulen wünschenswerth?" (Are Midwifery Schools Desirable?), which appeared one month later.[38] In both articles Zakrzewska promoted the cause of women physicians, challenging the biological, cultural, and legal arguments that were frequently put forth to justify women's exclusion from the medical profession. Both, moreover, continued the argument she had begun in her medical thesis, in which she had denied the existence of any significant differences between the sexes. But whereas in the second article Zakrzewska assumed the absence of difference and insisted as a result that women interested in medicine should be trained as physicians and not midwives, in the first article she tackled the question of difference head-on.

"Weibliche Aerzte" was a response to the arguments of the German physi-

cian Dr. C. Both, who had published a piece against women physicians in another New York City German-language newspaper, the *Familienblätter*. Dr. Both
had presented arguments typical of his day, questioning whether women had
the intelligence to practice medicine; whether their modesty prevented them
from carrying out dissections; whether the social cost of abandoning their roles
as wives and mothers was too high; whether women's physiology, particularly
menstruation and pregnancy, functioned as a deterrent; and finally whether
female physicians were necessary.[39] Zakrzewska did not know the author, but
this did not prevent her from ridiculing his claims; indeed, it may very well have
given her the desired freedom.

Herr Both, Zakrzewska told her readers, was one of those German pedants
who "come limping along to lay down their veto" after America has decided in
favor of women studying medicine. His objections, she contended, centered on
two questions: "1. do women have the right, and 2. do they have the ability, to
study and practice medicine." To Zakrzewska, even posing the problem in this
way seemed quintessentially German, for only in her native land did "the
police . . . tend to assign women the 'sphere' of her rights as well as of her
abilities." In America, on the other hand (and Zakrzewska was clearly identifying with her new country), there was no need to maintain a "female 'sphere'"
because "no laws dictate what we may learn and not learn; . . . we can be
educated according to our inclinations and abilities, as far as the opportunities
suffice, without having to ask an obscure German authority for permission."[40]

Turning, then, directly to the question of women's abilities, Zakrzewska challenged the "Herr Doctor" to come up with proof that men and women were
endowed with different "intellectual tendencies and abilities" and "to establish
these differences exactly and convincingly." She brought up for consideration
Justine Siegismundin, Madame Lachapelle, and Madame Boivin, three European women who excelled in medicine, earning national and international
reputations for their skills. Sarcastically, she went on:

> I do not know whether these "women doctors" had the necessary weight
> and the necessary number of meters. Herr Dr. Both shows us, through an
> extensive numerical proof, that, in addition to greater height, men also
> have greater body and brain weight than women. However, he withholds
> with surprising modesty the conclusions which one should draw from these
> differences in weight. Since, however, he cannot have shared all these num-
> bers only to prove that he has the expert knowledge of transcribing them, I

must take him by his word or by his number. I hope he will ascribe the same importance to the differences in weight among the men themselves as between the two sexes, and regret with me the death of the 600 pound man who died recently in New York and in whom we have certainly lost one of the greatest medical geniuses.[41]

Having ridiculed Both's association between body size and brain size, Zakrzewska went on to challenge his claim that female modesty made it difficult for women to practice medicine effectively. The critical problem, for Both as for many, centered on the image of women in the dissection room. Zakrzewska began by questioning the "brutal" nature of medicine, countering that when she had observed men and women in Germany and in America carrying out dissections, all she had recognized was "almost a solemn silence and a certain scientific dignity which, by providing enlightenment about the wonderful construction of the human body, satisfied the thirst for knowledge." But Zakrzewska also challenged the pristine nature of women's work in the home, adding that "the noble businesses of slaughtering, disemboweling and dissecting in the kitchen, which the Herr Doctor kindly designates as [our] 'sphere,' are more disgusting to me than the dissections in the anatomy room."[42]

Zakrzewska moved on from her criticism of "kitchen duties" to a dismissal of Both's concerns that women would be abandoning their social roles were they to choose a medical career over marriage and motherhood. She did not so much deny that this would occur, although she did relay the story of a friend who was managing to work as a physician and have a family. More important, she rejected Both's assumption that marriage should be a woman's ultimate goal. This is a theme Zakrzewska would address more fully when she sat down to write her autobiographical sketch the following year. Although her position on marriage would soften later in life, at this stage she could barely hide her disdain for the view that "woman has nothing else to study than the art of finding a man to support her. I do not know," she went on in "Weibliche Aerzte," "whether this concern for our happiness belongs to the male physician's profession; I do know that this concern will not be reciprocated from our side. I do not fear that the female sex will go bankrupt if the doctors of weight and meter-long height die as bachelors."[43]

Zakrzewska had two more points to make. As far as women's physiology was concerned, she declared the notion that "natural disturbances . . . make women 'irresponsible'" to be "mere fables." As she had done in her medical dissertation, she was challenging once again the claim that women's bodies rendered them unfit or even in need of special attention. "Either a woman is healthy or she is sick," Zakrzewska declared matter-of-factly. "If she is healthy, then all the functions of her body are in order without somehow taking on disease forms. If, however, symptoms indicate a diseased state, then the sick woman is merely on a par with a sick man who is likewise overcome, under such conditions, by mental disturbances." For Zakrzewska, pregnancy received so much attention only "because it is the most obvious" disturbance, not because it is the most serious. "Even if it were true that such conditions interrupt the functions of a female physician for days or weeks, isn't this just like what happens to male [physicians] who are held up for weeks or months through illness, etc?"[44]

Zakrzewska's denial of difference also shaped her response to Both's final assertion: that women physicians were unnecessary. What sense, she asked, does it make to ask why women doctors are here or whether "our prescriptions are better and more effective than those that men prescribe?" For Zakrzewska this question was just as silly as asking whether women wrote books because their books were better and more interesting than those men authored. "I have often written prescriptions for men and women because I have won their confidence through treating their families," Zakrzewska wrote in her conclusion to the article. "By this opportunity I learned that we women can have an effect on or through a man's stomach in a different way than through fine cooking."[45]

Zakrzewska wrote this article with the confidence of a woman who harbored no doubts that her arguments would demolish those of her opponent. "The reasons of Herr Dr. Both . . . are in general those one hears in any public saloon," Zakrzewska told her readers, designating his views as "low-brow" and, by implication, hers as educated and informed. But Zakrzewska's views were only in part the accepted ones, even of advocates of women's medical education. While in challenging men's intellectual superiority she was certainly joining others who were fighting for women's rights, her total denial of difference was not commonplace. Note that Zakrzewska rejected differences between the sexes on two grounds: she refused to attribute any significance to women's peculiar physiological functions, and she rejected the notion that women physicians had anything special to offer the field of medicine. This was an unusual position to defend.

At the time, most women who aspired to enter the medical field built their arguments on two central claims. The first emphasized that because of female modesty women needed practitioners of their own sex. How could one expect women to share their bodily and emotional troubles with men? Human decency and female delicacy worked against such confidences, with the result that many women avoided medical help until it was too late. The second claim built on woman's special nature as sympathetic and compassionate. Women, so the argument went, had much to offer medicine, which they defined as the caring profession par excellence, for they were uniquely positioned to combine "sympathy" and "science." No one, in fact, was more vocal in this regard than Zakrzewska's friend and colleague Elizabeth Blackwell, who believed that the maternal instinct—potential or realized—endowed women with a natural and singular capacity to heal.[46] Zakrzewska, in denying such differences, was distancing herself from the majority of her colleagues. Her argument for women physicians, unusual as it was, amounted to little more than the assertion that there was no justification for granting one sex privileges while denying them to the other.

Zakrzewska stood out not only because of what she was arguing but also because of her style. Thus, in contrast to her contemporary Ann Preston, the first woman to become dean of the Female Medical College of Pennsylvania, who refrained from displaying any behaviors that could be judged unfeminine, Zakrzewska engaged in a performance in which she intentionally inverted dominant gender stereotypes.[47] She did this by announcing her distaste for the preparation of food, certainly one of women's most traditional responsibilities, and by declaring a greater affinity for science (as a woman) than Dr. Both possessed. Her entire essay, in fact, focused on the illogic of his assertions, thus allowing her to claim for herself, as a woman and in opposition to her male opponent, the mantle of rationality. Using ridicule while displaying a biting wit, Zakrzewska showed little anxiety about how her gender transgressions would be received; on the contrary, she was clearly having a ball.

Zakrzewska's unusual performance does not mean that she shared nothing with her peers. Hannah Longshore, a member of the first graduating class of the Female Medical College of Pennsylvania and a successful practitioner, also claimed masculine-coded traits for herself, fashioning her autobiography around a heroic tale that highlighted her success at overcoming adversity by drawing on her own resources.[48] Mary Putnam Jacobi, who was certainly less brash than either Longshore or Zakrzewska, nevertheless matched Zakrzewska's disdain for arguments based on gender differences and engaged in scientific research designed to demolish the grounds upon which such arguments depended.[49] Finally, and perhaps most important, Zakrzewska was just one woman among many who were challenging gender stereotypes around midcentury simply by virtue of claiming space for themselves in the male-dominated medical profession.[50]

Thus it is best, as has been argued, to see these women as developing diverse strategies for securing a means to the shared end of opening the doors of the medical profession to women.[51] Why Zakrzewska chose her particular path to this end stemmed as much from her personal style—she clearly relished the opportunity to challenge traditional gender stereotypes—as from her political conviction that women's emancipation depended upon their willingness to replace what she eventually labeled "sentimental sympathy" with a scientific outlook. And this conviction, I argue, had much to do with her gradual immersion in the German radical community and the political meaning this group ascribed to science as a powerful weapon in battling arbitrary authority and promoting a radical democratic society.[52] As a symbol of reason, rationality, and objectivity, science seemed to these German radicals to promote the very mental attributes deemed critical in the battle against ignorance, superstition, and the church. At the time Zakrzewska penned "Weibliche Aerzte," she had evidently already felt the influence of this group, primarily through her friendship with Heinzen. Over the next few years, she would sharpen her attack on difference into a more coherent battle not only for women's right to study medicine but for women's rights more broadly conceived.[53]

· · ·

In the meantime, Zakrzewska also published "Sind Hebammenschulen wünschenswerth?" This article had a much more specific focus than "Weibliche Aerzte"; its purpose was to advise against the establishment of midwifery schools in the United States. It may seem odd that Zakrzewska would have chosen to write on this topic at a time when midwifery education was not actively being debated within the American medical community. By midcentury male physicians had emerged as the preferred birth attendants among white middle-class women, leaving primarily rural, especially black, and poor immigrant women in the hands of midwives. Few physicians challenged this division of labor until the last decades of the nineteenth century, when the arrival of millions of European immigrants greatly increased the number of midwives practicing in this country. Physicians, who were in the midst of an intense period of professionalization and specialization at that time, came to see these uneducated and unregulated practitioners as a serious threat. By the beginning of the twentieth century, a highly contentious "midwife controversy" was in full swing.[54]

But if, in the 1850s, little interest in this topic could be evinced from the American medical community, this was not the case among German émigrés. In fact, Zakrzewska's essay was a response to an article calling for the creation of just such schools.[55] That this topic should have generated greater concern within the German community is hardly surprising. Not only was there a long tradition among German women of using midwives as their primary birth attendant, but a significant number of midwives had emigrated, many of whom, like Zakrzewska, had received formal training at home. The question of whether—and if so, how—to train the next generation of midwives was thus of immediate concern. Zakrzewska, who felt strongly that the establishment of midwifery schools was a mistake, decided to weigh in.[56]

Zakrzewska built her argument around what she presented as a fact: that the education of German midwives "is the same as what the young men in obstetrics receive." In her previous article she had already tackled the question of whether any innate differences existed between men and women; here she focused on the absence of any differences in what German midwives and physicians learned about obstetrics. Given her unique position as a graduate of the Prussian school of midwifery and an M.D., it would have been hard to challenge her assertion. In fact, Zakrzewska did not spend much time defending this claim but turned rather to an analysis of the legal culture in her native land. There, she explained, the midwife's educational requirements as well as her rights and responsibilities were strictly laid down by law. Accordingly, despite her excellent training, she was forbidden from intervening in the birthing process. The state provided her with a superior education only to ensure that she could diagnose complications early enough to seek the appropriate help. Anyone who overstepped these boundaries risked a prison sentence of one to twenty years and a fine.[57]

Zakrzewska posed the question of whether such a system could ever work in this country, but she immediately declared that it would "be made into a farce, a caricature." She imagined two objections, one having more to do with the American character, the other with the legal system. If the midwife, she asked, knew exactly what to do when complications arose, "wouldn't it be, according to American ideas, a certain stupidity to ask someone else for help and perhaps to sacrifice, thereby, one's reputation and service?" But the more fundamental problem rested with the absence of any kind of restrictive legal code governing medical education and practice. At this point, Zakrzewska challenged her readers to consider whether such laws could ever be passed that would define the limits of the midwives' responsibilities or that would restrict the number of midwives permitted to practice in order to ensure that each one could make a living. Such laws existed throughout Europe, she admitted, but "can one introduce such laws in the United States, and would they, if introduced, be followed?"[58] Clearly, she expected her readers to respond with a resounding "no."

Whether Zakrzewska ever felt a sense of camaraderie with other midwives may be a reasonable question to pose, but certainly by the time she penned this article, she had exchanged whatever earlier identity she may have had as a midwife for one as a physician. Only in this way can one begin to understand why she did not propose establishing midwifery schools in the United States, modeled on the German system, that would produce high-caliber birth attendants. She could also have seen the absence of restrictive legislation as an advantage, for it would have removed the aspect of the German system she considered most unjust, that is, that despite their knowledge of how to handle complications, midwives were permitted to manage only normal births. But Zakrzewska herself was troubled by the prospect of producing midwives who would practice their skills in an unregulated environment. More than likely she feared that the line demarcating midwives and female physicians would be blurred, thereby jeopardizing her work to have women counted among the medical elite. Thus, whatever criticisms she may have had of Germany's medicolegal culture, Zakrzewska stopped short of embracing an open-market system. Not recognizing the inconsistency in her own thinking, she concluded her essay by denying the premise around which she had built her argument. Although she had begun by insisting that midwives knew every bit as much as medical students when it came to obstetrics, she ended by declaring that the responsibility of caring for other people's health, and especially their lives, was great enough to demand that birth attendants receive the best education possible. For this reason, she explained, "I am . . . in favor of making midwives superfluous in America through female doctors, in fact, in getting rid of them."[59]

• • •

It is worth noting that at the time Zakrzewska made this statement she had already accepted her new position at the New England Women's Medical College, an institution that trained midwives, nurses, and physicians. Small wonder she would soon become embroiled in battles with Samuel Gregory, the school's director. It matters little that Gregory probably never read this German-language article; Zakrzewska most certainly made her views known to him in other ways.

Zakrzewska still had six weeks before she would leave New York. Later in life she claimed that she had moved to Boston in order to be closer to Heinzen, but her reasons for leaving New York must have been more complex.[60] There can be no question that she was a highly ambitious woman, and while the offer from Boston was not to run her own institution, she was being asked to create and then take charge of a clinical department at the college. The new position thus promised a greater degree of independence than what she had at the New York Infirmary, where, she later explained, "the two Drs. Blackwells controlled the direction of efforts towards what seemed to them wisest and best."[61] Despite her full participation in the life of the New York Infirmary, she had, it seems, never felt as though she was a full partner.

There are suggestions, moreover, that tensions had been building between the three women. To some extent this may have reflected different personalities. There was already a hint of this in the letter Zakrzewska had written to Harriot Hunt just after the opening of the infirmary in May 1857. She had confessed at that time her puzzlement with "these two women," who had "all right to be satisfied with their work & efforts as it resulted, & they are, but still they won't acknowledge it either to [each?] other nor to themselves, they do persuade themselves, I believe, that they are not . . . or do they perhaps show their joy in their bedroom when nobody sees them? I really don't know, but one thing is certain they do wrong not to reward their friends by showing them a pleased countenance."[62]

Zakrzewska shows here the slightest hint of feeling unappreciated for all the work she had done, and although she went on to assure Hunt that "in spite of all I love them, and feel sad that nothing can cheer them up," by 1859 she may have grown tired of their more subdued demeanor. But she may also have become increasingly aware of a deepening rift when it came to their political views. According to Zakrzewska, at least, she preferred to travel in more radical circles. Indeed, she and Heinzen may have decided to move to Boston in part because of an expectation that that city would be more responsive to their goals. New York's Little Germany, according to one historian, was not even as reformist as the German American community in the Midwest, let alone the community in Boston.[63] In addition, Zakrzewska had come away from her many visits to Boston with the impression that the prejudice against women physicians was less palpable there than anywhere else she had lived.

In making her decision to move, Zakrzewska had also considered that the New York Infirmary was on sound financial footing; that she had fulfilled her two-year commitment to the Blackwells; that her experience had shown her that two physicians could run the hospital alone; and that she would make a greater contribution to the advancement of women's medical education in Boston. Still, if she found it easy to make the move for professional reasons, this was not the case where her personal life was concerned. More than anyone else, she had difficulty leaving Mary Booth, to whom she had grown extremely close during the years they spent together in New York. Zakrzewska described how Booth would often stay overnight with her at the hospital, sharing "my room and bed when she was out at night as reporter of the New York *Times* too late to return to her home in Williamsburg." Zakrzewska also spent the New Year's holiday in 1858 with Booth and her parents in Williamsburg rather than traveling to her own family in Hoboken. Later in life, thinking back over her friendship with Booth, Zakrzewska commented that "[i]t is not through blood kinship that we feel the strongest; nay, we may even feel no affinity at all towards the sisters and brothers we so love, while the few kindred spirits we meet fill our souls with life and inspiration."[64]

Carolyn Heilbrun once wrote that "the sign of female friendship is not whether friends are homosexual or heterosexual, lovers or not, but whether they share the wonderful energy of work in the public sphere. These, some of them hidden, are the friends whom biographers must seek out."[65] This would certainly describe the friendship Zakrzewska had with Booth. There is, in fact, little evidence that they were sexually involved, despite sharing a bed, which was, after all, quite common at the time. Physical contact between women in the Victorian period carried none of the meaning it would acquire after early twentieth-century sexologists began publishing tracts about the dangers of lesbianism.[66] If any additional proof of this were necessary, then Zakrzewska's willingness to state in print that she shared a bed with Booth would provide it. Often going to great lengths to protect her privacy, Zakrzewska would not have paraded her relationship with Booth publicly were it not considered normal by nineteenth-century standards.

The absence of a sexual relationship did not, however, mean a lack of intimacy. In an obituary Zakrzewska wrote after Booth's death in 1889, she explicitly used this term to describe the nature of their friendship. "Miss Booth," she wrote, "had many friends, but was intimate with only a few; therefore, the real depth of her nature was but little known. I am happy to say that I was one of those few, and our intimacy was only broken by death."[67] Theirs was an intense friendship, which the two women managed to sustain through a series of projects. The autobiographical sketch Zakrzewska published in 1860 actually began as a letter to Booth, undertaken after her friend had requested that she share some stories from her childhood. A few years later, they also set out to coedit a journal dedicated to promoting "the interests of women, and to furnish an impartial platform for the free discussion of these interests in their various phases."[68] And in the 1870s they traveled together, along with a few other friends, to Europe. This trip was the fulfillment of a wish Zakrzewska had earlier expressed to Booth that she would "be enabled some day to go with you to Berlin, to show you the scenes in which my childhood and youth were passed, and to teach you on the spot the difference between Europe and America."[69]

Zakrzewska's friendships with Harriot Hunt and Mary Booth, and the bonds she would forge with other women in Boston, provide evidence of what Carroll Smith-Rosenberg has called "The Female World of Love and Ritual," a world in which women's relationships with one another were marked by an emotional and physical (although not necessarily sexual) intimacy.[70] We will examine this world more closely in the next chapter, when we look at the forty-year-long relationship Zakrzewska enjoyed with Julia A. Sprague, a teacher and women's rights activist she met in 1862. The only caveat one must add is that Zakrzewska's circle of intimate friends included at least one man as well. Indeed, however strong her feelings may have been for Booth, she chose to leave New York in order to follow Heinzen to Boston and continue her political work side by side with him. Still, it was with mixed emotions and a heavy heart that she left Booth on 5 June for the city that would remain her home for the rest of her life.

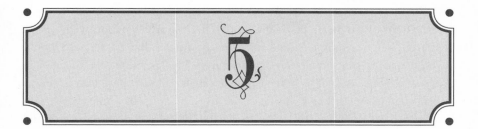

Fashioning a Home

Within a year of moving to Boston, Zakrzewska bought her own home. She saw home ownership as a mark of middle-class respectability, a sign of financial independence, and an indication that she could enter into any and all relations with others freely.[1] The home life she fashioned, however, had little to do with the idealized middle-class model, which by the mid-nineteenth century had become focused on a married couple, their children, and however many servants they could afford. Although in practice many middle-class households may not have fit the model exactly, in theory this nuclear family was ruled by a property-owning husband, whose responsibility it was to provide for and protect his wife and children. In return, the wife was expected to raise the children, manage the household, and, in the words of a contemporary advice manual, create "an elysium to which [the husband] can flee and find rest from the stormy strife of a selfish world," where he spent his days in productive labor.[2]

The family Zakrzewska ended up creating had, however, a radically different structure. Instead of radiating out from a central married couple, it consisted of several overlapping circles. Not only did her sisters Minna and Rosalia live with her when she first bought her home, but shortly thereafter Karl Heinzen moved in with his wife, Louise Henriette, and their sixteen-year-old son, Karl Friedrich. Two years later, Julia Sprague joined the household. Zakrzewska was, moreover, the primary breadwinner in her home. Although the members of the household contributed financially to its upkeep, neither Heinzen nor Sprague earned enough to live comfortably on their own. Still, financial necessity alone did not bring these individuals together; the Heinzens and Sprague were not "boarders" in Zakrzewska's home. Rather, shared political concerns and emotional ties bound them together as well. As Zakrzewska later commented, "Mr.

Karl Heinzen, Miss Julia A. Sprague, and my sisters formed the closer family circle in my affections."[3]

If the family is, in Karin Hausen's words, "the 'natural' location of the sexual division of labour," then it should come as no surprise that Zakrzewska would have created an alternative family structure.[4] The fact that she engaged in productive labor outside the home would not in and of itself have necessitated a radical change. According to one statistic, the percentage of women physicians who married in the nineteenth century was somewhere between one-fifth and one-third.[5] Yet it was one thing to practice medicine, which still took place in domestic settings and permitted flexible hours, and another to head the clinical department of a college or take on the directorship of a hospital. Zakrzewska was not in any position to assume the responsibilities traditionally expected of someone who wed.

Still, Zakrzewska's decision to create an alternative family structure—indeed, to fashion a home that bore little resemblance to that of her parents—was not simply a pragmatic move on her part, a way of making sure other people were managing her household while she was away at work. Like many others of her day, she viewed the institution of marriage critically. Indeed, in her autobiographical sketch, she went so far as to compare marriage to prostitution, describing how women frequently "sold" themselves to men in exchange for a home or to settle a family's debt.[6] The critics she joined spanned a wide spectrum. At one end were individuals like Lucy Stone and Henry Blackwell, who embraced the institution of marriage, favoring what many have called "companionate marriage," but challenged the institution's conventions; when they married in 1855, Stone retained her own name, the right to own property, and the power to control her own body. At the other extreme were "free lovers," who rejected marriage altogether, convinced that two individuals should remain together only as long as they felt a spiritual and emotional bond.[7] Zakrzewska's position appears to have been closest, at least in theory, to that of the "free lovers." Although there is no evidence that she was sexually involved with any of her housemates, criticisms she waged against the institution of marriage and the deep bonds she seemed capable of forming with both men and women indicate that the home she created was the one she believed would provide her with the greatest personal satisfaction. Zakrzewska may never have considered joining any of the alternative communities that were springing up around her, but it would not be going too far to say that she created a minicommunity, modeled on many of the same principles, within the walls of her own home.

. . .

The home Zakrzewska purchased in 1860 was at 139 Cedar Street in the town of Roxbury, on the outskirts of Boston. Roxbury would become annexed to Boston in 1868, but until that time, it was its own municipality. Originally a farming community, by midcentury it had already become a manufacturing and commercial center. Roxbury was also one of three "streetcar suburbs" to grow up to the southwest of Boston, its proximity to downtown (just two miles from its closest border) making it a popular location for those who worked in the city but wished to live in a somewhat more rural setting. Development was slow at first, but the establishment of a streetcar line in 1856 that connected Roxbury to downtown Boston encouraged growth. Although little more than a horse-drawn coach on iron rails (electric cars did not run until 1888), the streetcar permitted individuals like Zakrzewska to purchase property at the southern end of Roxbury and still be able to work within the city limits.[8]

At the time Zakrzewska purchased her home, Roxbury's inhabitants, numbering roughly twenty thousand, included a broad mixture of nationalities and classes. Although clear segregation by income would not occur until later in the century, distinct neighborhoods were beginning to form. The Tremont area, bordering on Boston's south end and closer to the Back Bay and Muddy River, was a manufacturing center and home to the lower middle class; Roxbury highlands, an area of steep hills at the far southeast corner of the suburb, was a predominantly residential section for people who were well-to-do. Zakrzewska's home on Cedar Street was not technically part of Roxbury highlands, but its possession of a "large garden with terraces" and "blooming pear trees" suggests that it was considerably more upscale than the brick row houses marking the Tremont district. Zakrzewska had been able to afford the house only because of a five-hundred-dollar loan she received from Samuel Sewall, one of the trustees of the New England Female Medical College and the father of the physician Lucy Sewall, who would help Zakrzewska run the New England Hospital for nearly twenty-five years.[9]

Most likely Zakrzewska felt compelled to purchase a home so soon after she arrived in Boston because of changes in her familial situation. Just six months after her move, she had received a letter informing her that her father had passed away. The news caused her particular pain because she and her father had not been on good terms. He had written disapprovingly of her decision to leave New York, where, he believed, the Blackwells had watched over her. In Boston, in contrast, she would be on her own, drawing more attention to herself than he deemed appropriate for a young woman. Annoyed by her father's criticisms, Zakrzewska had written a stern letter in reply, requesting that he either withhold his judgments or cease writing. She never learned whether he had read her letter and felt great sadness that she might have caused him unhappiness in his last days. "[T]hat year," she later wrote, "was one of the . . . most tragic, and . . . most conflicting, in emotion, in judgment and in making decisions."[10]

One of these decisions centered on who would take responsibility for her two youngest sisters, who were not yet on their own. More than likely, Zakrzewska bought her home in order to provide for them. Minna, who was nine years younger than Marie, posed less of a problem. Zakrzewska took her in and paid for her education as a language teacher, in exchange for which Minna managed the household. This arrangement lasted until 1863, when Zakrzewska's "favorite sister" was able to move out on her own. The deep affection that flourished between these two women probably stemmed from their considerable similarities: neither married, both pursued careers, and both supported many of the same politically radical causes. They remained close until Minna's early death from tuberculosis in 1877.[11]

Rosalia, the youngest child in the family, was more of a handful. Only sixteen years old at the time of her father's death, she suffered more than any of her other siblings from a lack of stability in her life. She had been aboard ship en route to America when their mother had passed away five years earlier. Whom she stayed with immediately thereafter is not known—perhaps she lived with her married sister, Anna, for a while. But by the spring of 1856, when Zakrzewska had returned to New York and was boarding with the Blackwells, Rosalia had joined her. Kitty Barry, an Irish orphan Elizabeth Blackwell had adopted, remembered Rosalia as a particularly tortured child. In her reminiscences, she described an incident in which Rosalia had locked her in a closet, refusing to free her until she agreed to say that she "hated Dr. Blackwell."[12] Zakrzewska, who must have had her hands full, took advantage of her father's remarriage to send Rosalia back to Berlin. Now, however, with their father's death, Rosalia was returning to the United States once again. Although at first she went to live with Anna, by April 1860 Anna had become ill and was sending Rosalia to Boston. It is not difficult to imagine Zakrzewska reaching the decision that it was time to provide her sister with a stable home. Unfortunately, we know very little about how long Rosalia remained with her. Zakrzewska made only one comment to the effect that her youngest sister "acts quite nicely as nurse," helping to tend to the ill who occasionally boarded in their home. Other than that, all that is known is that Rosalia eventually married a "John C. Steinebrey" and moved out as well.[13]

Zakrzewska's sisters lived in her home at most for several years. In contrast, Heinzen moved into Zakrzewska's home shortly after she bought it and remained until his death two decades later. The exact nature of their personal relationship is somewhat difficult to pin down, in part because neither wrote much about the other: Heinzen was virtually silent, and Zakrzewska did little more than repeat on several occasions that their bond stemmed from shared principles and a commitment to work together to promote social change.[14] But the difficulty in understanding their friendship stems as well from its unusual character: relationships of this intensity between a man and a woman that were not also romantic appear to have been uncommon at the time. At least, they have not been the subject of study in the same manner that marriages and same-sex friendships have been.

Zakrzewska was not, it should be noted, the only woman outside Heinzen's marriage with whom he formed a close friendship. The German émigré and political activist Clara Neymann also viewed him as a personal friend and even a father figure, addressing her letters to him with the salutation "Mein lieber guter Papa" (my dear good father).[15] Other women with whom he corresponded and whose work he admired and promoted included Mathilde F. Wendt, Mathilde Franziska Anneke, Marie Blöde, and Ernestine Rose. But whatever the nature of his friendships with these women, all of whom were deeply involved in radical causes, he was closer to no one (with the exception perhaps of his wife) than to Zakrzewska.

It was through Heinzen that Zakrzewska became deeply entwined in the German radical community, eventually sitting on the executive council of the Society for the Dissemination of Radical Principles, a group of German émigrés dedicated to abolition, suffrage, and a revision of the U.S. Constitution so that it would guarantee "equal rights for all citizens of the republic without regard to race, color, and sex."[16] She found within this community individuals who both shared and shaped her views on social justice, in particular her understanding of the place of science in radical political reform. More than a tool for acquiring information about the natural world, science represented for these radicals something akin to a worldview. Frequently describing society as a battleground between religion and arbitrary authority, on the one hand, and reason and political democracy, on the other, they linked science to humanitarian goals, convinced that the abolition of misery would not occur until individuals had the ability and the freedom to think for themselves. It is impossible to understand Zakrzewska's relationship to Heinzen, and her passionate defense of science, without first exploring Heinzen's political writings, in which he detailed his vision of a just society and what he believed would be necessary to bring it about. As William Lloyd Garrison II, a close friend of Zakrzewska's, once commented, Heinzen's "influence upon her life was deep and abiding."[17]

. . .

"There is no higher principle than that of freedom."[18] No statement of Heinzen's captures his convictions better than this; and no document inspired him more than the Declaration of Independence. Having transferred his hopes for a true democracy from Europe to his adopted land, Heinzen believed that the key to building a humane and democratic society rested in the Declaration's pronouncement that "all men are created equal; that they are endowed by their Creator with certain unalienable rights; that among these are life, liberty, and the pursuit of happiness."[19] Heinzen recognized that American society did not yet guarantee these rights for all, and he dedicated his life to fighting for such rights. Thus whether pronouncing his views on slavery, communism, religion, or suffrage, his starting point was that every human being, regardless of skin color or sex, had the right to be free and that the state had the obligation to protect this freedom. The domination of one group of people by another marked for Heinzen the height of barbarism.

Not surprisingly, Heinzen wasted little time after immigrating to America in joining the antislavery movement. Zakrzewska, we should remember, had once claimed that she had sought out Heinzen because of his commitment to abolition, declaring his position to be "equal to William Lloyd Garrison and Wendell Phillipps."[20] In 1851, when he assumed the editorship of a German newspaper, the *Deutsche Schnellpost*, he used it immediately to promote abolition, frequently blasting both the Fugitive Slave Law and, after 1854, the Kansas-Nebraska Act. Initially he also supported the Free Soil Party, and then the new Republican Party, though he turned against the latter when it refused to take an explicit stand against the Fugitive Slave Law in its 1860 platform. By 1864, he, along with many radical Germans, was supporting John C. Frémont in his challenge to Lincoln for the presidency. When Frémont withdrew from the race, convinced that he had no chance of winning, Heinzen still refused to back Lincoln, angry that he had failed to outlaw slavery throughout the United States. As for the Emancipation Proclamation, he dismissed it as a document inspired more by the need for a new military strategy than by moral and humanistic concerns.[21]

Heinzen alienated many of his paper's supporters with his harsh views of Lincoln, but he rarely worried about the popularity of his views, even when that translated into a loss of subscribers. After the war, Heinzen continued to lobby for the advancement of freed slaves. Although at times he suggested that blacks lacked certain abilities, he insisted that this reflected a history of lost opportunities rather than any inherent difference between the races. Consequently, throughout the period of Reconstruction, he advocated just as strongly for educational and employment opportunities as he did for citizenship and suffrage.[22]

Heinzen's hatred of slavery was matched by his distrust of communism, which he once branded "nothing more than a newly applied Christianity."[23] Zakrzewska, who declared herself "no friend of communism in any form," obviously shared this sentiment.[24] Well aware that Marx and Engels embraced materialism every bit as much as he did, Heinzen was nevertheless troubled by what he considered to be a dogmatic element in Marx's writings. Continuing his association between communism and religion, he accused Marx of playing "the pope" in a community in which "doctrines" substituted for "truth" and fanaticism replaced reason.[25]

As the last sentence suggests, Heinzen disliked and distrusted Marx intensely. But Heinzen's criticisms, despite his harsh tone, reflected more than a heated contest between two men with clashing personalities. Heinzen believed Marx to be mistaken in his assessment of where battle lines needed to be drawn in order to bring about a radical reform of society: the proletariat did not need to overthrow the bourgeoisie; rather, republicans needed to oust royalists. The enemy, in Heinzen's eyes, was the denial of freedom, not capital and private property. Rejecting Marx's prediction that the inevitable consequence of capitalism was the accumulation of capital in the hands of the few, Heinzen insisted that both capital and property were critical to the development of an individual's independence and sense of self-worth. Thus, rather than eliminate the right to property, Heinzen believed it should be protected for each and every one. And rather than criticize capital, he sought "to make every workingman as far as possible also a capitalist. . . . Not hatred against *capital*," he insisted, "but hatred against *oppression* is the saving watchword."[26]

Heinzen's fundamental fear was that communism would end up enslaving its citizens by empowering the state and thereby threatening individual rights. For this reason, he was convinced that communism and democracy could never coexist. Still, Heinzen embraced what he understood to be the ultimate goals of communism, that "of abolishing misery and of bridging the chasm between affluence and poverty." He simply favored the development of what he termed a socialist state, with an activist government that guarded individual rights—indeed, that refused to police the private affairs of its citizens—while funding "public streets, public fountains, public hospitals, public poor-houses, public insane asylums, public museums, public parks, public libraries, and public schools." As critical of the conservatives' emphasis on "self-help" as he was of communism, Heinzen insisted that it was the government's responsibility "to let no one sink below a minimum of human prosperity, and to secure for each one, by means of state-help, the general requisites that put him in condition to obtain by his own activity what his natural talent may enable him to obtain." Funding for the requisite "socialistic institutions" would come primarily from a progressive tax structure. "Every human being," Heinzen insisted, "is entitled to enough, no one has a right to too much; and if none have too much, all will have enough."[27]

Yet, however much Heinzen may have advocated for such social improvements, he remained convinced that the radical social reform necessary to create his ideal socialist state could never occur in the absence of a participatory democracy.[28] Thus he campaigned for nothing more vehemently than he did for freedom. Heinzen's criticisms of slavery and communism, as we have seen, stemmed from his conviction that both curtailed the legitimate rights of human beings and thus prevented the emergence of a democratic society. Nothing, however, in his opinion threatened human freedom more than the church.

Heinzen's hatred of the church knew, in fact, no bounds. Referring to priests as "spiritual wolves in sheep's clothing," he accused them of enslaving their followers, destroying their powers of reason and encouraging blind obedience.[29] Rather than fostering independence of thought, church officials used the fear of damnation to coerce people into subserviency, forcing them to focus on the afterlife rather than on the material conditions of their own lives and those of their fellow human beings. Reacting to a great extent to the dominant role the church played in European politics, Heinzen came to America suspicious of any signs of the power of this institution. "From a radical point of view," he wrote shortly after he arrived, "the church is not to be separated, but to be cut off and to be neutralized." He distrusted the suggestion of equality between the two institutions implicit in the U.S. Constitution's call for a separation of church and state. For Heinzen, the church was a hierarchical institution that was "constantly endeavoring to place itself *over* [the state]."[30] He feared that it would never rest content to remain a separate but equal partner.

Heinzen's diatribes against the church continued throughout his lifetime. Hardly an article or an essay that he wrote, regardless of the topic, failed to include an exegesis on the dangers of religion. Again and again, Heinzen declared religion and humanity absolutely incompatible, insisting that the only antidote to the marriage between "material misery" and "religious credulity" was atheism.[31] "When the believe [*sic*] in a God ceases," he announced, "then ceases also every obligation towards God which you would impose upon man, and only the duty of man to man remains."[32] For Heinzen, Zakrzewska, and other German radicals—and in contrast to most radical American reformers— atheism had to be embraced to pave the way for humanism.[33]

Atheism was key to the German radical program, but so, too, were science, reason, and rationality. Influenced by Ludwig Feuerbach and the so-called scientific materialists, Jacob Moleschott, Ludwig Büchner, and Karl Vogt, the German radical community sought to replace religion with an atheistic philosophy based on scientific materialism. In a pamphlet entitled *Six Letters to a Pious Man*, Heinzen portrayed the universe as nothing more than "a physical and chemical laboratory in which material powers carry on an unceasing change and transformation." Even the mind, Heinzen commented, "is nothing but the result of an organized combination and co-operation of physical and physiological powers."[34] These assertions were significant to Heinzen because of his conviction that one could not worship a divine being and still be capable of independent thought. "There is," he once exclaimed, "no greater contradiction than mind and God."[35] Adopting religious metaphors to convey his message, Heinzen spoke of the need for a new savior who would free his people from the earlier one. "His common name," Heinzen wrote,

is Reason, but he is not accustomed to sign himself with this name always, because now-a-days every rascal calls himself reason. The real name of the savior is Atheism or Unbelief, in other words, the belief in reason, the spirit of truth and the will to make these the ruling powers. . . . Yes, the new savior of the world is the spirit of truth—is radical heathenism—is the sovereign human nature. This armed with the besom of knowledge and science first sweeps the broad spaces of the universe clear of the spectres and harpies which have hitherto tortured poor mortals on this very tolerable earth, where no Lord God, and no devil, but only the reasoning, free, human being . . . makes its household arrangements as a democratic Republic and provides for all humanity, woman as well as man, food, lodging and education.[36]

It bears emphasis that Heinzen was insisting upon a link between science, social justice, and radical democracy. More than a rhetorical flourish, the link reflected a conviction among radical Germans (as well as more moderate liberals) that knowledge of the natural sciences would assist them in their struggles for political and social reform. It is crucial to note that most German states in the 1830s and 1840s lacked constitutions and were ruled by monarchs who derived much of their support from churches and a small but powerful landed elite. Those clamoring for change in the decades prior to the revolutions of 1848 sought to increase popular representation in the governing bodies; at the same time, they recognized the need to alter school curricula to educate future citizens of the state for their new responsibilities. In the eyes of these reformers, the method of the natural sciences, not religion or the classical languages, would best prepare the young for involvement in a participatory democracy by providing them with the mental attributes deemed critical in the battle against ignorance, superstition, and arbitrary authority. To nineteenth-century radical and liberal German reformers alike, science was fundamentally prodemocratic and antielitist, for in contrast to claims to power based on birth, talent, genius, or character, they believed that anyone could learn the method of the natural sciences.[37]

Did, however, "anyone" include women? For most Germans, the answer was no, but Heinzen drew a different conclusion. Although on occasion he shared his contemporaries' belief that women's minds were not as vigorous and logical as men's, he always insisted that women (and "negroes") should be granted the same inalienable rights and freedoms accorded to white men in the U.S. Declaration of Independence.[38] Their want of mental strength reflected, he believed, exclusion from such rights and responsibilities; the development of greater mental powers would follow their participation in a truly democratic society. For this reason, he was a staunch defender of women's suffrage throughout his lifetime and insisted that no one had any grounds for denying another human being the same rights that he possessed. To opponents of suffrage who argued that women had enough rights already without also needing the vote, he rejoined that one cannot speak of rights if someone has the power to give them to you or take them away. In that case, so-called rights amount to little more than "the conferring of permission and the granting of favors."[39] In adopting this stance, Heinzen found himself in a minority, even within the circle of German radicals. But he never wavered from this position. He even went so far as to portray suffrage as the sign of the most advanced society, arguing that at the summit of the "mountain of civilization . . . stands the free, independent woman."[40] He may very well have had Zakrzewska in mind as he penned this line.

· · ·

This brief synopsis of Heinzen's views sets the stage for an examination of Zakrzewska's own, subsequent writings: the introductory address she gave shortly after she assumed her position at the New England Female Medical College; her autobiographical sketch, which she published during her first year in Boston; and a lengthy lecture on hospitals she delivered six months after she founded the New England Hospital for Women and Children. In each and every one, she linked social progress to a rejection of religion and the church and an embrace of rationality and the natural sciences. Indeed, a vision of the world as a battleground between religion and arbitrary authority, on the one hand, and science and political democracy, on the other, colored most aspects of her life. An avowed materialist and atheist, she engaged in constant disputes with her neighbor William Lloyd Garrison, whose ideas of freedom derived precisely from his faith in a divine being. Many an afternoon she spent debating whether people had to feel directly answerable to God in order to be capable of true humanitarianism.[41] Her refusal to be converted led to the demise of friendships. She grew especially to hate Sundays at her hospital, where she had to "see a whole company sitting together doing nothing, saying nothing, and thinking nothing, because it is Sunday and they can't go to church, in order to hear nothing—but words and phrases." "The Golden Rule," she once exclaimed, "must be practiced every day and not merely formulated as a pious recital on Sunday." Her views also encouraged her later in life to refuse any religious ceremony at her funeral, even writing her own eulogy in which she told, or perhaps assured, her friends one last time "that the deep conviction that there can be no further life is an immense rest and peace to me. I desire no hereafter. I was born, I lived, . . . and I am satisfied now to fall a victim to the laws of nature, never to rise again."[42]

Zakrzewska's friendship with Heinzen was thus grounded deeply in their shared political commitments. Unfortunately we know little more about the nature of their bond. One of the mysteries when trying to understand their relationship is how little we know about Heinzen's wife, Louise Henriette. The daughter of a widow (Louise Schiller) with whom Heinzen had been emotionally involved, she and her three siblings were adopted by Heinzen when their mother passed away in 1835. Four years later they married, when he was thirty years old and she just sixteen. Although Heinzen's enemies in Germany—and he had made quite a few by then—accused him of marrying his own daughter, what evidence we have suggests that they had a good marriage. How Louise felt about moving in with Zakrzewska we will, however, never know. There does not seem to have been much closeness between the two women—it is noteworthy that Zakrzewska did not include Mrs. Heinzen within her "closer family circle"—but neither is there any record of tension. Mrs. Heinzen did leave the Zakrzewska household after her husband's death in 1880 in order to move in with the Prangs, whose daughter her son had wed five years earlier, but the two women remained in touch, even crossing the ocean together the year after Heinzen died.[43] They also continued to celebrate Christmas together long after he had died. Perhaps the most one can say is that while Zakrzewska may not have felt the same closeness toward Mrs. Heinzen that she did toward her husband or even toward many other women, by all appearances they sustained a cordial relationship over the years.[44]

Despite the appearance of propriety, at least one individual considered it morally questionable for two women to be living under one roof, both of whom felt a strong connection to the same man. That person was Adolf Douai, a radical German Forty-Eighter, who had once been a coeditor of Heinzen's *Der Pionier*. When the two men had a falling-out in 1859, ostensibly because Heinzen attacked Douai for being soft on slavery, Douai retaliated by casting aspersions on Heinzen's integrity. The two men carried on their feud in the German-language press, with everything escalating in 1869 when Douai published a small pamphlet entitled *Heinzen, Wie er ist*. After accusing Heinzen of considering himself as infallible as the pope, he turned to his opponent's personal life. "Our cause," Douai wrote, "needs morally clean and honorable characters. Whoever would defend woman's rights cannot be himself an adulterer. . . . Among men of honor, even that is adultery when a man, over fifty years of age, makes his faithful wife, who has loyally fulfilled all her obligations to him, boundlessly unhappy on account of a love affair. He who would champion the cause of labor must not live from the support that comes from women's skirts [Schürzen-Stipendien]."[45]

There was no question that Douai was referring to Zakrzewska. Such accusations angered many, not least among them Heinzen. In a rejoinder he published in the 10 November issue of *Der Pionier*, he challenged each and every claim Douai made, denied his financial dependence on anyone, and accused Douai in turn of being a liar and a slanderer. To further aggravate and alienate Douai he purchased one hundred copies of the pamphlet, offering them to anyone who wished to read its falsehoods. Louise Henriette Heinzen even urged her husband to take Douai to court, but he preferred to battle out their differences in the free press. After the initial uproar, however, things settled down quickly, and the entire affair faded into the background.[46]

Whether Douai was truly troubled by Heinzen's living arrangement is, of course, unclear. He may simply have hoped to destroy his adversary's reputation by accusing him of being both sexually and financially enmeshed with Zakrzewska. But Douai's motives matter less here than what this incident suggests about contemporary attitudes toward alternative living arrangements. No one appeared to be much concerned about the way the Zakrzewska household deviated from the idealized norm. The 1860s may have marked the beginning of increased legislation designed to preserve the institution of marriage, but at the local level considerable tolerance (or perhaps indifference) appeared to be the rule.[47] That said, it is possible that the deviations in Zakrzewska's household were not always so evident. At least initially, for example, she took in boarders (usually individuals who needed some medical care), a practice that was not uncommon in middle-class households.[48] Thus the cohabitation of unrelated individuals would not in and of itself have attracted any attention. But whatever the reason, we must acknowledge that none of the descriptions of Zakrzewska's home that have survived include anything about the makeup of the household other than to mention who resided there.

• • •

Perhaps it also helped to mute potential criticism that the permanent members of the household included not only Zakrzewska and the Heinzens. In the summer of 1862, the thirty-seven-year-old Julia A. Sprague also moved in, and she remained until the doctor's death forty years later.[49] How Zakrzewska first met Sprague is unknown; nor is it clear why she moved into Zakrzewska's home, although occasional references to the fact that she was an "invalid" suggests that she may have started out as one of Zakrzewska's boarders. The living arrangement was initially supposed to be temporary; indeed, some tension developed at first between Sprague and Heinzen.[50] By 1863, however, all signs of discord had disappeared. As Zakrzewska wrote Lucy Sewall, who was studying in Europe at the time, "Miss Sprague is now in Minna's place, and she heads the Roxbury house beautifully. I like her very much in this position, she takes such an interest in the whole affair."[51]

Not much is known about Sprague, although her name turns up frequently among Boston's leading women reformers in the immediate post–Civil War period. Apparently, she was a schoolteacher and one of the early architects of the kindergarten movement.[52] She was also a founding member and historian of the New England Women's Club, a largely social club designed to bring together women reformers in the hope that common events and the sharing of ideas would generate further good works. Other founding members, and thus her circle of acquaintances, included Harriot K. Hunt, Mrs. James Freeman Clarke, Abby W. May, Caroline M. Severance, Lucia M. Peabody, Lucy Goddard, Julia Ward Howe, and Ednah Dow Cheney. Most of these women had cut their political teeth on the abolition movement, moving quickly to the forefront of other reform campaigns, including the fight for women's rights. It was, in fact, a desire to keep alive the reform spirit, kindled both before and during the Civil War, that led them to form the New England Women's Club in 1868.[53]

The friendship between Sprague and Zakrzewska blossomed over the years. They vacationed together, including taking several trips to Europe; they worked together to advance women's rights; and they cared for each other during illnesses. Sprague once described how Zakrzewska, who "disliked being thought bodily weak or ailing," would claim Sprague was fatigued when she felt unable to accept an invitation to join an excursion. Like an old couple who learned to live with each other's quirks, Sprague added that she "had let it pass, because I understood why she did so."[54] When Zakrzewska passed away in 1902, Sprague grieved her death deeply. "Some day," she wrote Caroline Severance about six weeks after Zakrzewska's death, "I may be thankful for her release—but I cannot honestly say that day has yet come. I know it is selfish in me, I strive against the selfishness, but I cannot yet succeed. . . . You see, we had lived 40 years together sharing every thing, work, and leisure, travel, and home-life."[55]

Women's historians have radically altered our understanding of same-sex relationships by insisting that we study them on their own terms rather than forcing them into categories that did not become established until the post-Freudian era. Women lived, worked, and traveled together at a time when emotional attachments between women did not evoke suspicion of a lesbian relationship. Quite the contrary, as Carroll Smith-Rosenberg has argued, nineteenth-century women, whether single or married, young or old, frequently sustained loving, caring, and even romantic relationships with one another throughout their lives. This did not necessarily preclude whatever intimacy they might have had with their husbands (if they married); rather, female networks of love and support existed outside the marital bond, satisfying emotional needs that few expected to be met through marriage. Of course, the decision of two women to live together signaled a greater commitment than what was implied by the extended visits and constant letter writing that typically sustained female friendships. Yet within a climate that viewed strong emotional ties between women as normal, such relationships enjoyed a level of acceptance greater than what many experience today. Those of Sprague's letters that have survived, most of which date from the end of the nineteenth century and the beginning of the twentieth, attest to the love and affection that had developed between these two women over the forty-year period that they shared their home and their lives. "I know her," Sprague wrote to Kitty Barry in 1896, "better of course than any one else."[56]

The sharing of a household by two women, usually both middle-class professionals, had become common enough by the late nineteenth century to earn the label "Boston marriage."[57] Indeed, several of the women in Zakrzewska and Sprague's circle of friends and colleagues had female companions. These included Susan Dimock and Elizabeth Greene, Mary L. Booth and Anna W. Wright, and, for a short while, Lucy Sewall and Sophia Jex-Blake.[58]

There has been much curiosity about whether these female partnerships were sexual in nature, but several scholars have insisted that the focus on genital contact reveals more about our own understanding of companionship and intimacy than that of women in the past.[59] Zakrzewska, who had shared her bed with Mary Booth and now her home with Sprague, certainly did not worry that her relationships would be misunderstood. In 1862, in a letter she wrote to Lucy Sewall, she blurred the line between conventional marriage and same-sex relationships with great confidence and ease, providing further evidence that the anxieties that would surface later in the century about lesbians were not yet present. Sewall was at the time being courted, and Zakrzewska felt compelled to offer her some advice:

> Lucy, never marry a man with whom you do not agree on all points! I feel it more and more, the older I grow, that love grows stronger only towards those with whom we sympathize; and that we become more and more a burden to each other if we do not agree well. And although we may avoid

quarreling yet coldness is sometimes harder to bear than an absolute quarrel. I feel all this with Miss ——, and yet she is far more agreeable to me than a good many other of my acquaintances. I really feel an attachment for her, perhaps for the very reason that I feel we will not be obliged to be always together.[60]

Why the name of Zakrzewska's female friend is missing will be considered presently. What is most striking about this passage, however, is the seamless way in which Zakrzewska wove her own experience with a woman into a conversation about marriage. To her, whether one was talking about the bond between a man and a woman or between two women, the same advice held true: for the relationship to be a good one, it had to be based not only on a natural affinity between the two individuals but also on shared principles and interests. Only in one way did Zakrzewska draw a distinction between her relationship with a woman and a marriage, and that was to paint the former more favorably because of the freedom she enjoyed to end the relationship should it prove unsatisfactory. The same sentiment could be found among those who defended a woman's right to divorce because of their conviction that the only true union was one that both individuals entered and sustained without coercion.[61] It may not be going too far to suggest that Zakrzewska saw a relationship between two women as a kind of model for the companionate marriage. The proof, moreover, was in the pudding: the freedom she had to sever her ties to her female friend appeared to have strengthened her feelings of "attachment," not destroyed them.

Zakrzewska penned this letter roughly six months after Julia Sprague moved into her home, so the mysterious friend may very well have been her. We can only speculate about why the two women became lifelong companions. Women who formed Boston marriages did not always do so for the same reasons. While for some a Boston marriage may have signaled little more than a convenience, a way of sharing the many responsibilities and chores associated with running a household, for others the decision to become partners for life grew out of a romantic love they shared. Zakrzewska and Sprague's relationship may very well have fallen somewhere in between; what may have begun as a convenient arrangement seems to have slowly grown into a committed and caring partnership. There is, however, little evidence of any passion between them, although the dearth of documents makes it difficult to say anything definitive about the nature of their relationship, especially during the first two decades they spent together. Without a diary and with only a few letters from the years prior to 1880, the main source available to us is Agnes Vietor's biography. However, Vietor barely mentions Sprague, aside from noting that she "became [Zakrzewska's] faithful friend and home companion for life."[62] Of course, Vietor may very well have chosen not to include material Zakrzewska had left that was revealing of her relationship to Sprague. The omission of the woman's name from the letter cited above is possibly one case in point. Individuals of Vietor's generation, writing in the 1920s, had to contend with Freudian interpretations of women's expressions of love and intimacy for one another, and they often demonstrated a discomfort that had been absent decades before. But what seems equally likely is that Zakrzewska and Sprague censored the material they gave to Vietor. Not only were both extremely private individuals, but Sprague, while going through Zakrzewska's correspondence after her partner's death, confided to Severance. "I shall," she wrote, "lay aside what may be of use for a biography, and the rest are too sacred for preservation even, as they relate to such matters as should have warranted their instant destruction, lest death should lay them bare before strangers. I feel as if it were a lesson to us all, 'do not keep your letters'; much correspondence now published in connection with biographies seem[s] to me unwarranted. There have been 'love-letters' published, which were almost a desecration in my eyes, and gratify only a vulgar curiosity."[63]

It seems likely that Sprague destroyed much of Zakrzewska's correspondence, protecting their sense of privacy but also adding to the silence that surrounds women's relationships in the past. Perhaps it was she, and not Vietor, who removed the name from the letter cited above. Fortunately, however, letters she (and to a lesser extent) Zakrzewska wrote to Severance over a twenty-five year period have survived. The correspondence began in the early 1880s and continued, in Sprague's case, until several years after Zakrzewska's death. As we will discuss in the final chapter of this book, these letters may lack any mention of passion between the two women, but they do demonstrate the ease with which they viewed themselves as companions. "As the years pass on," Sprague wrote to Severance in 1893, "we feel that we need each other more and more; we have[,] you know, lived together over 30 years."[64] Sprague clearly had the expectation that others would view them as companions as well.

• • •

In trying to gain a deeper understanding of Zakrzewska's personal life, it is critical to keep in mind that however close her friendship with Sprague may have become, for the first twenty years they lived together they participated more in a "Boston family" than a "Boston marriage."[65] The evidence we have suggests, moreover, that after the initial tension between Heinzen and Sprague was resolved, the family became as tightly knit a unit as one might expect in any home. Perhaps the bond was in some ways even tighter, because unlike the division of labor characteristic of the traditional middle-class home, work bound the members of 139 Cedar Street together, and not simply the work of maintaining the household. For one, they all became invested in one fashion or another in Zakrzewska's hospital: Karl Heinzen kept his readers apprised of any and all events connected with the hospital; his wife helped organize fund-raisers; and Sprague even worked for three months gratis as the hospital's matron when Zakrzewska was in a pinch. They also all contributed to the production of Heinzen's newspaper, whether by writing an occasional article, looking for interesting material, again organizing fund-raising events or making their own financial contributions, or helping to distribute the paper when it came off the press. Once a week they also gathered together in the parlor to hear Mrs. Heinzen read aloud from the latest issue. Sprague, who had had little introduction to German radicalism before joining this household, claimed to have received an important political education through this weekly ritual. She eventually transformed this education into work, translating some of Heinzen's essays into English in order to further disseminate his ideas.[66] Clearly, the members of this household had little trouble blurring the boundary between the so-called public and the so-called private.[67]

Work in this household also mixed easily with play. Evenings were occasionally spent playing whist or chess, often with others. Doctors and interns were frequent visitors, as were some of the leading radicals in Boston. Louis Prang, for example, a German refugee who made a considerable fortune through his introduction of chromolithography to the United States, made up part of the household members' closer social circle, as did the Phillips and Garrisons. Within this group Zakrzewska appears to have been closest to William Lloyd Garrison II, whom she had met in 1857 during one of her visits to Boston. Heinzen favored the senior Garrison, with whom he frequently played whist. In addition to these local friends, political radicals from abroad occasionally stayed with Zakrzewska and her housemates when they came to the United States. The German radical materialist Ludwig Büchner may very well have been their most famous houseguest when he stayed with them in 1873 while on a lecture tour.[68] As the younger Garrison once commented, "although unmarried, the

Doctor rarely failed to have a house full of friends and relatives, making of her home a social center for her German and American acquaintances."[69]

One of the physicians who practiced at the New England Hospital for Women and Children recalled the "many pleasant out-of-door gatherings" that were held on Cedar Street. She described how the terraces were fully planted with grapes and how the parties always had an abundance of wine.[70] Heinzen's birthday, on 22 February, which he shared with George Washington, was one of the housemates' favorite days to celebrate. Combining politics with pleasure, they played joyfully with the similarities between the two men—Washington being responsible for establishing the Republic and Heinzen for helping to bring about "a purer democracy." On that day they had what Zakrzewska once described as "annual sociables," replete with dancing. In a tribute to Samuel Sewall, the man who had loaned her the money to purchase her home, she described how he had danced the "Virginia Reel" at one of these parties "as lively as possible and losing no step," despite his seventy-eight years of age. Twenty years after Heinzen's death, Zakrzewska, Sprague, and the Heinzen family were still commemorating this day.[71]

· · ·

Christmas of 1862 was a joyous time for Zakrzewska. She may have had little use for organized religion, but that did not translate into a dislike of holiday rituals. To create a festive mood, she and the other members of her household decorated the parlors with laurel and holly and covered the chandeliers with wreaths. They also put out apples, nuts, and plates of German gingerbread on tables they had dressed up with white tablecloths. When they returned from their evening meal, presents were awaiting them "which Santa Claus had brought to the room." Zakrzewska took it upon herself to call out everyone's name and distribute the gifts. "[L]ots of handsome little things came out of the brown and white papers," she wrote Lucy Sewall, "so that the room looked like a charming little fair, and we had ever so much fun, and many funny things, and I only wish that you had been here, too."[72]

Zakrzewska shared with Sewall a picture of domestic bliss. Surrounded by good food, white tablecloths, and chandeliers, she could have been describing the home of many middle-class families on Christmas Day. But there were some striking differences: most members of this family were not bound by blood or marriage, and a woman was the primary breadwinner. Zakrzewska even described herself once as "the head of a family," thus reinforcing the social importance of the family unit while simultaneously inverting the gender hierarchy upon which the family was built, assuming financial responsibility for the dependents with whom she shared her home.[73]

Zakrzewska had succeeded in translating her unconventional views on gender into an alternative family structure, creating a rich home life for herself that brought her considerable comfort and joy. Nevertheless, moments of doubt were not absent. In a letter Zakrzewska penned to Lucy Sewall in the winter of 1862 she wished for Lucy "all happiness that exists for us poor mortals—which is by no means in the single life."[74] Since Zakrzewska said nothing more about this, it is impossible to know what inspired her to make this claim. We do need to bear in mind that she wrote this before she and Sprague had grown close; perhaps she no longer felt this way after that friendship blossomed. But this letter also suggests that behind the bluster and bravado Zakrzewska sometimes struggled with what it meant to live her life—indeed, to maintain a consistent performance—in constant opposition to established gender norms.

In the end, Karl Heinzen, Julia Sprague, and Zakrzewska's sisters formed the inner of circle of individuals to whom she turned when she needed emotional support or simply wished to let down her guard. She also remained close friends with Mary Booth, despite the miles that separated them since her move to Boston. Outside this intimate circle were, moreover, others with whom she formed long and lasting friendships. Many, like the Prangs, she met through her engagement with the community of German radicals, but there was another group of individuals among whom Zakrzewska counted many friends and with whom she worked closely. This was the community of women's rights advocates. She had known Harriot Hunt and Caroline Severance since her days in Cleveland; Caroline Healey Dall, Abby W. May, and Ednah Dow Cheney she came to know well once she moved to Boston. Zakrzewska would grow extremely close to several of these women as she joined them in promoting their cause. Zakrzewska, whose primary contribution to the women's movement would be the founding of an all-women's hospital, made an earlier contribution when she published her autobiographical sketch shortly after arriving in Boston. In this sketch, as we will see, she applied German scientific materialism to a critique of gender relations, moving beyond even Heinzen in her insistence that "science has no sex."

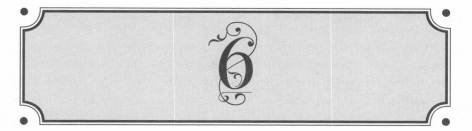

Writing Autobiography

Zakrzewska's determination to challenge social conventions about women's proper place informed not only her personal life but also her public activities. We have already discussed her attack on biologism in both her medical thesis and the articles she published in 1859 in the German-language weekly *Der Pionier*. Following her move to Boston she also became directly involved with the movement for women's rights. Indeed, her autobiographical sketch, entitled *A Practical Illustration of "Woman's Right to Labor"* and published shortly after she arrived in Boston, can best be seen as a conscious act on Zakrzewska's part to contribute to this movement. Throughout her years in Boston, she worked for this cause, participating in such organizations as the New England Women's Club and the Massachusetts Women's Suffrage Association. The idea of publishing the sketch had even originated with a women's rights advocate, Caroline Healey Dall, who believed that Zakrzewska's success in acquiring a medical degree—despite her sex, limited financial means, and language difficulties—offered proof that women, with the right spirit of determination and the appropriate support, could overcome obstacles and be successful in the public sphere.[1]

Like many other women's rights advocates at the time, Zakrzewska held that the problems women faced resulted not only from men's views of women but also from women's views of themselves. Women, Zakrzewska once commented, had to "make themselves useful not merely for others, but also for themselves ... because true satisfaction does not rest alone in the execution of an activity but also when the activity reflects our own plan and desire, when it is the fulfillment of our own idea."[2] Susan B. Anthony, traveling around the country trying to inspire women to stand up for themselves, could not have agreed more. She spoke of the "true new woman" who "will not be exponent of another, or allow another to be such for her. She will be her own individual self."[3] For these women, challenging formal barriers, even convincing state and federal governments to grant greater legal rights to women, was only part of what needed to be done in order to improve women's standing in society; they also attacked aggressively the image women frequently had of themselves as weak, sentimental, and dependent. As Dall remarked in her introduction to Zakrzewska's autobiographical sketch: "It is easy to rail against society and men in general: but it is very painful for a woman to confess her heaviest obstacle to success; namely, the *weakness of women*."[4]

An autobiography is, by nature, a highly constructed text, and while constructed does not mean fabricated, autobiography and fiction have much in common.[5] When Zakrzewska sat down to write her autobiography, she had already made the decision to move to Boston, where she was anticipating greater independence and a chance to work toward creating her own clinical unit, perhaps even her own hospital one day. The decision to record her life's story at this juncture must thus be understood as satisfying both a need to give meaning to past events and a desire to create an image of the kind of woman she wished to present for public viewing. To this end, Zakrzewska portrayed herself throughout the text as a fiercely independent person who exerted control over her own life. She did so, first of all, by employing what literary scholars have identified as a classic trope in the nineteenth-century autobiographies of middle-class men: that of the lone individual who struggles against all odds to achieve professional success.[6] In addition to this, she framed many of her stories around the tension that marked so much of the writing of the scientific materialists: that is, between science, rationality, and political democracy, on the one hand, and religion, sentimentality, and arbitrary authority, on the other. By positioning herself, a woman, so squarely in the first camp, she was utilizing this framework to disrupt the traditional gendering of traits in circulation at the time.

Zakrzewska hoped *A Practical Illustration* would help "to work a reformation" in women's lives, and to the extent that it challenged the sexual stereotypes that functioned to keep women out of the public sphere, it enjoyed considerable success.[7] Reviews of the book certainly hailed Zakrzewska as a model of what women who were equipped with a sense of purpose and the courage to persevere might accomplish. It bears mention, though, that however radical Zakrzewska's ideas on gender may have been, she did not show the same rebelliousness when it came to class. In focusing on individual empowerment rather than class relations she joined the vast majority of middle-class reformers who ignored the fact that all women did not have equal access to the resources that would make it possible for them to choose a different path. Without doubt *A Practical Illustration* threatened the sexual division of labor, but it did so largely within the confines of the existing class structure.

. . .

Zakrzewska would probably never have published her autobiographical sketch were it not for her acquaintance with Dall. A writer and reformer, Dall had just completed *"Woman's Right to Labor"; or, Low Wages and Hard Work*, in which she had argued for the necessity of improving employment opportunities for women. By her own admission, the reactions to her book were mixed, and she was looking for "a practical illustration" of the claims she had made in her work. Dall's primary focus had been on women of what she called "the perishing classes": those who had to work because they needed to eat. Influenced by the emerging field of social science, she filled her essay with statistics documenting the large numbers of women employed throughout the economy both in the United States and in England. She also engaged in more traditional forms of persuasion, offering anecdotes of women who often lost the battle to earn an honest living, struggling to support aging parents, invalid siblings, or dependent children on the paltry wages they earned sewing caps or tatting lace. These women, she argued, often turned to the streets, but only when they had exhausted all other possibilities. Quoting the French social scientist Duchâtelet, Dall challenged her readers to "Compare the price of labor with the price of dishonor, and you will cease to be surprised that women fall."[8]

In discussing the reactions to her book, Dall described how a handful of reform-minded businessmen felt inspired to hire young women as apprentices but found that women themselves often bridled at the idea of investing so many years in training for a job. Dall encountered, moreover, considerable resistance to her claims that working conditions in the city of Boston could be so bad. She thus came to believe that a specific example would help her to convince her readers of the seriousness of the situation.

In the introduction to Zakrzewska's autobiography, Dall admits to having originally considered some great personages, but she had rejected in turn Florence Nightingale because her "father had a title"; Dorothea Dix, who "had money and time"; Mrs. John Stuart Mill, who had never "wanted bread"; and George Sand, who "wasn't respectable." A conversation with Mary Booth, in which she learned that Zakrzewska had already penned a brief sketch of her life in the form of a letter to her friend, led her to believe that the young immigrant would make her case perfectly.[9] Booth, who was intrigued by the project, agreed to edit the autobiography should Zakrzewska be convinced to go along.

Dall had first met Zakrzewska in the fall of 1856, when the young physician had come to Boston to raise funds for the New York Infirmary for Women and Children. On that occasion, Dall had heard Zakrzewska speak of her experiences in the syphilitic wards at the Charité and had been most impressed by the young doctor's insistence "that the most sinning, suffering woman never passed beyond the reach of a woman's sympathy and help." "For the first time," she later mentioned, "I saw a woman who knew what I knew, felt what I felt, and was strong in purpose and power to accomplish our common aim,—the uplifting of the fallen, the employment of the idle, and the purification of society."[10]

Dall's language was common to antebellum middle-class female reformers, who frequently followed a familiar script when describing their work. Idealizing their own role as benevolent protectors, they saw themselves as extending a helping hand to those who no longer wished to be "fallen," "idle," or "impure." When Dall identified Zakrzewska as a kindred spirit, she saw her, of course, as a fellow reformer. However, the part Zakrzewska was to play in the autobiography was of the young immigrant who had to figure out how to survive in a city filled with peril. Only in this way could Zakrzewska's story verify first-hand Dall's claims about the dangers that awaited women who sought work in the cities.

Zakrzewska's success story was illustrative of several points that Dall hoped to underscore. First, she was living proof that the fate of a young immigrant could be influenced by women with power and connections. She may never have fulfilled her dream of studying medicine had Elizabeth Blackwell and Caroline Severance not supported her cause. But more than demonstrating the need for greater involvement on the part of the "higher classes," Zakrzewska's story provided a potent symbol for the power of self-determination. Here was a young woman who had faced countless obstacles, struggling to make her way in a strange land, to earn a livelihood, protect her younger siblings, and master a foreign language, and through it all she had never abandoned her dream of studying medicine. In short, for Dall, Zakrzewska was someone who could reach "ordinary women" because she had "a life flowing out of circumstances not dissimilar to their own, but marked by a steady will, an unswerving purpose." According to Dall, if nothing prevented women from succeeding more than their own weakness, then nothing could help them more than the story of a woman who persisted in the face of adversity. "I had felt, from the first," Dall wrote, "that her life might do what my words never could: namely, inspire women with faith to try their own experiments."[11]

Dall had wanted to set "an example before young girls," but why did Zakrzewska agree to tell her life story? At the time *A Practical Illustration* was published, autobiographies by women had not yet achieved the popularity they would enjoy by the end of the century. Instead they were considered a sign of an author's self-indulgence and egotism, a departure from the demureness and submissiveness expected of women at the time. Although Zakrzewska spent much of her life fighting this traditional image of women, she shared enough of her culture's discomfort with conceit in women to feel uneasy about placing herself at the center of attention. She thus claimed to have been reluctant when Booth and Dall first approached her and to have been persuaded only by Dall's argument that the publication of her life's story would benefit other women.[12] She also tried to diffuse any accusations of conceit on her part by emphasizing both her own humility and the usefulness of her story. Thus, as she explained at the beginning of her letter: "I am not a great personage . . . ; yet you may find, in reading this little sketch, that with few talents, and very moderate means for developing them, I have accomplished more than many women of genius and education would have done in my place, for the reason that confidence and faith in their own powers were wanting. And, for this reason, I know that this story might be of use to others."[13]

The use of such qualifiers was not uncommon among nineteenth-century female autobiographers, who struggled with the social impropriety of writing about themselves. But whereas most other writers also deemed it necessary to assure their readers that they were "feminine" and "ladylike," downplaying their accomplishments and the heroic nature of their lives, Zakrzewska further challenged gender stereotypes by portraying herself as strong, stubborn, and frequently alone in the battles she fought.[14] She may not have been alone in this endeavor—other women physicians, such as Hannah Longshore and Mary Dixon Jones, also advertised their accomplishments in public settings— but women who engaged in acts of self-promotion were clearly in the minority.[15]

Booth began editing the autobiographical sketch sometime in 1860. By October she was able to write to Dall that she had completed her task and was sending the final manuscript to Zakrzewska for approval. "I have preserved the simple letter form in which it was written," she informed Dall, "and endeavored to keep her own personality and phraseology in the whole, and to translate her pretty foreign idioms with equally idiomatic English." Booth had planned to see the work through to the end, but she decided that Dall could complete the project more efficiently "and in the way best calculated to be of use to the world and of credit to Marie."[16] Booth had figured correctly. By the beginning of December the letter was available in print under the title *A Practical Illustration of "Woman's Right to Labor"; or, A Letter from Marie E. Zakrzewska, M.D.* Zakrzewska, who had celebrated a birthday in October, was all of thirty-one years old.

• • •

"I do not," Zakrzewska wrote Mary at the beginning of her autobiographical sketch, "intend to weary you with details of my childhood, . . . I shall, therefore, only tell you a few facts of this period of my life, which I think absolutely necessary to illustrate my character and nature." The chapters on her childhood are, indeed, some of the sketchiest in the book. We learn very little, for example, about her parents, her siblings, or her experiences at school. Indeed, one reviewer commented that there was very little of Zakrzewska anywhere in this sketch (although he meant this as a compliment). To be sure, the book progresses through the important phases of her life, from her childhood to the study and practice of midwifery at the Charité, to her years in New York and Cleveland, and finally to her move to Boston. But this framework merely provides the structure for a series of stories, each of which seems to be carefully selected for a specific purpose. The "few facts" from her childhood, for example, which she promised to share with Mary, depicted a strong, willful, and courageous child, who walked nine miles at the age of two, staged funerals with her dolls, was not frightened when she found herself accidentally locked up with a corpse in a dissecting room for hours on end, and dominated the relationships she had with friends and siblings alike. She was, she explained, always making up stories for her younger sister, in which she "led [her heroes and heroines] into all sorts of adventures till it suited my caprice to terminate their career." When she played with others, she always "took the lead, planning and directing every thing; while my playmates seemed to take it for granted, that it was their duty to carry out my commands." Such strong-mindedness eventually led her, not surprisingly, into considerable trouble. When she went to school at the age of five, teachers noticed and disliked this independent streak. Except for the teacher of arithmetic, she explained, they all "called me unruly because I would not obey arbitrary demands without receiving some reason, and obstinate because I insisted on following my own will when I knew that I was in the right."[17]

Already in these first stories, Zakrzewska was portraying herself as a formidable force, confident and in control of her actions. That she was intentionally challenging traditional gender stereotypes becomes evident in subsequent stories when, for example, she informs her readers that as a child she preferred the company of boys, with whom she "was merry, frank, and self-possessed," whereas with girls she "was quiet, shy, and awkward."[18] Unlike other girls, moreover, she cared little about her looks. Once, upon seeing herself in the mirror, she "could not help laughing heartily" at the comical sight, "with one braid of hair commencing over the right eye, and the other over the left ear." Rather than fix her hair, however, she simply "hung a map" over the mirror and went back to her studies.[19] A woman's mind, she was insisting, must take center stage, not her appearance.

Zakrzewska's greatest challenge to the gendering of mental and moral traits came, however, when she claimed truth and reason for herself, as a woman. As in her battle with Herr Both, she wore the mantle of rationality throughout her many stories, which she repeatedly juxtaposed with arbitrary authority of any kind. Her account of the difficulties she encountered as a young child in school (except, of course, with the teacher of arithmetic) was just the first of many stories with this motif. She also took on more formidable opponents, most notably the great enemy of the German materialists—the church.

Zakrzewska's first encounter with the church, she tells us, occurred when she was just twelve years old. At that time, she met a quiet, melancholic, and sentimental girl who "won her affection." Elizabeth was a devout Catholic and destined to become a nun, and Zakrzewska, who felt such love for this friend, began attending church with her and even considered converting to Catholicism. Her own parents, she emphasized, were "Rationalists" and did not belong to any church, but they did not prevent their daughter from following "her own inclinations." Everything went sour, however, when Elizabeth, under pressure from her priest, explained that their friendship could not continue unless Zakrzewska became a Catholic. "Never in my life," wrote Zakrzewska, "shall I forget that morning. For a moment, I gazed on her with the deepest emotion, pitying her almost more than myself; then suddenly [I] turned coldly and calmly away, without answering a single word. My mind had awakened to the despotism of Roman Catholicism, and the church had lost its expected convert."[20]

Zakrzewska's strategy for discrediting the Roman Catholic Church was to link it with sentimentality, the very trait she deemed so harmful to her sex. That this and other stories may reveal some ambiguous feelings on her part toward her own gender identity is something we will return to later. For now what is noteworthy is the way Zakrzewska both embraced and extended the German materialists' attack on the church. Like them, she viewed this institution, and especially the Roman Catholic Church, as one of the greatest threats to personal and political freedom. Indeed, in almost every essay she published or lecture she delivered throughout her life, she found a way to blame the church for the passivity and ignorance that prevented individuals from taking control of their lives. But Zakrzewska was also especially concerned about the impact of the church on women; by associating this institution with sentimentality she was criticizing the growing feminization of religion, which she considered detrimental to the advancement of women's rights.[21]

Zakrzewska's animosity toward the church is evident as well in the story she told of spending the night in the dead house with a corpse, for she used it as an alternative conversion experience that mimicked the stories that female religious leaders, such as Mary Baker Eddy and Ellen G. White, told of the illness experiences that led them to embrace God.[22] Zakrzewska's account begins as well with a malady: she was having trouble with her eyes and wished to be close to her mother, who was training that summer at the Charité. However, instead of finding God, Zakrzewska found a corpse. God, moreover, did not heal her; rather, "a few days after this adventure," Zakrzewska wrote, "I recovered the use of my eyes," thus suggesting that the knowledge she had acquired of the human body had given her sight. Zakrzewska's conversion did not, finally, lead her to find religion but rather to her professional calling. "From this time," she claims, "I date my study of medicine."[23]

Zakrzewska's project—to present an alternative model of womanly behavior and activity—led her as well to distort certain evidence in her autobiographical accounts. Her story of her experience trying to secure the position of head midwife at the Charité is a case in point. As we mentioned earlier, Zakrzewska claimed that Schmidt wished to have her assume his position as professor of midwifery, even though he would never have considered bestowing a professorship upon a woman, let alone one who never attended the university. It is true that he wished to make her head midwife, but that was a position that had always gone to a woman. Thus, the resistance Zakrzewska encountered had little to do with her sex and everything to do with her age and lack of experience. However, by blaming her problems on the opposition of male physicians to the idea "that a woman should take her place on a level with them," she could make this a "question of 'woman's rights.' The real question at stake," she drove home, "was, 'How shall women be educated, and what is their true sphere?' "[24]

Notably, one reviewer of her autobiography was confused enough by Zakrzewska's discussion of her experiences in Berlin to describe her as "formerly at the head of the hospital charité."[25]

Taken together, the stories in *A Practical Illustration* all emphasize Zakrzewska's forcefulness, clarity, and sense of purpose. But what allowed her to forge ahead? How were her readers to understand the conditions that promoted her success? Zakrzewska gave some weight to the assistance she received from others, including Joseph Hermann Schmidt, Elizabeth Blackwell, and Caroline Severance. But however much importance she may have placed on the benevolence of others, the central message in *A Practical Illustration* is that her success derived from her own spirit of determination and sense of mission. Describing the powerful feelings she had when she first spotted land after her long voyage across the ocean, Zakrzewska told her readers in a heavy-handed fashion: "I had come here for a purpose,—to carry out the plan which a despotic government and its servile agents had prevented me from doing in my native city. I had to show to those men who had opposed me so strongly because I was a woman, that in this land of liberty, equality, and fraternity, I could maintain that position which they would not permit to me at home."[26]

Women, Zakrzewska was declaring, had to fight for what they believed in, but first and foremost they had to believe in something. "Something" could not, however, be the church, their teachers, or some other authority figure. No, they needed to believe in themselves, to determine what they wished their purpose in life to be, and then to find the inner strength to execute their plans. Women had choices, she was implying, and they needed to start taking action to improve their own lot.

· · ·

A Practical Illustration was not a text that encouraged women to acknowledge the many ways in which they were victims of forces beyond their control. Quite the contrary, to use a modern phrase, here were stories of empowerment. Given this, one may very well wonder who Zakrzewska and Dall imagined their audience to be, especially since Dall had selected Zakrzewska as a model for "ordinary women." But Zakrzewska had, after all, a bourgeois upbringing, and the women she cast as most worthy of help ended up bearing a marked resemblance to her. They certainly did not come from the uneducated poor who struggled to earn a living. Not that such women were absent from Zakrzewska's story line. Especially in her portrayal of the first year she spent in New York City, she wrote movingly of the plight of working-class women who slaved away for scant wages, often unable to keep their children fed. But as with other middle-class reformers, her class prejudices surfaced when she expressed her conviction that the parents were beyond help and should be left to their destiny; it was the children, who were still capable of being educated, who demanded attention.[27]

"Ordinary" also did not refer to the women who engaged in casual prostitution as a way of making ends meet. To Dall and Zakrzewska, as to other antebellum middle-class reformers, such women fit poorly into their own understanding of how women fell into prostitution. Accordingly, young prostitutes were cast as victims of duplicitous men who lured them with promises of love and riches, only later to be abandoned and left with nowhere to go but the brothel. This scenario differed considerably from one in which women calculated the advantages of exchanging sexual services for a fee. Revealing not only her class upbringing but also her anti-Catholicism, Zakrzewska suggested that such women were found most frequently among the Irish, who "resort at once to beggary, or are inveigled into brothels, as soon as they arrive," and the French, who "are always intriguing enough either to put on a white cap and find a place as *bonne*, or to secure a *private* lover."[28]

"Ordinary" women turned out, thus, to be a narrowly defined group. Modeled on Zakrzewska, they tended to be "chiefly Germans" from "good" families who had, for a variety of reasons, fallen on difficult times. Although Zakrzewska told several stories of women who fit this description—one, for example, was the "daughter of a physician"—the most poignant concerned a young German woman who had drowned herself because she had been unable to support herself and her ailing mother through piecework in embroidery. Offering a direct challenge to Dall's skeptics, Zakrzewska went on:

> Stories of this kind are said to be without foundation: I say that there are more of them in our midst than it is possible to imagine. Women of good education, but without money, are forced to earn their living. They determine to leave their home, either because false pride prevents their seeking work where they have been brought up as *ladies*, or because this work is so scarce that they cannot earn by it even a life of semi-starvation; while they are encouraged to believe that in this country they will readily find proper employment. . . . Not being able to speak English, they believe the stories of the clerks and proprietors, and are made to work at low wages, and are often swindled out of their money. They feel homesick, forlorn and forsaken in the world. Their health at length fails them, and they cannot earn

bread enough to keep themselves from starvation. They are too proud to beg; and the consequence is, that they walk the streets, or throw themselves into the river.[29]

Zakrzewska may well have written this with so much feeling because it came so close to describing her own situation. But Zakrzewska did not, of course, drown herself. This particular story is not her own but that of her shadow; it described what could happen to otherwise "good" women from "good" families who lacked the inner strength and the assistance they needed to take control of their destinies. For those readers who failed to grasp this message on their own, Dall commented in her conclusion to the letter: "[T]he possibilities of a Zakrzewska lie hidden in every oppressed girl. . . . Hasten to save those whom [the current] has not yet overwhelmed."[30]

Dall's and Zakrzewska's intent may have been to save the "perishing classes," but the focus on "good" education and "good" families reveals the extent to which the imagined recipients of their benevolent actions had middle-class origins or, at the very least, shared the values of this class. Indeed, who else would have been inspired by Zakrzewska's story, which was not, after all, so much about a "woman's right to labor" as it was about her right to labor in a man's world? In the end, *A Practical Illustration* had most to say about the obstacles that needed to be overcome by women who wished to be gainfully employed in the public sphere. And it was here, in challenging the sexual division of labor within the middle class, that Zakrzewska's radicalism came to the fore.

• • •

Zakrzewska promoted the transgression of gender norms by framing the stories in *A Practical Illustration* around two central motifs. The first she modeled on the German materialists' distinction between truth, justice, and science, on the one hand, and arbitrary authority, sentimentality, and religion, on the other. The second, closely related to the first, entailed subverting the gendered nature of these categories, something about which the German materialists, including Heinzen, showed some ambivalence. Indeed, Heinzen, who once claimed that women had "susceptible minds," did not totally abandon the idea of a special, woman's nature. Although at times he viewed this supposed weakness of mind as a product of women's upbringing, he was not consistent on this point. More often than not he wrote of gender differences as though they were fixed: women possessed "truly humane hearts" and "fine feeling"; men had stronger nerves and a more powerful intellect.[31] As a result, he occasionally defended the idea of separate spheres for women and men: women were better adapted to a life "infinitely richer in service to society," men to the life of "a scholar and philosopher."[32] Nor did Heinzen wish to blur the boundaries between the sexes. Claiming that "there is nothing more repulsive in this world than a masculine woman," he insisted that the goal of emancipation had to be "to establish the liberty and the right of women within the limits prescribed by the feminine nature."[33]

Zakrzewska left no documents directly criticizing Heinzen's comments, but her autobiographical sketch ultimately challenged such policing of gender boundaries. Indeed, she pushed these boundaries to the limit by embodying traits traditionally gendered masculine, portraying herself as a powerful woman whose courage, mental and physical fortitude, and self-determination allowed her to triumph over adversity again and again. At the time Zakrzewska wrote her autobiographical sketch, she did not yet talk explicitly of crossing gender lines, but later in the century she became more direct. Commenting on the antebellum period, she complained that when "a woman claimed the right of gaining intellectual power, it appeared as if she stepped out of her sphere. And this claim, so simple and natural, was perverted by a hostile spirit into the claim that she wished 'to become a man.'" This reached such an absurd level, she added, that some people, upon hearing about Elizabeth Blackwell's medical studies, fully expected "to behold a woman on whom a beard had developed."[34] Zakrzewska did not, however, wish for women to become men. In her battle to claim for women those traits that entitled one to power, she struggled instead to dissociate power from a person's sexual attributes completely.

Judging from the dozen or so reviews that came out just after *A Practical Illustration* appeared, Zakrzewska enjoyed some success in this regard. Considered by one author "better than many pages of theory," the autobiography was judged by others to be "exceedingly interesting" as well as "stimulating and encouraging."[35] While several commented specifically on its powerful depiction of the plight of young immigrants—thus vindicating Dall's claims about the deplorable working conditions women faced—most focused on Zakrzewska's unusual success in challenging gender norms.[36] The *Liberator*, for one, hoped that Zakrzewska's story would "stimulate many, now content to live and die mere females, to aspire to and attain the rank of intelligent and useful human beings." The *Portland Transcript* read *A Practical Illustration* as "a serious and successful protest against all those narrow philosophies which while allowing to men every variety of temperament, character, and activity, would restrict women to only one style of pattern and method of development." In the author's view, Zakrzewska accomplished this by showing how women often "establish themselves in the localities where they are forbidden to enter, and this, too, without lessening their womanhood." The *Christian Examiner*, as well, after commending Zakrzewska's "rare quality of unity and singleness of purpose," added that this story "shows a realization of the greatest obstacle in the way of the reform in which she [Dall] is engaged,—namely, the supineness of the sex whose 'rights' she advocates."[37]

With her "determined spirit," "inexhaustible invention and resources," "courage," and "brave endurance," Zakrzewska was considered by some of her reviewers to be a model for "every daughter of America."[38] To this extent, she had succeeded in providing an alternative image to that of the demure Victorian woman. Yet as the comment from the *Portland Transcript* suggests, some of the reviewers tried to downplay Zakrzewska's transgressions, assuring readers that women like her had not "lessened their womanhood." The *Boston Journal*, for example, cast Zakrzewska as an "illustration of woman's ability for patient labor and faithful perseverance," while the *Christian Inquirer* emphasized her "womanly refinement, culture, and sensibility." Other reviews went so far as to combine praise of Zakrzewska with an attack on the women's movement. The reviewer for the *London Critic*, for example, recommended *A Practical Illustration* "to the consideration of those who prate more loudly, but less logically, than Mrs. Dall, about those flimsiest of phantoms, 'Woman's Rights.'" Another, writing for *Harper's*, placed Zakrzewska among the "heroines without halos," adding that "one such life is worth a torrent of talk about woman's sphere."[39] Thus, despite the praise being lavished on *A Practical Illustration*, a fair number of reviewers felt the need either to restore Zakrzewska's femininity or to demonize women's rights advocates, suggesting thereby a considerable level of discomfort with the way Zakrzewska was attempting to blur the line separating the sexes.

The reviews' mixed messages may, however, also have reflected ambiguities in the autobiographical sketch itself. Indeed, despite Zakrzewska's attempt to explode gender stereotypes, it was not possible for her to fully escape the gendered tropes that marked nineteenth-century discussions and debates about human nature and individual rights. We have already noted the way she criticized religion by associating it with the weak, sentimental, and melancholic young Elizabeth. In other stories, she continued this depiction of women as sentimental and misguided, ridiculing, for example, antebellum reformers for supporting a cause by "knitting a baby's stocking" rather than going door to door to raise funds.[40] Wishing, moreover, to create an image of herself as diametrically opposed to these women, she ended up casting herself as more akin to men. Not only, as we have seen, did she proclaim her preference for the company of boys, but she also announced proudly that the male students at the Charité "never seemed to think that I was not of their sex, but always treated me like one of themselves."[41] By placing herself, as a woman, among the men, Zakrzewska may have been trying to remove gender from any discussions of power, yet these stories also demonstrate the difficulties women encountered in trying to come up with alternatives to the gender divisions that marked almost every aspect of Western culture at the time.

These difficulties may also have led Zakrzewska to struggle at times with her own gender identity. Although we are engaging in speculation here, it is possible that her total rejection of any traditional feminine markers, and her enthusiastic embrace of masculine-coded traits, signaled not only a strategic move on her part to model an alternative image for women but also a level of confusion about how to express her own femininity. Zakrzewska did not think of herself as an attractive woman. Indeed, in her autobiographical sketch she described herself as "neither handsome, nor even prepossessing," and claimed that one of her aunts would describe "plain people" by commenting that they were "[a]lmost as ugly as Marie."[42] To be sure, Zakrzewska's goal in telling this story was to emphasize that women should care about more important things than their looks, but there is a certain sadness in this story as well, especially when she goes on to describe the loneliness she felt when her peers, who cared for neither her obstinacy nor her looks, chose to avoid her. My suggestion is not that we view her political work as being driven by feelings of insecurity about her own womanly nature; her passion for justice had much deeper roots. Nevertheless, her stated preference for men and her characterization of women as sentimental and weak, both of which legitimized the very stereotypes she was trying to disrupt, may have been fueled in part by her own difficulties trying to embody a different type of femininity in a society that drew such clear lines between proper masculine and feminine behaviors. Small wonder the reviews of her book were ambiguous as well.

• • •

Whatever confusion we may recognize in *A Practical Illustration*, Zakrzewska considered it an unambiguous contribution to the woman's movement.[43] Nor was this sketch her only attempt to support this cause through the written word.

In the spring of 1862, she and Mary Booth declared their intention to establish a women's journal. Drawing attention to the great social and political changes that the Civil War was having on women's lives, they deemed it timely to publish a journal that would "centralize and give impetus to the efforts which are being made in various directions to advance the interests of woman." Announcements in both the *Liberator* and *Der Pionier* explained that the journal would "collect and compare the divers [*sic*] theories promulgated on the subject" but that its central motto would be "Equal Rights For all Mankind." They intended to cover "current social and political events, articles on literature, education, hygiene, etc., [and] a *feuilleton* composed chiefly of translations from foreign literature."[44] They had, moreover, already amassed an impressive list of contributors, including Lydia Maria Child, Caroline M. Severance, Elizabeth Cady Stanton, Wendell Phillips, William Lloyd Garrison, and William H. Channing. As it turned out, the war, although an inspiration to the founding of this journal, ended up acting as a deterrent because of the difficulty of raising funds. In September the *Liberator* and *Der Pionier* announced that the journal would be postponed until the end of the war.[45] By that time, however, Zakrzewska had become so involved in her hospital that the project was never taken up again.

In the early 1860s, Zakrzewska thus made two concerted efforts to contribute to the women's movement. The women's journal, however, never got off the ground, and *A Practical Illustration*, despite the positive reviews, soon ran into financial problems, perhaps because of its ambiguous message. In the fall of 1861, the publisher of the book, Walker, Wise, and Company, wrote to Dall, complaining about poor sales. It had sold only 500 copies, with 150 going to Dall and Zakrzewska. Thus despite Zakrzewska's assertion that "more than two thousand people read the book," *A Practical Illustration* was not a financial success, Dall ended up losing money on the book, and Zakrzewska had moments when she regretted ever having taken on this project.[46] As she wrote to Dall in 1867,

> The little book gives me daily annoyance, I am not made for being called famous nor to be so. It annoys me to have people know me. If I could have patients without seeing them, I assure you, I would have those alone. To be known is so painfully disagreeable to me, that I don't buy my shoes, till the toes really show through so as to avoid going in a store. I think it is even a monomania with me, to wish to be away from people. It is by force of will, that I follow my desires to work for women, as an example, and I feel it al-

most a blessing that the time has come, when it is not any more necessary to speak in Public. . . .

I cannot tell you how much I felt, and how hard it was when Mary Booth was willing to give to you my truest feelings for publication and only the idea that it may stimulate some better woman to come forward, has reconciled me to the constant annoyance I suffer whenever I am asked, where the little book is to be had.[47]

A Practical Illustration had not turned out exactly as Zakrzewska had hoped. When she had first sat down to write her autobiographical sketch, she had been intrigued by the possibility of using writing as a way of "stimulat[ing] some better woman to come forward." Recording her life story, although ostensibly a way of sharing "a few facts" about her past with her friend Mary Booth, had really marked Zakrzewska's attempt to continue her battle to dismantle the barriers preventing her and other women from claiming their place in what was being defined as a man's world.

Zakrzewska never, however, intended the written word to be her central contribution to the women's movement, despite her brief experimentation with this venue. She knew her strengths rested in her capabilities as both a teacher and an administrator, and it was here that she had been focusing her efforts since her graduation from medical school. Helping to found and then run the New York Infirmary for Women and Children had been only the first step. She had left this position in 1859 not only to follow Heinzen to Boston but also to assume a position at the New England Female Medical College as professor of obstetrics and diseases of women and children and to take on the responsibility of creating a new clinical department. The trustees of the college, who had recently been granted permission to award the M.D., had seen in Zakrzewska someone who would help raise the school's standing among the Boston elite. When she accepted the offer, Zakrzewska must have believed that she would be riding a wave of reform. She was, however, soon disappointed. As she was to learn, too many obstacles remained in place for her to succeed in building a medical curriculum around the natural and clinical sciences, ensuring that her female students received an education comparable to, if not better than, that available to men.

The Standard of the School
Was below Par

Zakrzewska spent most of the three years she was on the faculty at the New England Female Medical College fighting with the school's director, Samuel Gregory (1813–72). Gregory, who was critical of the way the basic sciences were beginning to alter the practice of midwifery, had founded the college in 1848 because of his hope that women's natural abilities to care, comfort, and nurture would keep medical science at bay. In contrast, Zakrzewska insisted time and again that, more than anything else, a capacity for scientific thinking had to mark the true physician. There is a certain irony to the battles they waged over the years: Gregory, a man, spoke disparagingly of medical science and hoped that female practitioners would help keep medicine a healing art, whereas Zakrzewska rejected any notion of special female virtues, insisting instead that all practitioners, whether male or female, had to receive rigorous training in the sciences. Put differently, where Gregory accepted the contemporary link between science and masculinity, even if only to argue against the masculinization of medicine, Zakrzewska rejected this link, challenging the gendering of science and rationality and casting them instead as universal traits.

The battles between Zakrzewska and Gregory had much to do with markedly different views of science and of the role women should play in medicine. Perhaps Zakrzewska should have anticipated running into problems with the school's director. Gregory had already earned a reputation as a controversial figure, largely because of several pamphlets he had published vociferously attacking man midwifery. In addition, he lacked a proper medical degree. Although he possessed both a Bachelor of Arts and a Master of Arts from Yale, his formal medical knowledge amounted to one summer of lectures on anatomy and physiology at that institution. (In 1853, the eclectic Penn Medical College granted Gregory an honorary medical degree, but he never practiced medicine.) All of this might very well have given Zakrzewska cause for concern. On the other hand, recent changes in the college, especially its receipt in 1856 of a state charter granting it the right to confer the medical degree, suggested that other reforms might soon be under way. Moreover, Gregory had initially been enthusiastic about her hire, sharing the trustees' belief that she would "add to the reputation and usefulness of our Institution."[1] Thus although Zakrzewska may have had reason to be cautious, there were also signs that Gregory, the board of trustees, and the board of lady managers were ready to implement pedagogical reforms that would place the institution on a par with the best medical schools in the country.

Indeed, the plan to found a teaching hospital, which led to Zakrzewska's hire, was evidence itself of the school's aspirations. As we have already discussed, medical schools did not as a rule offer clinical instruction until later in the century. Although they were often adamant about teaching only "practical" subjects, by which they meant topics such as anatomy, materia medica, therapeutics, pharmacy, chemistry, surgery, and obstetrics, instructors rarely deviated from the format of the lecture. Practical exercises or clinical instruction of the kind Zakrzewska had received at the Berlin school of midwifery, or that she had taught at the New York Infirmary, had not yet become a part of the American medical curriculum.[2] Thus the college's decision to incorporate a clinical department into its medical curriculum was an innovative move. One can only speculate that its commitment to training not only physicians but nurses and midwives as well may have inspired this decision. Certainly midwives, if they had any formal training at all, tended to acquire their skills through apprenticeship. Perhaps the clinical department was meant to replicate in a controlled setting the model of apprenticeship taking place outside its walls.

The idea for a teaching hospital had surfaced as early as 1848, but sufficient funds were not raised until the school altered its administrative structure in 1856, establishing both a board of trustees and a board of lady managers and giving the latter responsibility for establishing the hospital.[3] Among the lady managers were Abby May, Ednah Dow Cheney, and Zakrzewska's friend Caroline Severance, all of whom traveled in Boston's liberal circles. These women saw in this hospital an opportunity to further their social agenda, both by providing medical care for the poor and by advancing the education of women.

From the beginning it was intended to provide women of all classes "during sickness and in childbirth, a comfortable home, with medical attendance by their own sex." Free beds were planned for those without means, moderate accommodations for those who had some disposable income, and "private apartments" for well-to-do women. As far as educating female physicians was concerned, the lady managers, in reaching out to the Boston public for donations, made it clear that the issue "has been so long before the community, that it seems not necessary, now, to argue its importance, but merely to present its claims."[4]

In addition to founding a hospital, the New England Female Medical College was also seeking to move out of rented quarters into its own building. This finally occurred on 1 May 1859, when the college occupied new premises on Springfield Street. There was nothing grandiose about the new accommodations, but there was adequate space to set up a dispensary and a small pharmacy on the first floor. The rooms on the second floor were used for lectures, instruments, chemical work, a library, and meeting rooms and offices. The stationary clinic was on the third floor. Soon to be called the "clinical department," it had six rooms (two beds in each), three for paying patients and three for charity cases. The students lived on the top floor. (Zakrzewska lived there briefly as well before buying her own home.)[5]

The clinical department was clearly a small operation. The New York Infirmary, which Zakrzewska had just left, had twenty-four beds. The New England Hospital, which she would establish three years later, would expand to forty beds not long after it opened. Still, the arrangement at the college seemed large enough to serve Zakrzewska's pedagogical needs. Most important to her was the small group of highly motivated students she trained during her tenure at the college. Among them were Lucy Sewall, Emily Pope, Augusta Pope, and Helen Morton, all of whom would eventually join the staff of the New England Hospital. The strong camaraderie that developed among these women led one contemporary to refer to them as a "charmed circle, banded together for life, for the defense of the hospital."[6] Zakrzewska, who later in life often accused young interns of selfishly pursuing their own goals, spoke repeatedly and longingly of the spirit of loyalty that seemed to characterize the students she taught during the early years of her career.

At first, everything must have seemed rosy to Zakrzewska. She had, after all, come a long way toward fulfilling her dream of offering quality education to members of her own sex. In addition, she had a position with much greater independence than any she had occupied before. There were, of course, the lady managers and trustees overseeing her work, but since among them she counted some friends, more than likely she did not anticipate any difficulties. As already mentioned, she might even have expected to get along with Gregory, who had been championing women's entry into the medical profession for more than a decade. Zakrzewska had thus every reason to believe that the college would agree to implement the reforms she deemed necessary in order to place it among the better medical schools in the country.

That is not, however, what happened. During the three years Zakrzewska remained at the college, Gregory blocked many of her pedagogical reforms, including her attempt to introduce classes in microscopy and thermometry. The constant battles they fought have frequently been portrayed as disagreements over standards, which they were in part, but the two educators were also staking out radically different positions on two fundamental issues that were being hotly debated at the time: whether knowledge of the basic sciences should be a part of medical education, and whether women had a special role to play in the medical field.[7]

· · ·

One cannot understand these battles without taking into consideration the differences that existed between the German and American medical communities around midcentury. As we have seen, when Zakrzewska had been a student of midwifery in Germany, the vast majority of university-educated physicians had been united in their demands that greater attention be paid to the natural and clinical sciences in medical school. Thus when she arrived in America, she had brought with her both a conviction that more attention to the natural and clinical sciences would make better practitioners and an awareness that with this knowledge came cultural legitimation and authority. What she found in her new country, however, was a medical community that was neither organized nor in agreement as to what made a good practitioner. Indeed, an attempt on the part of the fledgling American Medical Association (formed in 1847) to institute such curricular reforms as a longer school year, along with increased emphasis on anatomical dissections and clinical training, proved largely unsuccessful. The problem was not simply that medical practitioners were endlessly divided among, in Zakrzewska's words, "the many schools of the Allopathists, Homoeopathists, Electropathists, yes even Indianopathists"; even regular physicians differed with one another over the kind of knowledge necessary to be a good practitioner.[8]

One of the most controversial issues was the relevance of the natural sciences for practice. By and large, Americans viewed with skepticism developments taking place in the European clinics and laboratories, which, they believed, too often placed the interests of science before the good of the patient. It is true that a small, powerful, and very vocal group of elite physicians advocated loudly for French clinical empiricism. From their vantage point, the French emphasis on the numerical method and on studying symptoms at the bedside and in the autopsy room provided a necessary antidote to the speculative medical systems, such as Benjamin Rush's heroic therapeutics, that had flourished around the turn of the century. But even this group did not look favorably at developments taking place across the Rhine. Indeed, only a handful of individuals joined Zakrzewska in promoting German approaches to the study of disease before the 1870s. In general, Americans were unable to reconcile the German emphasis on laboratory investigations—which, they felt, conceptualized disease as an abstraction—with their view of patients as individuals, each one suffering from his or her own peculiar diseased state. They were also troubled by the Germans' foregrounding of a rational approach to medicine, which, to them, brought back the specter of therapeutic practices being derived not from careful observations at the bedside but rather from vacuous theories.[9]

For a number of reasons, Zakrzewska did not share her American colleagues' anxieties about German approaches to medical practice. For one, the attack on theory-driven medical systems had taken place in Germany twenty years earlier. At that time, young physicians, trained in the school of natural history, had waged a battle against the highly speculative nature philosophers. By the time Zakrzewska had begun her midwifery training, the next generation of physicians was trying to distinguish themselves from the empiricism of the natural historians by emphasizing the necessity of grounding one's medical practices in knowledge derived not just from the bedside but also from the laboratory. They referred to this approach variously as "rational," "physiological," or "scientific" medicine. For Zakrzewska, in fact, and in contrast to her American colleagues, the term "empiric" was interchangeable with the label "quack."[10]

Zakrzewska would not, moreover, have accepted American characterizations of German medicine as insensitive to the peculiarities of the individual case. In fact, in promoting their approach to the study of disease, German physicians actually criticized the French on this very point, blaming them for placing so much emphasis on "counting" that they lost sight of the individual. My point is not that the Germans truly valued the individual, while the French did not, but that the accusation that the individual was being ignored flew back and forth in battles over the best way to practice medicine. Thus the Germans defended their "rational" approach to the study of disease by insisting that knowledge of the causes of disease and the laws governing the pathological process would allow a physician to determine the best course of treatment for each and every patient. This search for laws, they proclaimed, had nothing to do with the derivation of statistical norms (and certainly nothing to do with speculative system building). According to the German physician Carl Wunderlich, who founded a journal in 1842 entitled *Archiv für physiologische Heilkunde* (Archive for Physiological Therapeutics), "a law of nature cannot tolerate any exceptions."[11]

In the 1850s, when Zakrzewska first joined the faculty at the college, her defense of German medicine made her unusual, if not unique. Small wonder she and Gregory went head to head so quickly. But had she promoted French clinical empiricism instead, she might still have encountered resistance, for Gregory's concerns about the impact the natural sciences were having on medical practice were of a general nature, not directed at developments in a specific country. Nor was he alone. In fact, one of the more articulate critics of European medical science was the Harvard professor John Ware, who lamented the growing emphasis on anatomy, chemistry, microscopy, and pathology at the expense of studies that would educate good practitioners. The "habitual dissection of the dead body" worried him in particular, for he feared that through this practice the once revered human body would become nothing more than an object of study, akin to "the inorganic materials of the chemist's retort." Although vague about the exact nature of the studies he preferred, Ware stressed the importance of physicians possessing "a large fund of sound common sense"; "a natural talent for nice observation"; and "an intuitive quickness of perception."[12]

Ware's language highlights the extent to which the debates that flourished around midcentury over the kind of knowledge that should drive medical practice had a gendered inflection.[13] Indeed, in criticizing science, which was coded male, and praising intuition, which was coded female, Ware appeared to be opening the practice of medicine to women. That was not, however, his intent. He thus sought other traits that would allow him to gender medicine masculine and found them in both the physical hardships that medical practice entailed and the mental hardships that kept a physician from getting "carried away by his strong sympathies." Ware, who posed the rhetorical question of whether "the nature of woman [was] competent to this," went on to warn that women who did not live by their natures risked losing their gender identity. "Should we," he asked pointedly, "love her as well if it were? Would she not be less a woman?"[14]

In arguing against women's entry into the medical profession, Ware may have been representing a position that was widely held among his male colleagues, but neither Zakrzewska nor Gregory would have shared his fears or accepted his terms. To this extent, the two college professors perceived themselves to be fighting the same battle. But there the agreement ended. Before Zakrzewska's first year was up, she tried to fail two students who had performed dismally on their final examinations; to institute a Latin requirement for the students; and to include lessons in microscopy and thermometry in the curriculum. Gregory was not impressed. He is reputed to have dismissed microscopes as "another one of those new-fangled European notions which she tries to introduce" and to have claimed that thermometers were necessary only for those who could not otherwise diagnose illnesses.[15] By the year's end, the two professors were declared enemies.

In the battles that ensued, Zakrzewska may very well have confirmed Ware's suspicions that female physicians would upset traditional gender categories. She assumed, for example, that her appointment had come with authority and voiced her anger when this proved not to be the case. Complaining directly to a board member during her second year at the college, she expressed her frustration that she "could not even do what has been in my power heretofore, namely, discountenance as physicians those women who do not deserve that name." She found troubling the college's willingness to enroll students who lacked any preparatory education and to grant them a diploma after several years simply because they had attended the requisite number of classes. "Were it the intention of the trustees," she continued tartly, "to supply the country with under-bred, ill-educated women under the name of physicians . . . I think the New England Female Medical College is on the right track."[16]

Evidently, Zakrzewska did not hold Gregory alone responsible for the school's low standards; she blamed the trustees as well for refusing to limit admission to students with some preparatory education. But Gregory still received her harshest criticisms. Showing no inclination toward deference—or, for that matter, toward anything even approaching respect—she attributed most of the responsibility for the school's low standards to Gregory. "Had the originator of the school (Samuel Gregory), an ambitious man, originally a missionary, been a man of higher education and broader views," Zakrzewska lamented, "the school might have been taken up by the men standing highest in the profession." However, Boston's elite physicians, such as Henry I. Bowditch and Samuel Cabot, kept their distance and refused their support. One reason, as Zakrzewska recognized, was that Gregory had alienated many members of the medical profession by launching vociferous attacks on man midwifery. But more than anything else, Zakrzewska insisted, these physicians withheld their support because they believed "the standard of the school was below par."[17]

Gregory, together with many of the trustees, did seem willing to keep the school's requirements low in order to increase the number of students in attendance. Like many other schools of the time, the New England Female Medical College relied upon student fees, and this arrangement worked against strict entrance requirements and a rigorous course of study. Still, as Martha Gardner has recently argued, the institution's course of study was as rigorous as that of most other medical schools of the day. Moreover, Gregory's opposition to the Latin requirement Zakrzewska wanted to impose had more to do with an attack on the elitism of the medical profession than a disregard for high standards.[18] In short, we must avoid the temptation to permit Zakrzewska to set the terms of the debate and recognize that much more than a simple disagreement over standards was involved. The antagonists also held markedly different assessments of "woman's nature," of the nature of science, and of the relationship between the two. Where Gregory viewed women as more caring and nurturing than men, turning to them in the hope that they would help keep medicine a healing art, Zakrzewska promoted an image of women as capable of rational thought and mental and physical fortitude, hoping thereby to open doors that would allow them to engage in the pursuit of scientific knowledge.

· · ·

Gregory developed his views on the necessity of female practitioners most fully in two essays: *Man-Midwifery Exposed and Corrected* (1848) and *Letter to Ladies, in Favor of Female Physicians for Their Own Sex* (1850). Gregory's argument in both essays centered on the impropriety and "unnaturalness" of men's attendance at childbirth. Embracing and exploiting the image of women as chaste and modest, he decried the affront to "female delicacy" perpetrated by male physicians' entry into the birthing room. Their presence, he insisted, made women tense and nervous, with the result that contractions that had been occurring regularly often stopped. For this reason, physicians frequently had to intervene in the birthing process; drugs and instruments had become necessary in order to undo the damage male physicians had done when they stepped into the room. "If physicians . . . would pay some regard to the laws of propriety," Gregory admonished, "and refrain from unnecessary intrusion into the lying-in room, and permit the ladies to assist each other,—protracted, distressing, and exhausting labors would be less frequent, fewer stillborn children would be reported in the bills of mortality, much less need would there be of ether, and ergot, and ointment, and antimony; and knives, hooks, and forceps, perforators, excavators, and other obstetric implements, would for the most part be permitted to *rust* in peace in their green baize bags."[19]

Gregory filled both essays with horror stories of women whose babies were murdered in utero through the unnecessary and uneducated use of instruments; women who were physically damaged when physicians, in their haste, extracted the uterus, and even the intestines, along with the baby; and women who hemorrhaged to death because of the ruptures, tears, and lacerations caused by instruments. One cannot help but wonder whether his rejection of microscopes and thermometers may not have stemmed from his general distrust of instruments. Citing another physician, Gregory advised physicians who relied heavily on instruments "to practise butchery rather than midwifery, for in that case they could sell what they slay."[20]

The message may have been the same in both essays, but only in the earlier one did Gregory directly impugn the character of physicians who attended women in childbirth. In *Man-Midwifery Exposed* he accused them of greed, deception, and immorality. Searching for reasons why male physicians would continue to engage in practices that seemed to him so self-evidently calamitous for mother and child, he insisted that pecuniary benefits must be the main driving force. Physicians frightened families into believing that childbirth required a male attendant so that they could reap the monetary rewards; they even made "a difficult or instrumental labor out of a natural one" just so they could charge a higher fee. As if this were not serious enough, Gregory also accused physicians of seeking out midwifery cases in order to satisfy lustful desires. Arguing that the intimacy that develops between a male attendant and the parturient woman encourages sexual intimacy, Gregory blamed adultery, infidelity, and even the increase in prostitution on the tolerance of male midwifery, holding it responsible for the erosion of "domestic and social happiness, and the moral welfare of society."[21]

Gregory thus built his argument around a radical separation of the sexes, seeking to reverse a trend that had begun in the late eighteenth century when male physicians first developed an interest in replacing female midwives as attendants during normal childbirth. At that time, physicians realized that the greatest challenge they faced was overcoming charges of impropriety and immodesty. They countered these concerns by emphasizing that their knowledge and skills were superior to those of midwives and by insisting that safety must come before all else.[22] No wonder Gregory's writings infuriated so many of his professional colleagues. He was directly attacking their rationale for disrupting traditional gender boundaries by insisting that male physicians, their claims to the contrary, actually endangered the lives of mother and child. Moreover, while trying to reinscribe that boundary, Gregory was threatening to disrupt another one, namely, the boundary that kept women out of the practice of medicine.

They need not have worried too much, for throughout Gregory's career he remained highly ambivalent about the status of the female physician. Indeed, in *Man-Midwifery Exposed*, he mentioned female physicians only once—in a brief section in which he discusses the inappropriateness of male physicians attending women for their "female complaints."[23] This essay is thus largely an argument against male midwives and in support of a school at which female midwives could be "instructed and *diplomatized* [*sic*]"; it says little in favor of women's entry into the elite medical profession.[24] Perhaps this is not surprising. In its early years, the college trained many more midwives than physicians; not until 1856 did it formally receive permission to grant the medical degree. At the time he wrote *Man-Midwifery Exposed*, Gregory even promoted the kind of dual system that existed in Europe and Asia, where female midwives were trained to handle all normal cases, leaving only the problem cases to the more highly trained male physicians and surgeons.[25]

Letter to Ladies, written two years later, addressed in greater detail the need to train women as both midwives and physicians, yet even here Gregory failed to maintain a clear boundary between the two. Thus, although he tackled head-on the usual criticisms of female practitioners, insisting that they had the physical strength and could acquire, through proper education, the "coolness of judgment" and "firmness of nerve" necessary for handling difficult cases, he rarely discussed the practice of medicine outside midwifery.[26] Indeed, one of the strategies Gregory employed to convince his readers that women would make good practitioners was to sing the praises of the French master midwives (*maîtresse sage-femmes*) Madame Boivin and Madame Lachapelle. What he lauded was the small number of cases under these midwives' care in which some kind of instrumental or surgical intervention had been necessary. He also commended them for having "comforted, cheered, [and] sustained so many of their sex through their hours of fear and suffering as none but women can; for they have sympathies in common, a language and sentiments which seem to be made for the purpose; their sorrows and joys are the same."[27] Gregory seemed to care less about women's possession of medical knowledge. In fact, his most telling comment, aimed at convincing male physicians to abandon midwifery, was his insistence that "physicians of good intellectual and scientific attainments do consider it [midwifery] beneath their qualifications; and when circumstances permit they are glad to be rid of it, and devote themselves to departments better calculated to exercise their mental capacities."[28]

Despite his promotion of female physicians, Gregory pictured the medical profession as fundamentally hierarchical, with female physicians occupying not simply a separate but also an inferior position in that hierarchy. His obvious coolness toward the cause that most impassioned Zakrzewska remained evident as late as 1862, the last year Zakrzewska spent at the college. In an article entitled "Female Physicians," Gregory, who continued to blur the boundary between female physicians and midwives, showed no reticence at all in distinguishing sharply between male and female physicians. "The writer," Gregory stated, in reference to himself,

> has as little disposition to see women in men's places as men in women's. He is not one of those who take extreme views on the question of "women's rights," so called. . . . Even the matter of the *title* should not be disregarded: the masculine appellation of Doctor belongs exclusively to men, and the feminine correlative, Doctress, both convenience and propriety assign to the lady physician. But to take the ground that it is indelicate and unfeminine to study the structure of the human system, with a view to understand its conditions of health and diseases, and thereby to alleviate suffering and save life, is more fastidious than sensible.[29]

Gregory's final sentence was a direct challenge to the likes of John Ware, who insisted that women's nature rendered them incapable of practicing medicine. To Gregory, in contrast, this "nature" was exactly what qualified women for the practice of medicine. Yet exactly what would distinguish female from male physicians, other than their subordinate status and the patients they treated, remained totally unclear.

It is not difficult imagining Zakrzewska's reaction to the sentiments Gregory expressed in this paragraph. She would have challenged the subordinate position in which he wished to hold female physicians. She would have been just as troubled by his insistence that women practiced medicine differently than men because their gentler natures translated into greater compassion for their patients. For Zakrzewska, nothing mattered more than to ensure that women physicians receive an education every bit as rigorous *and scientific* as that of men, which would allow them to earn the respect that was their due. Thus her differences with Gregory were really twofold: not only did she have a less conflicted assessment of scientific training in and of itself, but she also sought to make women active participants in the development of a medical science, not protectors of the healing art.

· · ·

Zakrzewska addressed these themes immediately upon her arrival at the New England Female Medical College. The occasion was the opening address she was asked to deliver in November 1859, at the start of the school year. Speaking to friends of the college, physicians, students, and other faculty members, the newly appointed professor centered her talk on the question of what should be expected from a physician. First and foremost, she emphasized, a person must have the proper motives for studying medicine, and these, she insisted, could only be "an inborn taste and talent for the practice of medicine" and "an earnest desire and love of scientific investigations." Zakrzewska contrasted these objectives with those of a large number of women who, in her view, entered the medical field for no other reason than "to step out of daily domestic life" or to satisfy ambition. "To these two different classes of women," she went on,

> I must add a third, which belongs in part to both those already mentioned, but which is impregnated besides with a perpetual sentimentality, concealing these other motives, and which bears on its banner the inscription of *"Sympathy"*; sympathy with their fellow mortals of their own sex, with the suffering sisterhood. However absolutely necessary a certain amount of sympathy and compassion may be, to qualify the physician for success in practice, it will never be the right motive from which the student must start. This predominating, sentimentalizing sympathy, will dwarf or confuse the reason, the most necessary qualification for the study of human nature; and will be pernicious to logic, preventing even the most natural instinct from looking upon *every thing* [sic] *that is natural*, and that belongs to the well-being of the individual, from the right stand-point.[30]

Without doubt, this represented Zakrzewska's most explicit criticism of those who sought to open the doors of the medical profession to women by highlighting women's greater capacity for nurturing the sick. Indeed, the passage sounds as though her target was not Gregory alone but anyone who placed too much emphasis on women's compassionate natures rather than their capacity to engage in "scientific investigations." Note that Zakrzewska was not ignoring the importance of "a certain amount of sympathy," although she did not consider this to be a gendered trait. What troubled her—and it was the same message she communicated in her autobiographical sketch—was sentimentality. As she explained later in her talk, in comparison with sentimentalizing sympathy, "sympathy . . . never betrays weakness or timidity and . . . is firm and persevering, controlling every action that it may not become rashness."[31]

The condemnation of sentimentality was a strategy widely employed in the postbellum period as practitioners of the health and social sciences, seeking credibility and legitimacy at a time of rapid professionalization, sought to sever their ties with the early nineteenth-century tradition of female benevolence. This tradition had taken shape as female reformers across the political spectrum had eagerly embraced the casting of piety, purity, and domesticity as particularly feminine qualities. The new moral power they had thereby acquired legitimized their blurring of the supposed boundary between private and public and had inspired their involvement in what the historian Lori Ginzberg has called "the work of benevolence." Whether battling drunkenness, redeeming "fallen women," or reforming wayward children, female reformers had drawn strength from a rhetoric that emphasized their morally superior natures; they had also filled their writings with sentimental accounts of young women temporarily led astray by unscrupulous men whose salvation was made possible only through their own interventions.[32]

Zakrzewska's comments in her college address suggest that she stood at the beginning of the trend to replace the rhetoric of sentimental benevolence, maternalism, and salvation with the language of what was perceived to be a gender-neutral science. Later in the century, physicians would totally reject the notion of sympathy, replacing it with the concept of empathy, which they held to reflect more accurately the detached concern scientifically trained physicians needed to adopt toward their patients.[33] Writing in the early 1860s, Zakrzewska did not yet have such terminology, but her attempt to separate sympathy from sentimental sympathy, and to associate it with firmness and perseverance, suggests that she was groping her way toward a similar distinction.

INTRODUCTORY LECTURE

DELIVERED WEDNESDAY, NOVEMBER 2,

BEFORE THE

NEW ENGLAND

Female Medical College,

AT THE

OPENING OF THE TERM OF 1859-60.

BY

MARIE E. ZAKRZEWSKA, M. D.,

Professor of Obstetrics and the Diseases of Women and Children.

BOSTON:

J. M. HEWES, PRINTER, 81 CORNHILL.

1859.

Title page from Zakrzewska's *Introductory Lecture*. (Copied from the collection at the Boston Medical Library, Francis A. Countway Library of Medicine)

Scholars who have studied the consequences of the late nineteenth-century attack on the tradition of female benevolence have drawn most attention to the way the professions became defined as men's work, thus generating an antipathy toward women. In condemning not only this tradition but also female-coded traits, such as sympathy and sentimentality, aspiring professionals were undoubtedly expressing hostility toward certain definitions of feminine behavior in circulation at the time. Still, one must keep in mind that not all were in agreement as to what exactly defined woman's nature.[34] Even within Zakrzewska's immediate circle of peers, there was considerable variation. Thus while Elizabeth Blackwell, Sarah Dolley, and Ann Preston were inclined to ascribe to women nurturing traits, Mary Dixon-Jones, Mary Putnam Jacobi, and Zakrzewska had a greater tendency to downplay any differences between the sexes. All, however, were trying in their own ways to advance women's rights. For Zakrzewska, sentimentality conjured up images of mental confusion and excessive emotionality, both of which kept an individual subservient to others, whereas reason and objectivity stood for independence of thought and thus the ability to act on one's own and for oneself.[35]

Not surprisingly, then, Zakrzewska moved from her condemnation of sentimentality in her introductory lecture to the promotion of science. Painting a picture of the history of medicine, from ancient Greece and Egypt to the nineteenth century, as little more than a great battle between religion and rationality, she emphasized how the view of disease as a curse, the belief that the body's restorative power sprang from an unknown and intangible supernatural power, and the priests' use of secretive symbolic language to describe their remedies had all kept people ignorant and prevented medical progress. The consequences, she maintained, were often dire. Not hesitating to engage in melodrama when it served her own needs, Zakrzewska jumped from a criticism of the "mysticism of the oracles and astrologers" of ancient times, in which "everyone, except the priesthood," was prevented from studying medicine, to a nineteenth-century case, in which a priest sent a young woman to her grave by recommending "the praying of beads" when, in Zakrzewska's opinion, "a dose of quinine" would have been more appropriate. "This poor girl," Zakrzewska told her audience, "died soon after I saw her, when she might have been saved, had she been less faithful to her priest and more faithful to a surgeon."[36]

There is perhaps no other passage Zakrzewska wrote that so fully captured the worldview she adopted from the German scientific materialists. Religion versus reason, secretive versus public knowledge, backward versus modern, the priest versus the surgeon, death versus life—the contrasts all work to promote science not simply as the best foundation for the practice of medicine but also as the surest way to bring about a just and open society in which informed individuals made good choices. Until this point in her lecture, Zakrzewska had not, however, directly taken on Gregory's contention that women had no place in this world of science and surgery, but she now turned specifically to the history of obstetrics to make her case.

Zakrzewska, who cast the history of obstetrics as a long battle to return to the principles of Hippocrates and integrate medicine with the other natural sciences, presented the eighteenth century as the critical turning point, when obstetrics finally achieved scientific footing. From that point on, she asserted, "the complaint has ceased to be heard, that abuse is the main demonstration of the practice of midwifery." In other words, in stark contrast to Gregory, she was insisting that medical abuses were attributable not to the embrace but rather to the neglect of science. The individuals whom Zakrzewska named as contributors to this transition included the French master midwives Madame Lachapelle and Madame Boivin. This was a shrewd move on her part. Not only did it raise her own standing, given her own training in European midwifery, but these were, after all, the same midwives Gregory had lauded for their sympathy, compassion, and noninterventionist approach to medicine. Thus, where Gregory had cast the master midwives as the embodiment of women's natural inclination to nurture, Zakrzewska has them defying traditional cultural stereotypes, indeed reaching "the heights of logical development." This did not, she insisted, render them brutal; on the contrary, they remained "in every respect humane." As far as Zakrzewska was concerned, their humanity developed not despite but because of their scientific training.[37]

Zakrzewska not only cast other female healers as rational human beings but also promoted this image of herself, frequently displaying her German roots and aligning herself with the style of scholarship that marked mid-nineteenth-century German medical science. "[W]orks like Kölliker's *Comparative Anatomy*, later Virchow's *Cellular Pathology*, and works on biology, embryology and histology became really the foundation upon which I built my practice," she once announced. This allowed her to ignore the endless advice about how to treat specific cases and how much of which remedy to give. Instead, she explained, "I did my own reasoning, I made my own deductions, in as logical a method as possible as the cases revealed themselves to my understanding through physical or psychical symptoms."[38]

In promoting and embodying an image of women as logical and assertive, Zakrzewska was continuing to battle assumptions about women's relationship to science and medicine from two sides. On the one hand, she fought to counter claims by the likes of Carl Mayer, Dr. Both, and John Ware that women lacked both the stomach and the intelligence to study medicine. On the other, however, she denied that women had something special to offer medicine. In this way, she was trying to break the link between science and masculinity while also challenging the claim that women had greater affinity for sympathy and compassion than men. Women, she told her audience, had every bit as much ability as men to develop their faculties of reason and logic; this was the path they had to pursue if they wished to succeed as physicians. Indeed, much of what Zakrzewska wrote in these early years was aimed specifically at reclaiming for women traits that had been gendered masculine by her culture.

One is, of course, left with the question of why Zakrzewska would have found it necessary to educate female physicians at all. If they had nothing special to offer medical practice, why not leave the field of medicine in the hands of male physicians? It seems surprising that Zakrzewska did not, at the very least, make an appeal to female modesty and insist that women, because of the delicate nature of many of their complaints, needed to have access to medical practitioners of their own sex. But Zakrzewska did not yet countenance any defense of women physicians that began from a position of difference. As she implied in her challenge to Dr. Both, she believed women had the right to study and practice medicine by virtue of being members of the human race. There were simply no grounds for excluding women from the practice of medicine or, for that matter, from any other traditionally male field of activity.

• • •

Clearly Zakrzewska did not share Gregory's anxiety that too great an emphasis on science would lead the young physician astray, teaching him (or her) to care more about the results of scientific investigations than about tending the sick. On the contrary, she embraced a vision of science, articulated most clearly in Germany around midcentury, that imagined an intimate relationship between scientific studies and medical practice. Seen in this light, the disagreement between Zakrzewska and Gregory over the value of microscopic studies was clearly about more than just standards. Indeed, Gregory's dismissal of microscopes as "new-fangled European notions" was just the beginning of a larger point he was making about the relationship between science and practice: "It is my opinion," he went on, "that we need a doctor in our medical department who knows when a patient has fever, or what ails her, without a microscope. We need practical persons in our American life."[39]

"Practical persons" of the sort Gregory lauded did not, however, impress Zakrzewska. From her vantage point, they lacked the ability to think for themselves and make their own judgments. They were, in fact, the "empirics" and "quacks" she so looked down upon, focused on "curing disease" rather than on studying the scientific foundations of medicine.[40] By no means did she wish to see anyone educated in this fashion, least of all women.

The antagonisms between Zakrzewska and Gregory finally escalated to such a degree that Zakrzewska informed the board of trustees in June 1861, just two years after she joined the faculty, that she would be leaving the college when her term of appointment expired the following spring. "My work as teacher in the college and as physician in the medical department," she wrote to the board, "has not . . . given me satisfaction. Not one of my expectations for a thorough medical education for women has been realized."[41] Zakrzewska's list of complaints covered almost every aspect of the school: she found it impossible to work with the director; the vast majority of her students lacked "superior educational training" and thus failed to show any interest in expanding their medical knowledge through clinical work; and neither the dispensary nor the hospital was flourishing, something she blamed on the hospital's location in a "demi-fashionable" section of town, which reduced the demand for dispensary services among the local population. In short, Zakrzewska had come to believe that the New England Female Medical College could not provide her with the proper setting to carry out her goals. Thus in March 1862, at the close of the winter semester, she resigned her professorial position, and three months later she left her clinical position as well.[42]

Zakrzewska's harsh assessment of the college was echoed in the years to come by other women physicians. Indeed, in her review of the history of women in medicine, Mary Putnam Jacobi characterized the institution's curriculum as having been "so ludicrously inadequate for the purpose, as to constitute a gross usurpation of the name."[43] By and large, the emerging medical elite among women physicians—Elizabeth Blackwell, Emily Blackwell, Mary Putnam Jacobi, Ann Preston, Mary Thompson, Eveline Cleveland, and others—all feared that a substandard school would produce graduates whose skill level would reinforce the accusation that women physicians could never be more than second-rate practitioners. Few among this elite (with the clear exception of Jacobi) may have offered as unabashed a defense of science as did Zakrzewska, but they all insisted that scientific instruction be part of any medical school curriculum. Indeed, the all-women's medical colleges founded in the 1850s and 1860s frequently stood at the forefront of curricular improvements. Thus the Female Medical College of Pennsylvania offered clinical training to its students at the newly founded Woman's Hospital as early as 1861; eight years later it instituted a curriculum that surpassed the requirements at many all-male institutions, including a three-year graded curriculum and mandatory clinical instruction. In 1867, the Woman's Medical College of the New York Infirmary had done the same, years before similar changes were adopted at Harvard and the University of Pennsylvania.[44] Clearly Zakrzewska was trying to make an early move in this direction when she fought for curricular changes at the New England Female Medical College.

Significantly, Gregory closed the clinical department as soon as Zakrzewska left. From his perspective, the experiment had also not worked out well. The constant battles were detracting from the school's central mission, which remained, in his eyes, the training of female practitioners who could wrest midwifery out of the hands of male physicians and thereby protect the women and children entrusted to their care. The college continued on under Gregory's directorship until his death in 1872. One year later, it merged with Boston University to form a coeducational homeopathic institution, a move Gregory would probably never have made. Ironically, he would have found common ground with Zakrzewska on this issue, but once again for vastly different reasons. Where Gregory would have objected to educating men and women together, Zakrzewska opposed the merger because of its association with homeopathy. In her estimation Boston University Medical School was "an inferior school and a homeopathic one, which has no other merit than that it admits men and women on equal terms to all its advantages; therefore, it does not injure the movement for women any more than it does the profession at large."[45]

By the time of the merger, Zakrzewska had been directing the New England Hospital for Women and Children for eleven years. She had founded the hospital immediately upon leaving the New England Female Medical College in 1862, when she was just thirty-six years old. Zakrzewska had finally achieved what she had been working toward since her arrival in the United States: the establishment of an institution committed to training female physicians at the bedside in modern medical techniques and, most important, one that was almost completely under her control.

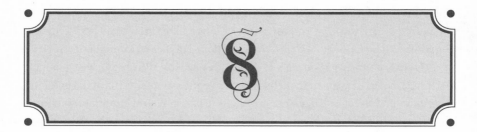

On Hospitals

On 22 June 1862, Zakrzewska founded the New England Hospital for Women and Children, one of only a few institutions in the United States at which women could receive clinical training. Not much had changed in the nine years since Zakrzewska had begun her medical studies. Women continued to be denied admission at most medical schools, and those fortunate enough to receive an education often had difficulty acquiring clinical training. Zakrzewska and Blackwell had set out to redress this when they founded the New York Infirmary for Women and Children. Four years later, in 1861, the Woman's Hospital of Philadelphia opened its doors. Now, in 1862, Zakrzewska followed suit, creating only the third institution of its kind.[1]

There can be no question that Zakrzewska most wanted to create a teaching institution. Indeed, when she first contemplated leaving the New England Female Medical College, she had explored the possibility of establishing her own medical school rather than a hospital. She had envisioned a coeducational institution, although one run by women that catered primarily to female students. She had also imagined male professors on the faculty and dreamed of luring Jacob Moleschott, one of the premier German scientific materialists, to the faculty of her school. However, the lean years of the Civil War turned out to be a bad time to start experimental projects, and Zakrzewska had difficulty attracting donors. She thus redirected her focus and succeeded in generating support for a hospital run by and for women. As she informed an audience that came to hear her speak about her hospital seven months after she had opened its doors, the plans for a school having fallen by the wayside, she had founded a hospital that would "set an example that women understand how to run a hospital, and that they can practice medicine just as well in such institutes as they do in private practice. In this way we cultivate public opinion through facts and bring the public, through examples, to the realization that women are just as well cut out for the medical profession as men."[2]

Zakrzewska recognized that the tepid response she had received from donors to the idea of a medical school required that she shift her focus away from the pedagogical aims of her institution and toward the benefits the hospital would provide poor women in need of quality care. For the first ten years of the hospital's existence, this is exactly what she did. Her first love may have been pedagogy, but her experiences at the Charité and the New York Infirmary for Women and Children had had a great impact on her, and with the political education she had acquired from both the women's rights movement and her contact with the radical German community, she approached the founding of her hospital with the zeal of a social reformer, intent on and committed to improving the lot of the poor.

The New England Hospital was, in fact, founded at a time of steady growth in the number of social welfare institutions. In Boston alone, Boston City Hospital, the Children's Aid Society, and the Children's Hospital were all founded in the 1860s, followed in the next decade by the reopening of the Boston Lying-In Hospital and the founding of the Dispensary for Diseases of Women and the Dispensary for Children, the Boston Society for the Relief of Destitute Mothers and Infants, the Free Hospital for Women, the Cooperative Society of Volunteer Visitors among the Poor, and the Associated Charities of Boston.[3] These institutions and associations marked a concerted effort on the part of both public and private organizations to gain control over the rapidly increasing population of urban poor. Historians of social welfare have long argued that nineteenth-century reformers frequently drew their inspiration from a mixture of Christian stewardship and Victorian moralism, combining a sense of obligation toward the poor and needy with a reformist impulse that sought to discipline them. Whether establishing a female asylum, an orphanage, or a hospital, reformers sought to offer a respectable alternative to the almshouse for the "worthy" poor: those individuals who did not abuse alcohol, who were engaged in or sought honest work, and who seemed to have fallen on hard times through no fault of their own. Such compassion for the poor did not, as historians have illustrated, usually translate into an acceptance of different lifestyles, values, and habits. Administrators set out to educate, rehabilitate, and reinforce middle-class values and a Protestant work ethic every bit as much as, and sometimes more than, they concentrated on providing adequate financial support or medical care. Those deemed "unworthy" of such charity were still destined for the poorhouse.[4] The New England Hospital was no exception. Zakrzewska understood her responsibilities as director of a new charitable institution to be a blend of medical care and moral education. She also shared with other reformers the conviction that she could distinguish between the "unworthy" and the "worthy" poor.

Still, among nineteenth-century reformers important differences existed in where one drew the line between these two groups and in how one evaluated the roots of poverty. At one extreme were those who linked urban poverty to an individual's character. As a result, they focused their reform efforts on moral education. At the other extreme stood individuals who believed that socioeconomic conditions limited one's choices more than individual character, and they thus paid greater attention to improving the material conditions of the poor.[5] In the early 1860s, Zakrzewska clearly stood among the latter. Convinced that one's "vices" were often a reaction to unjust social and political conditions rather than a matter of choice, she viewed herself as an advocate for the poor, especially for poor women. Women, she insisted, were caught in a particular bind, trapped in a political system that discouraged and sometimes prevented them from achieving financial independence and then abandoned them when they became ill or pregnant. The hospital Zakrzewska imagined would mark a significant step toward remedying this injustice, for one of its central goals was to provide poor, needy women with medical assistance and a "respectable" environment that would guarantee them the honor and dignity she claimed they deserved. Nowhere did she lay out her vision more clearly than in a public lecture she delivered almost seven months to the day after the New England Hospital for Women and Children opened its doors.

· · ·

Entitled "On Hospitals," the lecture gave Zakrzewska an opportunity to showcase her hospital and to generate much needed financial support. Radical Boston newspapers, including William Lloyd Garrison's *Liberator*, provided lengthy descriptions of the event in subsequent days, praising "the good thoughts and wise suggestions of the accomplished lecturer."[6] Heinzen's newspaper, *Der Pionier*, went one step further, translating the lecture into German and reprinting it almost verbatim in a five-part series, extending to twelve long newspaper columns. If *Der Pionier*'s account reflected the actual structure of her talk, Zakrzewska was not the most disciplined public speaker. Still, although disorganized, she filled her lecture with powerful anecdotes and images, all of which allowed her to communicate clearly the patient population she wished to serve and the kind of hospital she believed would provide the best care.[7]

Zakrzewska recognized that her greatest challenge was to distinguish the New England Hospital from other Boston institutions that were already catering to the poor. Why, in other words, in the midst of the Civil War, should anyone donate funds to yet another hospital when the city already had an almshouse, was about to open a municipal hospital, and could lay claim to Massachusetts General Hospital, a privately endowed voluntary hospital that had been in existence since 1821? Zakrzewska's strategy was to invoke her audience's worst fears about large institutions, especially public ones, in order to set the stage for her promotion of a small hospital with the "character of home." She conjured up images of patients being treated worse than "a herd of cows," left to wallow in their own filth, and housed in buildings so deteriorated that "snow and ice . . . covered the floors." She even invoked the dangers of medical science in the hands of those who felt no compassion for their patients, describing how the deaths of the poor are "often awaited with impatience in the cold months when, after expelling their last breath, they can be useful again—on the dissection table of the students who naturally long for a rich selection of 'objects' which can still their craving for science." Small wonder, Zakrzewska remarked, that the poor have come to fear the hospital. Ostensibly recounting a case from her past, she described the great anxiety experienced by the family of a young man who had been brought to the Charité with a broken leg, fearful that young physicians, interested in practicing amputations, would remove this young man's leg without regard for the severity of his case. Although she ridiculed the belief that "soup for the patients was then cooked from the amputated limbs," she accepted that such fears might be grounded in actual abuses, reflective of the disdain many felt toward the poor. "Hospitals, like almshouses," Zakrzewska emphasized, "are the horror of the poor, for whose well being they were founded."[8]

That Zakrzewska chose to highlight the potential abuses of medical science at the beginning of her lecture may seem odd, given her otherwise marked enthusiasm for science. Yet what better way to cultivate her audience than to play off their fears of the cruelties that could take place in large institutions lacking in effective supervision. In that setting, nothing prevented unscrupulous medical personnel from turning hospitals into sites for "medical study and experiment." Zakrzewska seems, in other words, to have made a calculated choice, hoping that the vision of such horrors would compel members of her audience to support her hospital. Perhaps she had learned more than she liked to admit from Samuel Gregory, who had used a similar strategy. It is, however, also the case that a closer reading of her lecture suggests that the true villain in her story was the large public institution, with its "spirit of disdain for the poor that . . . degrades those for whom I register a complaint." One might have had to listen closely to catch this nuance, but the individual who read Zakrzewska's lecture in *Der Pionier* may very well have realized that her true contention was that the setting, not medical science per se, hardened the young physician's heart.[9]

Having set the stage, Zakrzewska turned to the advantages of small hospitals, including the ease of oversight, which prevented abuse, and the more direct influence donors could have on those they were helping. But far and away what she emphasized most was the "*Häuslichkeit* [homelike nature]" of a small hospital, which allowed patients to feel as though they were being cared for in their own homes. This was, in fact, a recurrent theme during the hospital's first decade of existence. The institution's directors constantly reminded their subscribers of the role their hospital played in protecting women from "the publicity of the crowded wards of a public institution." Its small size allowed it, moreover, to "adapt circumstances to individual cases much more than can be done in public institutions."[10] Such claims appealed to the hospital's supporters. Garrison, for example, who promoted the New England in the *Liberator*, focused less on the medical interventions available at the hospital than on the existence of a unique environment absent "of all disturbing causes . . . of a large general hospital."[11] Significantly, in the early years of Massachusetts General's existence, it too used the language of the home. However, by the mid-1860s, when it had 180 beds and provided in-house care to more than 1,500 individuals a year (compared with 10 beds and about 130 individuals at the New England), the hospital's trustees focused more on "improved forms of hospital economy" than on the virtues of the home.[12]

It bears emphasis that Zakrzewska was by no means alone in her attack on large public institutions or her praise of the home. By midcentury, reformers from across the political spectrum engaged in a similar rhetoric as they grew concerned that traditional forms of poor relief, high among them almshouses, were proving ineffective in either caring for or controlling the rapidly increasing population of urban poor. Motivated by a combination of fear, arrogance, and benevolent stewardship, reformers tried to ensure that those capable of working did not live off the public dole, while digging deeper into their pockets to help those they considered truly needy. In their eyes, almshouses only fostered long-term dependency and sheltered those too lazy to work. Many of the reforms thus sought to distinguish between those deserving and undeserving of assistance, to deny access to anyone capable of work, and to steer children, single mothers considered capable of redemption, and the sick poor into the newly founded orphanages, maternity homes, and voluntary hospitals. These alternative institutions were frequently promoted as respectable environments, promising to replicate the virtues and values of the middle-class home.[13]

The valorization of the "home," touted almost universally by the founders of social welfare institutions, built on the tradition of female benevolence we have already mentioned.[14] Lauding domesticity, piety, and purity as particularly feminine traits, female reformers had justified their transgression of traditional gender boundaries by recasting the solution to many social problems within a language of domesticity. To these women, the home promised refuge from the hardships of the street, encouraging an intimacy that cemented bonds between those providing care and those receiving it, while permitting increased surveillance. Among nineteenth-century reformers, no site could compare to the middle-class home as a symbol of virtue in and of itself.[15]

When Zakrzewska had delivered her introductory lecture at the New England Female Medical College, she had chosen to distance herself from this tradition. Now, however, her needs had changed, and in an attempt to generate enthusiasm and financial support for her hospital, she emphasized the *Häuslichkeit* of her institution, even at one point challenging her audience to consider whether a hospital is "anything other than a representative home for the sick."[16] She also promoted the idea that such a home should be reserved for the worthy poor, denying entry to "paupers in the true sense of the word." Indeed, despite her attack on large state institutions, Zakrzewska insisted that some individuals deserved nothing better than the almshouse. Reflecting the same prejudices she had revealed in her autobiographical sketch, when she had written so disparagingly of the Irish and the French, she defined paupers as "those whose feelings are dulled, whose mental capacity for understanding is not much above that of animal life."[17] In contrast, she assured her listeners, the individuals to whom she intended to provide a homelike environment during times of need consisted of the "true poor." They marked, she explained,

a different class of needy, who become ill either through all kinds of misfortune (no matter whether they are responsible or not) or by the effort to earn their livelihood. . . . There is, moreover, among these individuals a class for whom the opportunity to secure their own existence is either curtailed or totally denied, and who, neither through upbringing nor through birth[,] belong to the class of paupers. However, by their efforts to escape from this fate, either through bad luck or through the fault of others, they nevertheless fail—I am speaking of women.[18]

Zakrzewska's confidence that she could distinguish between deserving and undeserving women situates her among middle-class reformers who frequently spoke disparagingly of the very people for whom they claimed to be advocates. This attitude was certainly typical of nineteenth-century hospital trustees.[19] Yet despite her limits, she belonged without doubt to what Michael Katz has labeled "the left wing of respectable reform,"[20] and it was to those on this end of the political spectrum that she directed her talk. This is evident in the trenchant critique she offered of a social system that denied women the means of supporting themselves financially, and then held them solely responsible for their situation. "Shame upon those who deny them their help," she preached to her audience.[21]

It is also evident in the analysis she provided of the relationship between labor and poverty. Unlike, for example, many evangelical Christian reformers, who viewed poverty as necessary in order to encourage individuals to rise above it, or even to provide the wealthy an opportunity to act magnanimously, Zakrzewska argued that the true reason the wealthy needed the poor was for the labor they provided. For this reason the wealthy had an obligation to care for those "who work for us and to whom we owe so much." Indeed, part of her critique of large public institutions was that rather than acknowledging this obligation, which, in her view, should translate into creating institutions that served the needs of the poor, state hospitals and almshouses served the wealthy by basically removing those individuals who had become a burden because of "their poverty, their dirt and their sickness."[22]

Even Zakrzewska's embrace of the rhetoric of home represented an interesting twist because, unlike evangelical reformers, who adopted a sentimental vocabulary when they spoke of the "spiritual" and "redemptive" power of the home, Zakrzewska emphasized the feelings a home conveyed of "authority, independence, and security." Thinking perhaps of her own role as a home owner, she established a link not between domesticity and morality but rather between home ownership and power or status. This is a country, she elaborated, "where even the middle classes are not considered 'respectable' if they do not possess their own homes, where they can find refuge in old age and sickness; [a country] where the ability and respect of a person are determined by his independence from his friends. In such a country knowing one is homeless must necessarily create a feeling of degradation."[23] Zakrzewska's choice of words suggests that she did not fully approve of the association made between the ownership of private property, social independence, and respectability, but she believed strongly that in a culture that attached so much meaning to the home, to offer the poor anything less than at least the feeling of home was to treat them as though they were less than human.

Finally, the way Zakrzewska spoke of the patient populations she intended to care for places her among the more radical nineteenth-century reformers. She may have joined her contemporaries in deciding for herself who was worthy of care, but she definitely drew her lines more loosely than most. Indeed, the last section of her lecture focused specifically on the patient populations she deemed most vulnerable and thus most in need of a caring hand. After defending the needs of foreigners, especially the wives, mothers, and daughters whose men were fighting in the Civil War, she turned to a much more controversial group: unwed mothers, whom she declared "most needy, but also most cast off." To the frequently heard charge that such women deserved to be punished, Zakrzewska cautioned her audience, "Let he who is without sin throw the first stone."[24] She also insisted that poverty and the feelings of abandonment and helplessness that accompany bringing a child into the world alone were punishment enough; the claim that coddling such women would lead to repeat offenses she considered simply erroneous. But her radicalism truly showed itself when she condemned making admission to a hospital dependent upon possession of a marriage license. Not only did she deem the practice ineffective—married women were known to loan their marriage licenses to unmarried friends—but she balked at the notion that a marriage license should determine whether a woman was treated humanely. "[T]rue charity and humanity," she told her audience, "consists of examining each person individually and either rejecting their admission because it is unnecessary, or permitting it and giving the admitted every kindness, so that she either gets better or is prevented from sinking even further down."[25]

The lecture of 1863 was not the only time Zakrzewska addressed the particular dilemma faced by unmarried mothers. As we will see later, it was a constant theme in the hospital's early annual reports. Indignant that a different set of standards often applied to women of means, Zakrzewska saw the New England as leveling the playing field, providing women the opportunity to live their lives with respect, regardless of their financial situation. One should note, however, that there was nothing unusual in Zakrzewska's decision to draw attention to the problem of unwed mothers; they had been a focus of Christian moral reform societies for decades. But such reformers frequently advocated punitive measures, standing behind the decision on the part of most lying-in institutions to deny access to anyone who could not produce a marriage certificate. It may be that unwed mothers did occasionally find refuge in these institutions, thus suggesting that practices did not always follow policy statements. Nevertheless, at a time when Massachusetts General Hospital refused to take any maternity patients at all for fear of attracting "women of notoriously bad habits . . . whose inheritance has been sin" and the Philadelphia Woman's Hospital's stated policy was to admit only married women to its maternity wards, Zakrzewska's public defense of the rights of unwed mothers stands out.[26]

Punishment was not, however, the only approach to illegitimacy proposed by antebellum moral reformers. Many, inspired by sentimental and melodramatic tales of seduction and abandonment, cast unwed mothers as innocent victims of unscrupulous men and thus capable of repentance and redemption. As a result, they occasionally reached out to single mothers, at least during the first pregnancy (a second pregnancy implied culpability).[27] Still, Zakrzewska's approach differed from theirs in two important respects. She did not speak out against single women who had had previous pregnancies. (As we will see in the next chapter, the New England Hospital also did not necessarily turn them away when they sought care during childbirth.) And, picking up a theme she had developed in her address at the New England Female Medical College, she eschewed most forms of sentimentalism. Although at other times in her life she did not hesitate to portray poor women as objects worthy of pity, the unwed mothers she wrote of in this lecture did not seem capable of being duped. On the contrary, they knew how to work the system, producing marriage certificates, for example, with ease. Zakrzewska's message was not, however, beware of sly women. Instead, she seemed determined to portray them as equal to anyone sitting in the audience and therefore entitled to the same care as those who had money. As she once explained, her goal was to dispense justice, not charity. "Charity," she elaborated, "is what an opiate is to a patient: it soothes for the time but the same bad consequences result as follow the drug. We must teach ourselves that the Golden Rule must be actually practiced in order to reach and raise those who need to be helped."[28]

In significant ways, then, Zakrzewska's vision of the population the New England Hospital would serve differed little from that of other founders of voluntary hospitals and social welfare institutions. Her harsh comments about paupers, even her emphasis on domesticity, all signal the way middle-class values shaped not only the rhetoric she used but also her image of the institution she was creating and the population she hoped it would serve. In other ways, though, Zakrzewska's vision was far more radical than that of many nineteenth-century moral and social reformers. Importantly, in the age-old debate about the extent to which the poor are responsible for their own living conditions, she tended to blame poverty and disease on social and political inequalities rather than on an individual's behavior.[29] As a result, she reached out to many women whom others would have condemned to the almshouse. For these women, receiving medical, surgical, or obstetric care at the New England Hospital rather than at a large public institution may very well have made all the difference in the world.

·   ·   ·

Zakrzewska realized that for strategic purposes she needed to keep her lecture focused on her institution as a site of care, but she still dedicated an entire section to the question of how the hospital should be staffed.[30] Founding a hospital at which female physicians could receive clinical training had, after all, been her primary intent. In her lecture she expanded her discussion to include the need for female administrators and nurses as well. As she had done in her autobiographical sketch, Zakrzewska charged right into an attack on standard definitions of what it meant to be a woman. "The great error," she told her audience, "is the expectation that women should play the sacrificing role everywhere. Wherever they take part, whether in charities or other enterprises, their participation is always considered as a duty toward others." Zakrzewska insisted instead that women should work "directly for their own goals and their own satisfaction." Doing charitable work was all well and good, but true satisfaction came only when actions marked "the execution of our own ideas." For this reason she encouraged women's employment as hospital directors and administrators, insisting, in fact, that women be allowed to direct Civil War hospitals. To those who raised the question of decorum, she replied that women "of upbringing and purity of the senses [Reinheit des Sinnes]" would never have problems and that such an argument was simply a ruse to keep women away. Drawing once again on the domestic ideology of female reformers, she insisted that since the hospital was just like a home and no one questioned women's ability to run their own homes, their directorship of hospitals should follow naturally.[31]

When Zakrzewska turned to the question of female physicians, she continued to tackle assumptions about women's nature, but she did not waste time pointing out the fallacies of the standard claims about women's inferior intelligence, delicacy, and physical liabilities. Perhaps she suspected that she was preaching largely to the converted. Whatever her reason, she chose instead to challenge directly men who considered themselves to be liberal in their views of women but who nevertheless prescribed limits for them. Thus, she told a humorous anecdote of a well-known Episcopal minister who could not understand the resistance to female physicians. In fact, he could not imagine anything more natural than for a woman to care for the sick and suffering. Yet when Zakrzewska suggested that women would also be good priests, he insisted that the ministry was no place for a woman because it demanded "a masculine power of mind, experience, and power of influence." Zakrzewska then turned to a man of the law, who begged to differ with the minister, expressing his belief that a woman could minister just as well to the soul as to the body. But when Zakrzewska provoked him by expressing her regret that she had never studied the law, he exclaimed that that would be impossible, because " 'a woman would never be able to handle the strain and discomfort of an advocate's practice.' . . . So we see," Zakrzewska drove home to her audience, "that even those men who consider themselves very liberal in their judgements of women, usually flatter themselves with the belief that at least for their own special subject they can only acknowledge the aptitude of their own sex."[32]

These criticisms did not prevent Zakrzewska from acknowledging the considerable support she received from male physicians, especially from those "who have achieved a reputation and standing in their subject." In contrast, those who have stood in greatest opposition tended, in her opinion, "to have the least understanding, the most deficient education, and the worst practice." Zakrzewska may well have been thinking of Samuel Gregory as she recited these lines. Indeed, she went on in her talk to lambast the arrangement at the New England Female Medical College, where most of the lectures were given by male professors and those who ran the school had very little understanding of medicine. As she told her audience, her experience there had led her to rethink her position on separate education for women, concluding that a school primarily for women must be directed by women as well, lest the students always be treated as subordinate beings. "If we are supposed to be capable of prescribing for and helping others," Zakrzewska contended, "then we are also capable of helping ourselves."[33]

Zakrzewska said little more in her lecture about the importance of educating female doctors, most likely because her potential donors had made it clear that they preferred to support a hospital for poor women than to contribute funds for clinical training. Still, what is surprising is her absolute silence on the advantages that an all-women's hospital would offer patients in providing them with physicians of their own sex. This omission is difficult to explain given that the hospital's bylaws listed as the first of its three aims "to provide women medical aid of competent physicians of their own sex."[34] Moreover, as we will discuss in the next chapter, there can be no question that the opportunity for women to be treated by women was one of the hospital's singular features and much of the reason for its subsequent success. Zakrzewska's silence is, therefore, all the more puzzling. It is possible, since *Der Pionier* did not reprint the entire lecture, that the pertinent section was cut out, but that hardly seems likely. More probable is that Zakrzewska felt highly ambivalent about this aspect of her hospital in the early years of its existence.

We must remember that four years earlier Zakrzewska had published an article on female physicians in which she had insisted that women did not practice medicine any differently than men. The medical school she had wanted to open was, moreover, supposed to be coeducational. Even when it came to founding her hospital, she was not initially opposed to having male physicians on the staff. In fact, a few months after giving her lecture, she hired Dr. Horatio Storer as attending surgeon at the New England. When challenged as to "whether it is not an inconsistency to have a gentleman in attendance, as it has always been stated that the advantage of our Dispensary is that women can be attended by physicians of their own sex," Zakrzewska quipped that it is well known who is in attendance on what days, "so that patients can have their choice."[35] A woman's dignity need not, in other words, be compromised through attendance by a male physician. Zakrzewska may have stood at the head of an all-women's hospital, but she was ambivalent about its identity as a separatist institution. This would change over the years, but certainly for the first twenty years that she ran the New England, she joined other regular women physicians in voicing her preference for coeducation, viewing her hospital's status as an all-women's institution as a temporary arrangement at best.[36]

Thus, the vision that Zakrzewska offered her audience in January 1863 was of a hospital that resembled a home, where highly qualified female physicians provided medical care in a dignified setting for poor women who had nowhere else to go when they became sick or pregnant. The vision was almost romantic, perhaps even a bit sentimental, an indication that Zakrzewska was not always adverse to employing the rhetoric of female antebellum reformers. At the same time, however, the picture she painted of women was anything but sentimental. Both her physicians, who were charged to work "for their own goals and their own satisfaction," and her patients, whom she portrayed as willing to lie about their marital status in order to receive the care they needed, promoted an image of women as capable of taking charge of their lives if given the opportunities. And that, of course, was exactly what Zakrzewska wanted her hospital to do. By providing women physicians with a clinical setting where they could perfect their skills, and poor patients a respectable environment where they could recover from their ailments and avoid sinking further into poverty, the New England would level the playing field for all women, whether middle class or poor.

•   •   •

The hospital Zakrzewska created did not reflect her vision alone. It was also shaped by the individuals who gave considerable time and money to ensure its success. The New England Hospital's first board of directors numbered nineteen and consisted of several of the trustees and most of the Board of Lady Managers of the New England Female Medical College. Frustrated by Samuel Gregory's stranglehold over the college, they had chosen to leave with Zakrzewska when she handed in her resignation, inspired by her plans to create a hospital by and for women. Many of these individuals came, in Zakrzewska's words, from the "liberally inclined part of the community."[37] George W. and Louisa C. Bond, Ednah Dow Cheney, Lucy Goddard, Edward E. Hale, Frederick W. G. May, the Honorable Thomas Russell, Caroline M. Severance, Samuel E. Sewall, and John H. Stephenson were only the most prominent. Several of the New England's consulting physicians, most notably Henry Ingersoll Bowditch and Walter Channing, were also part of this community. Other activists, such as William Lloyd Garrison, Karl Heinzen, Julia Ward Howe, Lucy Stone, Mary Livermore, Abby May, and William F. Weld, although not officially affiliated with the hospital, were strong supporters. All these individuals were active in the abolitionist movement and the battle for women's rights, all of them leading social reformers.[38]

Although not as close knit or insular as Boston's Brahmins, this community of liberal and radical social reformers nevertheless had its own cohesiveness. Several, for example, followed the teachings of the Unitarian minister Theodore

Parker or attended James Freeman Clarke's Church of the Disciples. Of the latter, Zakrzewska once wrote that "it was among the members of his church that the idea [of the hospital] was materialized, and that funds for the beginning of the experiment were provided."[39] Both Parker and Clarke were heavily influenced by Emerson's transcendentalism and engaged in their own reform efforts within the Unitarian Church. Critical of the formalism of established church doctrine, with its focus on biblical miracles and contemplation of an external god, they preached instead a more personal religion, one that heralded the divine powers within each person and posited the possibility of a direct intuition of God. Zakrzewska, as we have already mentioned, was an avowed atheist by this point in her life and never joined any church. But her ties to these men stemmed from their shared political views. Importantly, both Parker and Clarke paired their religious radicalism with social activism. Indeed, Clarke, founder of a church well known for the power it invested in the laity, believed that the glue that bound his congregants together rested in a "coincidence of practical purpose" rather than a "coincidence of opinion." This entailed not only the way they worshiped but also their devotion "to the relief of the poor" and "to doing away with social abuses."[40]

Deep friendships also bound many of these individuals together. Traveling together, attending the same religious meetings, visiting one another's homes, and occasionally marrying, they tended not surprisingly to support many of the same political causes as well. The New England Hospital clearly benefited from this. With the exception of a handful of people, the majority who donated funds to the hospital probably did not do so out of any particular commitment to the institution; rather, they must have viewed it as one of many good causes deemed worthy of support, such as women's rights, abolition, poor relief, and medical reform. They may not have shared exactly the same vision of the New England's central purpose, but by and large they were convinced that the hospital's mission dovetailed with their broad efforts at reform.[41]

A closer look at a handful of Zakrzewska's most prominent supporters demonstrates the variety of interests that led individuals to support the hospital. Certainly no person committed as much time and energy as Ednah Dow Cheney, secretary of the New England from 1862 to 1887 and then president from 1887 to 1902. Born in Boston in 1824, she was raised by reform-minded parents and counted herself among the "band of devoted adherents and friends" who went to hear Theodore Parker preach most Sundays. Inspired by Parker and other transcendentalists, Cheney became involved in a variety of reform causes.

In 1851, she helped found a school of design, intended to provide women with skills that would help them achieve financial independence. She also became involved in abolitionist work and then, after the war and throughout the 1870s, served as secretary of the teachers' committee of the New England Freedmen's Aid Society. In this capacity, she traveled to the South, visiting and evaluating schools and helping to coordinate the hiring of teachers from the North. Later in the century, she returned to her focus on women's issues. She was a founding member of the New England Women's Club; she, along with Abby W. May, founded the Massachusetts School Suffrage Association; and she was an active member of the New England Woman Suffrage Association, the Association for the Advancement of Women, and the Massachusetts Women's Suffrage Association.[42]

The New England Hospital's appeal to women's rights advocates has been well documented by other scholars. It was, to use Estelle Freedman's phrase, an example of the "female institution building" that took place in the second half of the nineteenth century. Indeed, Freedman argues that most progress in women's rights in the nineteenth century occurred not through women's entry into the male-dominated spheres of politics and the professions but rather through the creation of all-female institutions, such as colleges, reform societies, and clubs. These female networks provided the social, emotional, financial, and institutional support that helped women in their efforts to challenge traditional gender roles. In addition to the publicity the New England received in the pages of the *Woman's Journal*, a journal founded by Lucy Stone, Mary Livermore, and Julia Ward Howe as the spokespiece of the American Woman Suffrage Association, it was also actively supported by the New England Women's Club, which was formed in 1868 to further women's place and power in society. In fact, many of the club's founding members joined Cheney in taking a seat on the hospital's board of directors over the years.[43]

Cheney's attraction to the New England Hospital must also have been because of its position on race. Although Zakrzewska made no mention of it in her 1863 lecture, the hospital was on record as providing medical assistance to "colored" patients. In the 1866 annual report, for example, Cheney emphasized that a "noble woman, of the race to whom we owe so much, came in for a surgical operation. No sign of prejudice here. All met on the common ground of humanity." And in her memoir of Susan Dimock, who served as resident physician from 1872 until her untimely death in 1875, Cheney highlighted the fact that Dimock's first maternity patient at the hospital was "colored" and that

Dimock was named godmother of the newborn girl. In addition, William F. Weld, a Boston shipbuilder and regular contributor to the New England, gave five thousand dollars in the late 1860s for mothers-to-be "without regard to color or nationality." Not surprisingly, as we will see in the next chapter, this never translated into anything more than the occasional woman of color receiving care, but it is significant that it mattered rhetorically to Cheney and others to promote the hospital as a color-blind institution.[44]

Cheney first met Zakrzewska in 1856, when Zakrzewska was in Boston soliciting funds for the New York Infirmary for Women and Children. Their mutual friend Harriot K. Hunt had arranged this meeting, suspecting that the two women would take to each other immediately. She had guessed correctly. Cheney, a recent widow and mother of a one-year-old girl, later credited Zakrzewska with helping her to get out of her own misery and to think again about "the claims of duty outside of my own home."[45] Cheney ended up joining the board of lady managers at the New England Female Medical College; in 1862, she left with Zakrzewska to found the New England Hospital, where she remained for forty years.

Cheney was not alone among the longtime officers of the New England Hospital who bridged the abolitionist and women's rights movements. Samuel E. Sewall did as well. Father of Zakrzewska's close friend and pupil Lucy Sewall and originally a trustee at the New England Female Medical College, he left with Zakrzewska in 1862 and went on to serve at the New England Hospital as a member of the board of directors, a vice president, and one of the hospital's two legal counselors until his death in 1888. A well-known abolitionist and Garrisonian, he provided legal counsel in countless slave cases. By 1851 he had earned enough of a reputation to win election to the Massachusetts Senate as a Free-Soil candidate, where he continued to fight for the passage of antislavery laws, particularly one to render unenforceable the Fugitive Slave Act, which he considered to be "as void in law as it is in the forum of conscience." Later in the decade, Sewall also became involved in John Brown's case, first preparing legal arguments in Brown's defense and then, when the conviction stood, turning his attention to the raising of funds for Brown's family.[46]

As a senator, Sewall showed himself to be a champion of other radical causes as well, petitioning the legislature to grant "aliens" greater rights, to accept legal testimony from witnesses regardless of their religious views, and to abolish capital punishment. But after abolition, no theme drew his attention more than the legal rights of women. As both a senator and a citizen, Sewall fought for women's suffrage, for women's right to hold office, to be justices of the peace, to sit on juries, to retain their right to property after marriage, and to be able to end marriages more expeditiously.[47] He had, it should be recalled, loaned Zakrzewska the money she had needed to purchase her home, thus translating into practice his belief that women should be encouraged to own property. Committed to removing any and all obstacles that prevented women's entry into the public sphere, he demonstrated a particular interest in women's medical education that predated his involvement with the New England Female Medical College. Zakrzewska recalled how "profoundly interested in the subject and kindly disposed" he had been toward her when she had come to Boston in 1856. When he died in 1888, she refused to attend his funeral, fearful that her grief might lead her to make a spectacle of herself.[48]

In their promotion of radical reform, Sewall and Cheney were joined by Henry Ingersoll Bowditch, consulting physician at the New England from 1865 until his death in 1892. One of the most accomplished medical personalities in Boston, Bowditch earned his medical degree from Harvard in 1832, spent two years refining his medical skills in Paris, was on the faculty of Harvard Medical School from 1859 to 1867, and enjoyed an association with the prestigious Massachusetts General Hospital from 1838 until his death. According to Bowditch's own account, he became involved in the abolitionist movement the day he encountered an angry mob on the streets of Boston, intent upon attacking William Lloyd Garrison for his antislavery speeches. Already opposed to slavery on principle, Bowditch reacted to this lynch mentality by assuming an active role in the Garrisonian camp of the abolitionist movement.[49]

Known for his strong sense of justice and commitment to principles, Bowditch translated his beliefs into practice, ending an affiliation with the Warren Street Chapel, an institution dedicated to assisting children of the poor, when it closed its doors to black children. He similarly threatened to resign his position as admitting physician at Massachusetts General when the trustees, troubled by the number of "colored persons" Bowditch had been granting admission, passed a law restricting his freedom to admit whomever he considered needy. Disturbed by this turn of events, Bowditch informed them that he had "always regarded the colored man or woman in the same light that I looked upon other men and women," making it impossible for him "to remain any longer in a situation where I may be obliged to violate thus my views of justice."[50]

Like Sewall, Bowditch showed an early and sustained interest in promoting women's rights. He had, along with several other prominent physicians, encouraged Zakrzewska as early as 1860 to take the examination for admission to the Massachusetts Medical Society. (She had not been permitted to do so, the society being steadfastly opposed to the admission of women.)[51] Later in the decade, he took on the American Medical Association, actively promoting women's admission to the national organization. As he wrote his wife at the time, he "disgusted the Association" by speaking out in defense of women doctors, but he was unable to sit still "and see an honest cause abused and spit upon without at least protesting." Linking this cause rhetorically to that of abolition, he informed his audience that having been born "under the atmosphere of Northern liberty," he did not believe that anyone, man or woman, should be kept from studying or pursuing a trade.[52]

Joining Bowditch in his support of the New England Hospital were other members of Boston's elite medical establishment. Indeed, the list of the institution's consulting physicians and surgeons reads like a veritable who's who of the city's most prestigious physicians. Most of these men had received their medical degrees from Harvard; several subsequently served as faculty members at Harvard Medical School; and most had affiliations with Massachusetts General Hospital. Their support of the New England Hospital, as other historians have shown, stemmed in large part from their appreciation of Zakrzewska's commitment to regular medicine. Yet what is often overlooked is that most of these men also traveled in Boston's liberal and radical circles. In addition to Bowditch, Edward Jarvis left a job in Lexington, Kentucky, because of his opposition to slavery. Walter Channing and John Ware, both members of the faculty at Harvard Medical School, supported the admission of black students in 1850; they were also both actively engaged in poor relief. Channing's 1843 *Address on the Prevention of Pauperism* blamed social conditions and politics for the plight of Boston's poor, not the poor themselves, a perspective, as we have already seen, that Zakrzewska shared.[53] The New England Hospital must have appealed to these men not simply because it promoted scientific medicine but because it paired this commitment with a program of social reform. Not all the consulting physicians supported women's rights directly—we have already mentioned John Ware's skepticism that women had the fortitude to succeed as physicians— but the New England Hospital's role as a "homelike" refuge for poor women and as an emblem of modern scientific medicine made it attractive enough that even male physicians who questioned women's ability to practice medicine could support its cause.[54]

An intriguing example of this is Edward H. Clarke, best known for his now (in)famous work, *Sex in Education; or, A Fair Chance for the Girls*, in which he argued that women could not stand the strain of engaging in academic studies on a par with men. The very year he published this study, Clarke joined the consulting staff of the New England Hospital, where he remained for five years. Zakrzewska had known him since her days as head midwife at the Charité. He had come to Europe to further his education, and she claims to have helped him out. When she moved to Boston in 1859, Clarke became one of her earliest supporters, sending patients to her in her private practice and offering to consult with her should she need his advice. He even joined Cabot and Bowditch in supporting her application to the Massachusetts Medical Society. According to Zakrzewska, Clarke never believed *in principle* in the medical education of women and viewed her as an " 'exception' to her sex," but other sources suggest that Clarke had begun his career in favor of women doctors and only gradually changed his mind. It is, of course, possible that Clarke was doing little more than repaying a debt for the help Zakrzewska granted him when they were together in Germany. Whatever may have been the case, Clarke's willingness to begin consulting at the New England at the very moment he went on record advocating a less intellectually rigorous academic program for women deserves a closer look.[55]

What is possible is that Clarke's interest in Zakrzewska's cause reflected as well the vision he shared with her of the path medicine should pursue. In 1864, in an article entitled "Recent Progress in Materia Medica," Clarke came out strongly in support of "rational therapeutics," which he described as the application of scientific methods in the pursuit of "an exact knowledge of the physiological action of remedies" and "an equally exact knowledge of the natural history of diseases." Significantly, sprinkled throughout this essay were references to American, British, French, and *German* sources. Quite evidently, Clarke did not share the skepticism of most his colleagues toward German methods of studying health and disease. Using language that harkened back to the battles fought in Germany in the 1840s and that would have been familiar to Zakrzewska, Clarke warned that unless rational methods are embraced, "[t]herapeutics in the future will be what they have been in the past—empiricism."[56] In short, Clarke's support of the New England Hospital, and Zakrzewska's decision to reach out to Clarke despite his criticism of higher education for women, may have resulted from a bond they forged over their shared condemnation of "empiricism" and their positive evaluation of "rational therapeutics."[57]

It bears mentioning that Bowditch also expressed respect for German developments in scientific medicine, suggesting that at least a few of Zakrzewska's consulting physicians may have lent their support because of their positive assessment of European, including German, approaches to health and disease.[58] Zakrzewska may have studied only midwifery in Europe, but as we will see, the first generations of women who assumed positions as resident and attending physicians had all studied medicine in one or more of the major European centers of medical training (Zurich, Paris, London). Thus for those physicians committed both to medical and social reform, the New England Hospital would have had a particular appeal.

• • •

Zakrzewska, who was not used to public performances, was exhausted by the hospital lecture. "I am tired and worn out," she wrote Lucy Sewall, five days after giving the talk. Sewall was in London, training in that city's hospitals as a way of improving upon the education she had received at the New England Female Medical College. "I felt miserable all last week," Zakrzewska added, "so miserable that I had to give up my work and my lessons for the last three days and rest." Her exhaustion stemmed in part from the talk but also from the demands of private practice. In addition to her hospital responsibilities, Zakrzewska held office hours for her private practice from twelve to two, six days a week. Moreover, for those too sick to make it to her home or to the dispensary, she made house calls, and in 1863, a good two years before she purchased a horse and buggy, this frequently meant long walks. That winter was also a particularly busy time. Not only was her home filled with patients, but her private practice had really taken off. "If you could see my office day after day," she wrote Sewall, "full of school-teachers, dressmakers, mill operatives and domestics, all too proud to go to the dispensary and yet not rich enough to pay a large fee, you would agree with me that the prescription for good meat, wine or beer would be a farce if I took the money with which they ought to buy these instead of taking the small fee which allows them to keep their self-respect."[59]

Zakrzewska was succumbing under the strain. Matters were not helped when her sister Anna, who lived in New York and had been caring for their youngest sister, became ill and had to send Rosalia to Boston. But the final straw seems to have been the resignation of Mary E. Breed, the hospital's first resident physician, which left Zakrzewska with no choice but to assume the position herself, spending nights in the hospital and supervising the day-to-day care. Zakrzewska collapsed under the stress, becoming so ill that she had to suspend her practice for a week. When she did not recover, she packed a bag and, along with a friend, "went to New York on a 'spree.' "[60]

Zakrzewska returned refreshed from her trip and immediately tried to make some changes to prevent a relapse. She began by offering Sewall the position of resident physician upon her return from Europe, an offer that Sewall accepted. Zakrzewska also decided not to take so many patients into her home. "I would rather live by myself and pay more for the comfort of having a free home," she wrote to Sewall, "than to make a little profit." Her decision to simplify her life did not last long, however. Soon she was complaining that a year had passed since she had been able to read a newspaper, joking that her dependence on patients for news was giving her some queer opinions on the war and slavery. By November 1865, Elizabeth Blackwell was describing Zakrzewska in a letter to her family as "looking haggard."[61] Zakrzewska, who until this time had continued to give public lectures, decided once and for all that she had to end this activity. Thus, when Caroline Dall asked her to lecture at the Lowell Institute the following year, she responded with a remarkably frank letter, explaining that her strength was as "a logical practising physician," and not as a public speaker. Wishing no longer "to increase the number of mediocrity which we have so plentiful to endure on the Platform," she informed Dall of her resolution "to refuse any such work."[62]

Zakrzewska appears to have kept this resolution. Moreover, in 1869 she redefined her role at the hospital. In 1863, when Sewall had assumed the position of resident physician, Zakrzewska had been the primary attending physician at the hospital, doing her rounds and carrying ultimate responsibility for the care of the patients but no longer playing a part in the actual day-to-day care. Now, six years later, C. Annette Buckel became resident physician, Sewall became a second attending physician at the hospital, and she and Zakrzewska decided to alternate this position every three months.[63] Zakrzewska hoped this would allow her increased time for her private practice, which provided a necessary and important source of income, but it also permitted her to focus more of her time and energy on both her administrative and pedagogical responsibilities. Directing a rapidly expanding hospital was proving to be considerably more work than Zakrzewska had anticipated. It was one thing to imagine a hospital that benefited women, whether physicians or patients, and another thing entirely to execute one's plans, particularly given the changes that took place over time as the hospital outgrew its cozy setting in a small rented home and gradually assumed the trappings of a modern hospital complex.

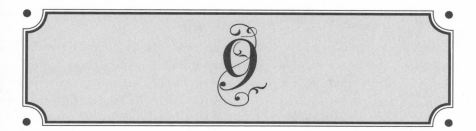

The Hospital in Transformation

When the doors of the New England Hospital for Women and Children opened in June 1862, it was a small, charitable operation. Located in a rented house in central Boston, it had just ten beds at its disposal, one resident physician, two consulting physicians, and two student interns. The New England admitted an average of about 130 patients a year in the first years of its existence, the vast majority for childbirth or "diseases of women," and attended to approximately 1,500 patients more through its dispensary practice. The annual reports of the hospital in these early years repeated much the same message Zakrzewska had spelled out in her 1863 lecture, keeping their focus on the necessity of providing a safe haven for the poor and destitute, including unwed mothers. Declaring "absurd" the idea that a lying-in hospital could ever foster immorality, Zakrzewska insisted that every laboring woman, with no exceptions, "must in the hour of trial be sheltered and cared for." Clearly not having lost any of her radicalism, she urged her supporters to consider the plight of the destitute and respond not only with "sentiment or sentimental sympathy" but also with "gold."[1]

By the end of the century, the New England Hospital was a totally different enterprise. With a capacity of roughly ninety beds, it averaged just over 800 patients a year in the first years of the new century and another 17,700 through its dispensary. It had also abandoned the inner city in 1872, moving out to the suburbs of Roxbury close to Zakrzewska's home. Over the years it expanded to include a new maternity building (1892), a new dispensary (1896), a new surgical building (1899), and a renovated central building, which housed the medical wards. The dispensary, which remained in the inner city, was divided into six separate clinics, one each for gynecology, medicine, surgery, skin, eye, and throat, nose, and ear. The staff consisted of one resident physician; twenty-four advisory, attending, and assisting physicians at the hospital; another thirty attending and assisting physicians at the dispensary; and thirteen consulting physicians.[2]

With this expansion came a change in the rhetoric of the annual reports as well. Gone was any explicit concern with poor unwed mothers, even though they continued to make up roughly 20 percent of the maternity patients. Instead, the hospital proudly announced that the vast majority of its maternity patients were married; indeed, many of them owned their own homes but preferred to deliver in the hospital because they lacked the "quiet and freedom from responsibility" they needed during childbirth. The reports on the medical and surgical wards followed a similar trend; whereas earlier ones emphasized the importance of a dignified setting for "the wives of clergymen in the country" and "school teachers, worn out by their arduous labors," later ones focused on creating an environment where "those who have good homes and the command of all that wealth can procure still find their best chance of recovery."[3] The New England Hospital had been almost completely transformed.

As the century drew to a close, such changes were taking place throughout the country as hospitals reconsidered their obligations to the poor. As their numbers grew—from 178 hospitals in 1870 with a capacity of 50,000 beds to 4,000 in 1910 and 400,000 beds—hospitals changed from largely charitable institutions, offering both medical and custodial services primarily to the chronically ill poor and infirm, to acute-care institutions, defined increasingly by new technological developments and surgical interventions and catering increasingly to the middle class and wealthy. Abandoning its identity as a home for the "worthy" poor, the hospital became defined instead around its clinics, laboratories, and efficient dissemination of care to a paying clientele.[4]

Still, few hospitals had started out with as radical an agenda as the New England Hospital, and thus few had been so utterly transformed. As we will see, financial concerns, a growing disillusionment with the changing nature of the patient population, and the realization that poor, chronically ill women did not best serve the needs of a teaching hospital all contributed to a new understanding of the institution's obligation to the poor. Zakrzewska, whose true passion had always been to open the doors of the medical profession to women, proved unwilling to do anything that would possibly jeopardize that cause.

· · ·

"Our beds have been filled and our dispensary thronged with wives, mothers, and children whom want and anxiety have sent hither, for bodily and mental relief," wrote Ednah Cheney in the hospital's first annual report. Only one year in operation and the small house on Pleasant Street was already inadequate to meet the needs of the poor. By 1865 the directors had managed to raise sufficient funds to triple the size of the hospital's properties and increase the number of available beds from ten to forty, but the New England Hospital still had difficulty keeping pace with the demand. By the fall of that year, the medical staff had seen a total of almost 400 patients since it had opened; it had attended to more than 6,400 people in the dispensary; and it had treated almost 400 patients in their homes. Three years later the numbers had grown to 1,500 hospital patients, more than 18,000 people in the dispensary, and more than 1,000 patients in their homes. Just six years after the New England had opened its doors, the directors were looking once again for a way to expand the hospital in order to accommodate the large numbers of individuals who continued to seek their care.[5]

Hospitals all over the country were experiencing similar patterns of growth. Certainly the exigencies of war propelled this trend; with so many sons and husbands away from home, family members who became ill often had no one to care for them. The end of the war did nothing, however, to stop this trend. On the contrary, a combination of factors, including humanitarian sentiments, a rapidly growing urban population, and concern for the health of industrial workers, led to the founding of ever more and ever larger hospitals that could provide care for the sick and infirm. The pressures the New England Hospital was experiencing were thus typical of hospitals founded in this period. Although many started out small, most soon found that they had to expand in order to meet the needs of the populations they were trying to serve.[6]

Much of the New England Hospital's particular appeal stemmed from the opportunity it provided women to be cared for by physicians of their own sex. Like the small number of other all-women's hospitals, it was satisfying a need, Victorian sensibilities having long rendered problematic the physical intimacy that marked the relationship between a male practitioner and his female patients. As resident physician Lucy Sewall wrote in the hospital's 1867 annual report, women who had evidently been suffering for some time with "what are commonly called 'female diseases,'" when asked why they had not previously sought care, responded, "Oh, I *could not* go to a man." Aside from the obvious power such a story had for soliciting funds from the hospital's subscribers—what were the annual reports, after all, if not a means of generating and sustaining the interest of their readers in the good work of the institution—there is little reason to question the validity of this appeal. The year Sewall wrote this report, almost 63 percent of the women receiving care in the hospital were maternity cases, and another 30 percent among both the hospital and the dispensary populations were diagnosed as suffering from "diseases of women." A vague category, it referred to a host of ailments that included everything from prolapsed uteruses to nervous ailments, conditions that many women often found difficult to discuss openly with men. Such feelings of propriety contributed at least in part to the popularity of unorthodox medical practices, as a woman would be more likely to find female homeopaths and hydropaths than female practitioners of orthodox medicine. Zakrzewska was, of course, trying to alter these statistics, and although she herself tended to downplay the separatist nature of her institution, for the women seeking care this was certainly one of its greatest draws.[7]

The experiences at other all-women's hospitals confirm this. Indeed, the New York Infirmary for Women and Children had moved shortly after Zakrzewska's departure from its residence on Bleeker Street to Second Avenue because of its need for larger accommodations. The Woman's Hospital of Philadelphia, which opened in 1861 under the direction of Ann Preston, also found its services much in demand. By 1875 it had grown from twelve to thirty-seven beds and was attending 2,000 patients in their homes annually and seeing another 3,000 through its dispensary. Other women's hospitals, such as Clemence Lozier's homeopathic New York Medical College and Hospital for Women, Mary Thompson's hospital in Chicago, and Charlotte Blake Brown's in San Francisco, showed similar signs of success. Quickly outgrowing their initial accommodations, they had to expand both their physical space and their staff in order to treat the large numbers of women and children who showed up at their doorstep.[8]

Unfortunately, too little is known about the specific policies and practices at most of the all-women's hospitals to assess the reasons, beyond Victorian sensibilities, that may have contributed to their popularity. However, if the New England Hospital is representative, the appeal may have extended beyond gender to class. At least in the New England's early years, the hospital did not require those who were attending the dispensary to pay anything for either their visits or their prescriptions, although other Boston hospitals, such as Massachusetts General Hospital, charged a nominal fee. In fact, charging the poor a modest amount for their care was a widespread practice, promoted as a way of discouraging dependency and encouraging a work ethic that linked financial independence with self-respect and handouts with humiliation. Zakrzewska and her staff, it should be emphasized, shared these values, but after addressing the possibility of screening their patients to determine who might be able to afford a small fee, they decided that "no test . . . will suffice to separate these from others who need all for daily support." Zakrzewska, who was especially concerned about the psychological impact such scrutiny could have on the poor, refused to require dispensary patients to submit proof of their neediness because she did not wish them to receive "the impression of being considered a pauper." She chose to trust instead that only those individuals who had no other options available to them would seek free medical attention.[9]

The New England's policies regarding admissions were similarly lenient. To be sure, as at other hospitals, medical, surgical, and maternity patients were expected to pay for their care: four dollars a week for full board (which was increased to eight dollars in 1864 and to ten dollars in 1869). Those with little or no means of meeting this expense had the options of reduced board or no charge at all. However, unlike other hospitals where a lay board of trustees handled admissions and evaluated an applicant's "worthiness" for care, the New England Hospital placed admissions squarely in the hands of the resident physician. In fact, Zakrzewska had made it a condition of her directorship that the medical staff retain the right to determine care based on an individual's need. To be sure, this did not mean that resident physicians ignored nonmedical issues when determining whether to admit a patient; an applicant's presumed morality was part of their calculus of admission as well. Nevertheless, investing the resident physician with the power to weigh medical and pedagogical needs over moral concerns meant that the level of scrutiny would vary depending on the judgments of the person who occupied this position.[10]

This may help to explain why the New England Hospital was able to reach out to unwed mothers when so many other hospitals turned them away. As already mentioned, most other hospitals with maternity wards refused admission to anyone without a marriage certificate. Tellingly, one member of the medical staff at the Woman's Hospital of Philadelphia tried to alter her institution's policy in order to offer refuge to unwed mothers; her request, however, was not heeded, presumably overruled by the lay board of trustees, who did not believe that helping these women would serve the best interests of the hospital.[11]

This is not to suggest that medical personnel were necessarily more sympathetic to the plight of unwed mothers than were lay trustees. We simply know too little to make such a claim. What is clear, though, is that Zakrzewska's insistence that admissions remain ultimately with the medical staff created a situation in which it was easier for those who were so inclined to show openness to a class of women whom others turned away. Thus both Zakrzewska, as attending physician, and Lucy Sewall, as resident physician, came repeatedly to the defense of pregnant women, regardless of their marital status. In the 1867 annual report, for example, Sewall announced proudly that the New England had saved "many a poor girl, at the very crisis of her fate" from the almshouse, being "the only institution, in the great city of Boston, for the reception of indigent women in the pangs of labor." Zakrzewska, moreover, repeating much the same message she had communicated in her hospital lecture, issued a lengthy report the following year, insisting that women in labor be treated with respect and chastising those who recommended sending unmarried mothers to the almshouse for subjecting them to a "greater debasement than an illegitimate pregnancy entails." To those who continued to condemn maternity hospitals for encouraging illegitimacy, she responded curtly that no woman, "(to her honor be it said), however degraded, thinks, in the beginning of her love-affair, of the consequences and of the probably existing charities of which to make use in case a child is born." After all, she explained, we are talking about roughly twenty dollars' worth of charity, which cannot possibly compensate for the "long months of deprivation and anxiety" that mark illegitimate pregnancies. But what also troubled Zakrzewska was the unfairness of meting out punishment based solely on one's financial status. "A woman in labor must be taken care of," she insisted as she had in 1863. "Whether this is done by means of her own money, by private charity, or by public institutions, has no effect upon her morality."[12]

This should not be taken to mean that the New England Hospital set no limits on the women it was willing to help. As in her hospital lecture, Zakrzewska once again coupled her impassioned defense of unwed mothers with a promise that her hospital did not welcome just anyone who showed up at its doorstep, turning away those who had been "recognized as absolutely perverted." Similarly, her insistence that a homeless mother deserved shelter after being discharged from the hospital did not apply to the "very few really bad women, bad in every way," who were granted temporary refuge only because they had arrived at the hospital in an advanced stage of labor. Thus, Zakrzewska flouted social conventions only to a certain degree, but she still went further than most. She seemed, in fact, to care less about the specific actions a woman had taken and more about whether the woman was capable of feeling shame for what she had done and, conversely, whether she understood the honorable

TABLE 1. Unwed Mothers at the New England Who Had Previous Pregnancies

	1872	1873	1878	1883	1888	1893
Number	1	11	1	4	1	2
Percentage	6.2	27.5	3.6	7.8	3.6	5.7

Source: Calculated from New England Hospital for Women and Children, *Maternity Case Records* [B MS b19.3], Boston Medical Library in the Francis A. Countway Library of Medicine, Boston, Mass.

thing to do. In one of her more radical statements in the 1868 annual report, Zakrzewska defended unwed mothers of multiple births by insisting that they knew the difference between honor and shame and that frequently these women chose, on their own, not to return to the hospital during their confinements because of the shame they felt. While others, such as Mary Delafield DuBois of the Nursery and Child's Hospital in New York, also reached out to single mothers during their first pregnancies, few went as far as Zakrzewska when she spoke kind words in public about mothers who had had more than one child out of wedlock.[13]

Unfortunately, the absence of any maternity records prior to the New England Hospital's move to Roxbury makes it impossible to assess the relationship between rhetoric and practice. We simply do not know how many unmarried women gave birth in the hospital while it was still located in central Boston and, of these women, how many had had a previous pregnancy. In 1872, however, the first year following the move, sixteen out of twenty-nine maternity patients were listed as single (55.2 percent), with one having had a previous pregnancy. The number of unmarried mothers may, of course, have been higher, given the likelihood that some unwed mothers may have lied about their marital status. The following year forty out of eighty-eight maternity patients were listed as single (45.5 percent), with eleven having had a previous pregnancy. Such a high number of multiparae was, however, unusual and probably reflected the unwarranted poverty and devastation that resulted in 1873 from a national economic depression combined with a citywide fire. As Table 1 demonstrates, in no other year did the number of unwed mothers who had had previous pregnancies exceed more than a few a year.

One must, of course, be cautious about extrapolating backward to the 1860s from data collected in the 1870s. Still, given that the patients who came to the

TABLE 2. "Colored" Patients at the New England (All Wards)

	1873	1878	1883	1888	1893/94
Number	3	0	2	1	0
Percentage	1.2	0	0.6	0.3	0

Sources: Calculated from New England Hospital for Women and Children, *Maternity Case Records* [B MS b19.3], *Surgical Case Records* [B MS b19.1], and *Medical Case Records* [B MS b19.2], Boston Medical Library in the Francis A. Countway Library of Medicine, Boston, Mass.

Note: Because records for 1893 are missing for the medical ward, the data under 1893/94 are drawn from 1894 for the medical ward and from 1893 for the maternity and surgical wards.

New England Hospital once it was located in Roxbury tended to be somewhat better off financially than their predecessors (more on this later), chances are that the percentage of single mothers had, if anything, been higher than 50 percent while the hospital was still in the inner city.[14] As far as the multiparae are concerned, there is simply too little evidence to speculate whether a higher percentage may have found refuge in the 1860s than after the move. The most one can say is that the rhetoric of the early years suggests that it was at least Zakrzewska's intent to create an environment that would be welcoming to second-time single mothers as well.

Similar problems arise when trying to determine whether the New England Hospital's rhetoric of color blindness led to the admission of patients of color. Again, since we lack any patient records for the years prior to the move out to Roxbury, we are limited in what we can conclude. The data we have for the years after 1872, as Table 2 shows, demonstrates that the New England Hospital never had more than a few patients of color at any given time, although given the small size of Boston's African American population throughout this period (1.3 percent of the total population in 1860; 1.2 percent in 1870; 1.6 percent in 1880; and 1.8 percent in 1890) this may also have reflected a lack of demand for services.[15]

We know, in fact, hardly anything at all about the patient population prior to the hospital's move to Roxbury. Although records exist from the medical and surgical wards, they never mention whether, or how much, an individual paid, so we do not know the percentage of patients who received charity. The records also did not start including the individual's occupation until 1873. We are thus dependent upon the annual reports to paint a picture of the patient population,

TABLE 3. Percentage of Foreign-Born at the New England's
Dispensary and Hospital Compared with Massachusetts General

	1863	1864	1865	1866	1867	1868	1869	1870	1871	1872
NEH-D	54.1	52.9	55.1	55.1	58.0	61.5	57.6	60.7	60.7	58.4
NEH-H	59.3	n.d.	n.d.	n.d.	59.6	54.2	42.4	58.2	55.4	49.4
MGH	60.7	59.1	52.4	52.0	53.7	52.3	51.0	55.1	54.5	57.0

Sources: Calculated from the annual reports of the New England Hospital and Massachusetts General Hospital and from New England Hospital for Women and Children, *Records of Patients Who Received Prescriptions* [B MS b19.5], Boston Medical Library in the Francis A. Countway Library of Medicine, Boston, Mass. *Records of Patients Who Received Prescriptions* were used for 1864, 1865, and 1866, the only years for which the annual reports of the New England Hospital contained no information on the nationality of the dispensary patients.

Notes: The data for Massachusetts General Hospital are for its female patients alone.

NEH-D = New England Hospital, Dispensary; NEH-H = New England Hospital, Hospital; MGH = Massachusetts General Hospital; n.d. = no data.

and the only reliable information they provide concerns the patients' nationality. Our picture is thus highly sketchy, but we learn, as Table 3 shows, that for most of the decade the populations in both the dispensary and the hospital consisted predominantly of the foreign-born. This remained the case at the dispensary, where the percentage increased over time. At the hospital, in contrast, despite some fluctuations, the percentage of foreign-born gradually declined, until the year of the hospital's move to Roxbury, when it dipped below 50 percent for the second time. As will see later in the chapter, this dip marked the beginning of a trend toward ever greater Americanization of the hospital population that eventually distinguished it not only from the dispensary population but also from other hospitals in the city that catered to the poor. Until the move, however, as row 3 of the table demonstrates, there was basically no difference between the hospital populations at the New England and Massachusetts General when it came to the percentage of the foreign-born receiving care. If nationality was any indication of socioeconomic status during that time, then as long as the hospital remained in the inner city, its patients were every bit as poor as those who sought care at Massachusetts General.[16]

All in all, then, Zakrzewska seemed intent on fashioning a hospital around a radical social agenda, whether by providing physicians of their own sex to poor women, by instituting policies that relieved the financial burden on the poor during times of illness, or by extending an open hand to single mothers. This was, moreover, the reputation her hospital enjoyed among Boston's social reformers. The *Liberator*, which kept its readers apprised of developments at the New England, emphasized the hospital's "continued reception of unmarried women needing humane and friendly care in confinement" and its focus on "the relief of sickness which was complicated with poverty and distress."[17] Zakrzewska, whose deep sense of justice had been honed by years of involvement in the German radical community and the American women's movement, had created an institution that sought to level the playing field, providing poor women with both the comfort and the care that women of means could take for granted when they became ill or brought children into the world.

• • •

The radicalism of the early years did not last. Indeed, looking back, one can see signs of fracturing almost from the beginning. The greatest problem Zakrzewska faced was the large number of chronically ill individuals turning up at her doorstep. Needing comfort more than medical care, this population posed a serious challenge. As Zakrzewska wrote as early as 1865: "Providing good homes and care for [the poor and unfortunate] in their hour of need and trial, is not the sole proof of [the hospital's] necessity; another proof, more striking can be brought forth, namely, that of absolute saving of life, to say nothing of its scientific test and value."[18] Zakrzewska's goal of demonstrating the clinical and scientific acumen of women physicians could not, in other words, be put to the test on patients whose ailments were chronic rather than acute. Portraying the New England Hospital as a home for the needy was all well and good, but she also needed patients who required short-term medical and surgical interventions in order to prove her case, for it was their lives that could be saved quickly and heroically.

Early on, then, Zakrzewska came up against the problems inherent in trying to serve two different populations: her patients and her students. Other hospitals that permitted clinical instruction experienced this tension as well, but at least at those hospitals a lay board of trustees usually guarded its role as protector of the patient population, frequently thwarting attempts by the medical staff to put pedagogical interests before the well-being of the patients. As a result, the two populations had different authoritative bodies representing their interests.[19] That was not the case at the New England Hospital, where, despite the existence of a lay board of trustees, Zakrzewska retained most of the decision-making power. She thus struggled to find a balance between the good of her students and the good of her patients. As time went on, she tended to favor the former more and more.[20]

The chronically ill posed another problem above and beyond their slow recovery rates. They also drained financial resources, occupying the limited number of beds for long periods of time, often unable, moreover, to contribute much toward their care. This was a burden the hospital could hardly afford. Although the charity cases in the maternity ward were paid for largely by the Lying-in Hospital Corporation (an association that had funded the Boston Lying-In Hospital during its brief existence in the mid-1850s), for those who needed charitable assistance in the medical or surgical wards, the hospital had to scramble about for donations from year to year.[21] In addition, the expansion in 1865 had been expensive, and although the New England had received a five-thousand-dollar matching grant from the Massachusetts legislature, it had encountered difficulties raising funds for both the match and its operating expenses. As a result of these financial concerns, the hospital ultimately changed its policies toward the poor. First, in the summer of 1866, the board of directors passed a resolution refusing a bed in either the medical or surgical ward to anyone who could not pay the full price of eight dollars a week. Not wishing to make this a permanent measure, it next turned to the dispensary. Thus, in 1868, just a few years after Zakrzewska had refused to scrutinize dispensary patients, the New England Hospital began charging twenty-five cents for each prescription unless an individual could produce a certificate authenticating her poverty. By the end of the year, Cheney could announce that "the result has exceeded our expectations" and that the fees almost covered all the dispensary's expenses. What she did not mention was that this policy also effectively reduced the number of individuals seeking help. From a record-breaking 4,576 individuals who were treated in the dispensary in 1867, the numbers dropped to 3,236 in 1868 and to 2,854 in 1869. Zakrzewska, who approved of this new arrangement, insisted at the end of the decade that she no longer wanted to see in the dispensary anyone "who is not so poor as to have a charity certificate signed."[22]

Zakrzewska never explained her dramatic switch from refusing to humiliate her dispensary patients by insisting on a "card of introduction" to demanding "a charity certificate." Circumstantial evidence suggests, however, that two factors were probably at play. We have already noted that for Zakrzewska the hospital mattered most as proof that women could manage their own hospital. As interested as she may have been in the charitable dimension of the institution, she was more committed to the role the institution played in challenging

TABLE 4. Percentage of Foreign-Born and Irish at the New England's Dispensary

	1863	1864	1865	1866	1867	1868	1869	1870	1871	1872
Foreign	54.1	52.9	55.1	55.1	58.0	61.5	57.6	60.7	60.7	58.4
Irish	26.3	30.5	38.1	40.6	44.1	41.2	45.3	47	44.9	40.9

Sources: Calculated from the New England Hospital's annual reports for 1863, 1867–72, and from New England Hospital for Women and Children, *Records of Patients Who Received Prescriptions* [B MS b19.5], 1864–66, Boston Medical Library in the Francis A. Countway Library of Medicine, Boston, Mass.

stereotypes about women's ability to hold positions of power. As in her auto-biographical sketch, gender once again trumped class. Thus when the New England faced the possibility of financial debts, which, she believed, marked "the commencement of the undermining of an institution," she implemented policies for the good of the institution that resulted in the curtailment of benefits to the poor. Over the decades Zakrzewska would repeatedly relax some of her principles when the survival of her institution was at stake.[23]

But financial concerns alone did not lead to Zakrzewska's change of heart. She also showed signs of growing disillusionment with the women attending the dispensary. Indeed, by the end of the decade, the annual reports no longer portrayed the typical dispensary patient as "a respectable woman" who was "too proud to ask charity of a physician" but rather as someone who needed to be taught how to "dispel ignorance, promote temperance, banish licentiousness and other vices." Evoking images of the undesirable as unclean and contagious, Zakrzewska even went so far as to blame the dispensary patients, who came "from the poorest quarters of the city," for adding "to the impurity of the atmosphere" of the hospital, even though she acknowledged that the two structures were "almost entirely shut off" from each other.[24] A look at changes in the dispensary population over the first ten years reveals why this may have been the case. As Table 4 indicates, the population was becoming not only increasingly foreign but also increasingly Irish. One need only remember Zakrzewska's anti-Catholicism as well as her disparaging remarks about the Irish in her auto-biographical sketch to recognize that she harbored little affection for this immigrant group.[25] It bears mention, as Table 5 shows, that a similar shift in national identity did not take place in the hospital population, which became both less foreign and less Irish as the decade wore on.

TABLE 5. Percentage of Foreign-Born and Irish at the New England's Hospital

	1863	1864	1865	1866	1867	1868	1869	1870	1871	1872
Foreign	59.3	n.d.	n.d.	n.d.	59.6	54.2	42.4	58.2	55.4	49.4
Irish	33.1	n.d.	n.d.	n.d.	33.3	29.6	18.5	32.2	23.5	23.1

Sources: Calculated from the New England Hospital's annual reports for 1863, 1867–72, and from New England Hospital for Women and Children, *Records of Patients Who Received Prescriptions* [B MS b19.5], 1864–66, Boston Medical Library in the Francis A. Countway Library of Medicine, Boston, Mass.

Note: n.d. = no data.

Alongside this growing distaste for the dispensary population, Zakrzewska also began to show an increased interest in attracting a more affluent patient population. This shift was evident in the annual reports, which retained the image of the hospital as a home but which began to make it over into a home with middle-class accoutrements. Thus subscribers read about the hospital's need for more private rooms, a "patients' parlor," "more ground around the house," and, above all, respite from the "noise and dust and crowded condition of the streets [which] make our present place quite unfit for nervous chronic patients."[26] Not surprisingly, by this time, Zakrzewska and her board of directors had decided that it was in their best interest to move the hospital out of the inner city.

No doubt this decision was spurred on by the New England Hospital's need for more space. The 1865 renovations had, in fact, proved inadequate almost immediately. But there can be no question that the move was also part and parcel of a drive to attract a different patient population and to create a different image for the hospital. Significantly, there was never any plan to move the dispensary to Roxbury with the hospital.[27] Although this made sense, both because the poor lacked the time and money necessary to take the streetcar out to Roxbury and because the hospital's interns learned medicine in part by attending to the sick poor in their homes, more was clearly going on. Zakrzewska's characterization of the dispensary population as carriers of impurities and thus a threat to the salubrity of the hospital patients reveals the dense connections between ideas of cleanliness and contagion and notions of class and ethnicity that historians of disease have long described.[28]

In fact, Zakrzewska and her staff had been voicing their concerns for years that the noxious airs of the inner city were detrimental to the convalescence of their hospital patients. In doing so, they were embracing a view of disease that

went virtually uncontested in the days before the germ theory and that imagined disease, and especially infection, to be intimately linked with the environment; bad air, whether emanating from people or places, and not germs per se,
could cause an infection to spread out of control through the hospital wards. As
a result, standard practices were to increase ventilation through open windows
and specific architectural design, as well as to vacate wards where the infections
began for purposes of purification.[29] Indeed, Zakrzewska explained that much
of her motivation for wanting a larger facility was in order to leave some wards
"always in reserve for change and purification, thus fulfilling all the hygienic
laws demanded by hospital life." Writing this in 1869, she estimated that the
New England Hospital had two years before its current conditions would be
considered "not merely undesirable, but really injurious to the health of all,
both patients and officers."[30]

Zakrzewska, however, did not simply want more room; she also wanted to
move the hospital out of the inner city and thus as far away as possible from the
individuals who frequented the dispensary and made the already bad air cours-
ing through the hospital even worse. Her desire for a "better" class of patients
surely reflected both her hope for more revenue and her conviction that individuals of means had a better chance of recovering from a serious illness.[31] What
better way, after all, to convince the world that women physicians should be
encouraged to practice medicine than to sit at the helm of a hospital whose rates
of cure surpassed those of comparable institutions? Indeed, an intern who
studied at the hospital later in the century accused the institution of turning
away seriously ill patients because their deaths "would make the Hospital report look badly."[32] But Zakrzewska's increased indifference toward the plight of
the poorest of the poor, among whom the Irish were well represented, also
reveals the limits of her radicalism and her growing willingness to accept, for at
least certain populations, the tight links between poverty, filth, contagion, and
ethnicity that flourished in her day.

Zakrzewska's pleas for a new hospital were heard, and adequate funds were
raised to start construction. By September 1872 the new premises were ready to
be occupied. Located on Codman Avenue in Roxbury, the New England Hospital now had the "benefit of country air and quiet." With a capacity of ninety
beds—fifty-seven for the patients and another thirty-three for nurses, students,
and other staff—the hospital had more than doubled its occupancy. Twenty-
three of the beds were in the medical ward, another twelve in the surgical ward,
and another six earmarked specifically for children. The remaining twenty pa-

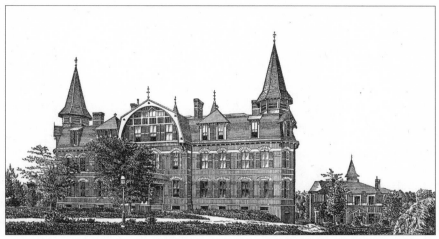

New England Hospital for Women and Children. (Courtesy of
Sophia Smith Collection, Smith College)

tient beds (twelve for mothers and another eight cribs for infants) were housed in
a separate maternity cottage on the premises. The 1872 annual report drew
particular attention to the hospital's new physical arrangement, which allowed
it to prevent the spread of infection to parturient women. It also advertised the
"light, airy, sunny wards" found throughout the main building and the presence
of a "pleasant Patients' Parlor" on the west side of the building. (In subsequent
years, the annual reports also conveyed news about piano recitals and carriage
rides.) Finally, it mentioned the addition of a few private rooms on the first floor
for those women "whose means enabled them to pay for superior accommodations." Anyone paying twenty-five dollars a week had the benefit of "a nurse
exclusively devoted to her,—board, medical attendance, and washing." According to Emma Call, who joined the medical staff in 1875, the changes brought
about the desired effects, with the result that "the class of patients was . . . a
much better one," no longer including "any considerable number of the most
undesirable cases, which inevitably gravitate to an institution located in the
midst of a dense population." The institution certainly still catered to the sick
poor, but it had taken a big step toward assuring that "the moderately well to
do" would also find a home within its walls.[33]

• • •

Patient information for the years following the New England Hospital's move to
Roxbury is rich compared with the data available for the first decade of the

TABLE 6. Percentage of Charity Cases at the New England, the Boston Lying-In, and Massachusetts General, 1877–1886

	1877	1878	1879	1880	1881	1882	1883	1884	1885	1886	Avg
NEH	57.2	54.2	55.5	54.1	45.1	34.6	25.6	41.5	39.9	47.2	45.5
BLI	71.8	68.5	76.1	80.2	70.6	66.4	61.8	56.2	70.3	74	69.6
MGH	83.1	82.0	82.9	81.7	72	n.d.	72.4	80.6	84.7	84.2	80.4

Sources: Calculated from the annual reports of the New England Hospital, the Boston Lying-In Hospital, and Massachusetts General Hospital. See also Bowditch, *History of the Massachusetts General Hospital*, 702, and Vogel, "Patrons, Practitioners, and Patients," 290.

Notes: The data for Massachusetts General Hospital are for its female patients alone.

For 1877 and 1878, the New England Hospital provided joint statistics for those who paid nothing and those who paid part board. To derive an estimate of the number who paid absolutely nothing (necessary in order to make a comparison with the other hospitals), I calculated the relationship between full charity and part charity for 1879, 1880, and 1881; took the average of the three (which was 72.33 percent for full charity, compared with 27.66 percent for part); and used that to estimate the number of full charity cases for 1877 and 1878.

NEH = New England Hospital; BLI = Boston Lying-In Hospital; MGH = Massachusetts General Hospital; n.d. = no data.

institution's existence, allowing one to evaluate the validity of Call's claim. For one, hospital records regularly included the patient's occupation and nationality. In addition, the maternity wards recorded the patient's marital status and the number of previous pregnancies and children. In 1877, the annual reports also began to include information on the financial status of the hospital's patients: from 1877 to 1886 they offered data on the number of patients who paid full board, half board, or nothing at all. Beginning in 1887, they switched to calculating the number of free days compared with paid days.[34] Taken together, the reports suggest that the hospital did indeed attract a "better" class of individuals; at least they came from a slightly higher socioeconomic class than those who received care at either Massachusetts General or the Boston Lying-In Hospital, which reopened its doors in 1872.

This is evident, for example, from the data on the hospital's charitable work. Table 6 covers the years 1877–86, when the New England, Massachusetts General, and the Boston Lying-In all recorded the number of patients who received free care. Table 7 covers 1887 to 1893, when the New England switched to recording the number of free days (versus paid days).

TABLE 7. Percentage of Free Days at the New England Compared with Percentage of Charity Cases at Massachusetts General and the Boston Lying-In, 1887–1893

	1887	1888	1889	1890	1891	1892	1893	Avg
NEH	45.2	n.d.	43.2	52.7	52.5	49.9	52.3	49.3
BLI	80.7	77.3	76.2	84.7	79.1	77.2	69.5	77.8
MGH	83.7	81.9	83.6	76.7	79.7	77.0	n.d.	80.4

Sources: Calculated from the annual reports of the New England Hospital, the Boston Lying-In Hospital, and Massachusetts General Hospital. See also Bowditch, *History of the Massachusetts General Hospital*, 702, and Vogel, "Patrons, Practitioners, and Patients," 290.

Notes: The data for Massachusetts General are for its female patients alone.
  See Table 6 for abbreviations.

It is clear from both tables that following its move to Roxbury the New England never served quite as poor a population as Massachusetts General or the Boston Lying-In. The contrast is, in fact, quite marked. And while the data from 1887 to 1893 must be used cautiously, since we are comparing free days at the New England with the numbers of patients who received free board at the other hospitals, it may very well be that the gap was even greater than indicated: between 1897 and 1901, when the New England provided information on both free days and the number of patients receiving free board, the former indicated a higher level of charitable care than the latter.[35]

The claim that the patient population at the New England was somewhat better off than the populations at other Boston hospitals is further supported by an analysis of occupational structure. Table 8, which covers the years 1873 to 1894, demonstrates that the percentage of white-collar workers at the institution was, with the exception of 1873/74, higher than at Massachusetts General or Boston City Hospital. In addition, although the percentage of blue-collar workers dropped in all three institutions, the drop at the New England was more precipitous (down 40.4 percent compared with 32.7 percent for Massachusetts General and 32.5 percent for Boston City).

The shift in the makeup of the patient population is significant for several reasons. First, scholars who have studied the New England Hospital's patient population have claimed that it differed little from what one would find at other private hospitals in Boston. This has been used to argue that any differences in medical practices between the hospitals would most likely be attributable to the

TABLE 8. Percentage of White- and Blue-Collar Patients at the New England, the Boston City Hospital, and Massachusetts General, 1873–1894

	1873/74	1878	1883	1888	1893/94
NEH-White	7.2	10.0	8.3	10.5	9.7
MGH-White	0.9	1.6	4.2	5.0	5.6
BCH-White	9.2	4.3	5.3	3.8	6.1
NEH-Blue	47.5	40.6	44.0	38.6	28.3
MGH-Blue	48.5	48.0	44.3	31.8	32.6
BCH-Blue	54.4	57.1	55.8	43.1	36.7

Sources: For the New England Hospital, calculated from New England Hospital for Women and Children, *Maternity Case Records* [B MS b19.3], *Surgical Case Records* [B MS b19.1], and *Medical Case Records* [B MS b19.2], Boston Medical Library in the Francis A. Countway Library of Medicine, Boston, Mass. For Boston City Hospital and Massachusetts General Hospital, calculated from their annual reports.

Notes: The data in the first column are drawn from 1873 for the New England Hospital. Since Massachusetts General Hospital and the Boston City Hospital lack records for that year, the data were drawn from 1874 for those two institutions.

To determine whether an occupation was white collar or blue collar, I adapted the classification scheme Stephan Thernstrom developed for male occupations (see *Other Bostonians*, app. B). Under white collar, both high and low, I included teachers, nurses, physicians, asylum attendants, saleswomen, governesses, proofreaders, actresses, bookkeepers, stenographers, journalists, musicians, ministers, writers, artists, peddlers, canvassers, librarians, printers, hotel keepers, clerks, photographers, managers, and cashiers. The remainder of the patient population consisted of blue-collar workers, housewives, children, those for whom no occupation was registered (unknown), and those who fell outside these categories, such as students.

BCH = Boston City Hospital. For all other abbreviations, see Table 6.

gender of the physicians, since the other Boston hospitals had all-male medical staffs. We will explore in greater detail in the next chapter the scholarly debate over whether any significant differences in practice actually existed. Of importance here is the realization that since the patient population at the New England came from a higher socioeconomic bracket, any differences in practice could just as easily be attributable to class as to gender. The issue remains, in other words, unresolved.[36]

None of this is to suggest that the majority of the patients at the New England came from the monied classes. Nothing could have been further from the truth.

Despite evidence of the kinds of changes that would ultimately transform the charity hospital into a middle-class institution, the New England Hospital in the last decades of the nineteenth century continued to cater to the poor. Still, all signs indicate that however poor these women may have been, they were somewhat better off than the women who sought care at Massachusetts General, Boston City Hospital, or the Boston Lying-In.

More directly, the changes in the patient population also signify Zakrzewska's loss of interest in charity work. The dispensary, for example, which she had once described as the department where "the usefulness of the whole institution is called forth," became for her "not merely centres where the ailments of the indigent are attended to, but . . . sources of instruction, giving the young practitioner chances for observation and investigation of diseases and their causes." It also helped "to develop the manners as well as the ingenuity of the young physician." The dispensary continued, of course, to carry on charitable work, adding, for example, a "Diet Kitchen" that provided "wholesome and strengthening food" to the sick poor. But what Zakrzewska cared about most were the educational opportunities it provided her students.[37]

In addition, the radicalism of the early years, as it pertained to the poor, was gone. The scrutiny of patients, for example, which had begun in the late 1860s, was intensified in the early 1880s when the New England Hospital turned to the Associated Charities of Boston for assistance in evaluating "the worthiness of applicants for help." Founded in 1879, this organization set out to coordinate the city's poor relief by establishing a registry of those receiving aid. The New England took advantage of this by requiring all applicants to "sign a statement, giving the name and address of some responsible person as reference." This the hospital filed away so that, should a question arise concerning the patient's financial situation, it could be submitted to the Associated Charities for investigation. The hospital's dispensary physician believed that the new practice was deterring those "who might otherwise seek free medical aid, although able to pay a small fee," but it is also possible that some individuals stayed away simply because they refused to be scrutinized in this way. Whatever the reason, the numbers of individuals seeking care dropped from a high of 5,235 in 1886, when the New England began requiring the signed statement, to 3,859 the year Zakrzewska retired.[38]

The dispensary was not the only department that evinced signs of marked change. The maternity ward, which Zakrzewska had long promoted for its radicalism, also underwent a significant transformation. Shortly after its move,

TABLE 9. Percentage of Single Mothers in the New England's Maternity
Wards Compared with the Boston Lying-In, 1872–1897

	1872	1873	1878	1883	1888	1893	1897
NEH	55.2	45.5	29.5	46.4	26.4	22.9	19.1
BLI	n.d.	n.d.	54.6	46.5	53.4	38.5	35.1

Sources: Calculated from New England Hospital for Women and Children, *Maternity Case Records* [B MS b19.3], Boston Medical Library in the Francis A. Countway Library of Medicine, Boston, Mass., and from *Annual Reports of the Boston Lying-In Hospital*.

Note: n.d. = no data. For all other abbreviations, see Table 6.

the hospital established a policy refusing to admit unwed mothers "a second time," unless circumstances were deemed extenuating.[39] That this determination was occasionally made was evident in Table 1, which showed that four multiparae were admitted in 1883. Nevertheless, it is significant that the hospital decided to go on record as formally opposing the presence of second-time unwed mothers in its wards.

At the same time, the New England Hospital also prohibited "the admission of unmarried women upon the free beds." Since single mothers were least likely to be able to afford the twenty dollars for a confinement, this could well explain the drop in the percentage of unwed mothers in the maternity wards from 55.2 percent in the year of the hospital's move to 19.1 percent in 1897. As Table 9 indicates, this downward trend took place at the Boston Lying-In as well, but not quite as precipitously.

In 1891, the resident physician announced in the annual report that 111 of the 161 maternity patients that year were married. She went on to describe the two populations to which they now catered: married women who, because they were boarders, lacked proper care, and women who had their own homes but were "prevented by a family of young children or moderate circumstances from enjoying the quiet and freedom from responsibility that a hospital offers them." Although 31.1 percent of the mothers that year were single, notably absent from this report is any mention of "unmarried women" who, as Zakrzewska had written in 1865, needed to be "saved from moral and physical ruin." Indeed, by the year of her retirement, Zakrzewska had so changed that she could write to a board member about the hospital's maternity cases: "I don't care for the Charity & I don't care for working in that line any longer, than what we do.

That kind of work brings us not a step forward in the great evolution of women's work in the profession."[40]

. . .

The New England Hospital may have started out as an institution of charity, proudly promoting an image of itself as serving the poor and needy without regard to race, class, or marital status. Several decades later, however, that was not the public face Zakrzewska wished to present. The move to Roxbury had marked the turning point. While the hospital was in central Boston, it had embraced many of the goals she had spelled out in her 1863 lecture: small and homelike, it defined its mission in terms of the care it offered poor, immigrant, and frequently single women and mothers. In addition, in terms of rhetoric and to some degree policy, it displayed understanding for human frailty and respect for the poor. After the move, the hospital catered to a somewhat wealthier, definitely more American patient population, and new policies reflected a desire for greater scrutiny of those seeking charity. In the hospital reports, moreover, one read more often about the institution's ability to provide safe and comfortable accommodations to *all* who needed care. To be sure, this continued to include the "poor, lonely wanderer, who know not where to lay her head," but increased attention was paid as well to "the woman of wealth and refinement, who finds that intelligent ready service which money cannot always provide elsewhere." Money could, however, guarantee service in the hospital: thirty dollars a week secured a private room and private nurse; twenty-five dollars a week, a private room and the half-time services of a nurse; fifteen dollars a week, a room with two beds; and ten dollars a week, a room with four beds. The level of care had become dependent on one's ability to pay.[41]

The dominant script in the annual reports of the 1870s and 1880s was not, however, the improved accommodations available to patients seeking care. Instead, one read much more frequently about the important inroads the institution was making in advancing the cause of women's medical education. Certainly, this had been one of the central goals of the hospital from its inception, but in most of the early annual reports it had played second fiddle to the importance of the work being carried out in the name of charity. Not so in the annual reports following the hospital's move to Roxbury. Rather, the focus came to rest on the hospital's objective "to aid in the medical education of women by affording them opportunities for thorough clinical study."[42]

Zakrzewska's reasons for gradually abandoning the radical and charitable dimension of her institution can only be surmised, since she never addressed this change directly. We have already considered her growing disillusionment with treating the poorest of the poor, especially if they were Irish. It is also possible that by the time of their move to Roxbury, Zakrzewska and her board had no longer felt a need to fill this niche. Boston City Hospital had opened its doors in 1864 with the clear intent of catering to the city's poor, and the Boston Lying-In reopened its doors in 1873, after a sixteen-year hiatus. With other alternatives to the almshouse now available for the "worthy poor," Zakrzewska may have seen an opportunity to transform her creation into the kind of institution she had always wanted. One need only recall that her first choice had been "a college primarily for women" but that she had been unable to generate enough funding to bring that to fruition.[43] By the early 1870s, however, there were sufficient signs that women's medical education was becoming more desirable. Not only were the number of all-women's medical colleges increasing, but more and more medical institutions were opening their doors to women. Most noteworthy was the University of Michigan Medical School's decision in 1870 to accept female students. Zakrzewska may very well have decided that she could now risk refocusing the hospital's central mission on the pedagogical role that she had originally coveted.

Scientific Medicine at the
New England Hospital

Zakrzewska may have waited until the move to Roxbury to focus attention on the New England's role as a teaching hospital, but she had been working to advance this cause from the outset. Disturbed by the persistence of barriers blocking women's entry into the medical profession, she had envisioned an institution that would once again do its part to level the playing field, this time by providing opportunities for women both to acquire medical knowledge at the bedside and to showcase what they had learned. Zakrzewska, who was determined that her institution not be a failure, set out to create a hospital that would meet the standards of Boston's elite medical community.[1] This translated into an emphasis on the practice and teaching of scientific medicine. Medical educators may not have agreed precisely on what scientific medicine entailed, and divisions may have been growing between those who drew inspiration from Paris and those who had begun to favor Germany.[2] But however scientific medicine was defined in the 1860s and 1870s, no one was yet building the large laboratories and research hospitals that were becoming part of the German university landscape. Indeed, the Johns Hopkins Medical School, which was modeled on the German university, was not founded until 1893. Thus, in the immediate postbellum period, those who sought to base clinical instruction on scientific medicine usually promoted smaller-scale practices such as autopsies; the charting of a patient's temperature, pulse rate, and rate of respiration; and the chemical and microscopic analysis of bodily fluids. Most hospitals at the time did not, however, even go this far when they instructed students in clinical techniques.[3] The New England Hospital, as we will see, was among those that did.

The teaching hospital would eventually emerge as the mainstay of medical education. That was not yet the case in the 1860s and 1870s, when hospitals, although frequently allowing medical faculty access to their wards for clinical instruction, severely restricted student contact with patients. In response, some medical schools established their own small clinics and hospitals, but by and large the expense of founding and running a hospital was prohibitive. This was, to be sure, one of the main reasons formal clinical instruction remained so poor in the United States right up to the turn of the century.[4]

Zakrzewska's situation differed from that of most other medical educators of her day because she directed an institution created in part to provide clinical instruction. As we have already noted, the New England Hospital was also basically run by the medical staff, not a board of trustees. Zakrzewska thus had a level of freedom most other medical educators lacked, and she used it to put in place a clinical program grounded in orthodox medical practices that provided her students with knowledge of the latest scientific techniques.

· · ·

As soon as Zakrzewska decided to found a new hospital, she sought the support of Boston's elite physicians. In November 1862, at the hospital's first annual meeting, she was able to announce that "[t]wo of the best medical men in the city, Dr. [Samuel] Cabot and Dr. John Ware, are our consulting physicians, and a dozen more are willing to give their assistance whenever it is asked."[5] Many of these physicians had withheld their support from Zakrzewska when she had been affiliated with the New England Female Medical College, convinced that Samuel Gregory was running a second-rate institution. Now, however, Zakrzewska stood at the head of a hospital committed to promoting the highest standards of medical orthodoxy, and they threw their weight behind her.

Zakrzewska's determination to create an elite medical institution was characteristic of the directors of other all-women's regular colleges and hospitals, the vast majority of whom had founded their institutions only after trying unsuccessfully to integrate all-male institutions. By and large these women viewed their creations as temporary measures, necessary only until coeducation would become standard policy. Acutely aware that until that time their institutions would be scrutinized closely for any signs that women were unfit for the practice of medicine, they maintained, as we have already mentioned, the highest standards.[6] They also went to great lengths to distance themselves from unorthodox

practitioners and institutions. Thus the Female Medical College of Pennsylvania, which initially had a few eclectic physicians on its faculty, fired these individuals as early as 1853 and restricted its appointments thereafter to graduates
of orthodox medical schools. Similarly, Elizabeth Blackwell refused to have
anything to do with Clemence Lozier, who had founded an all-women's homeopathic medical college in New York City in 1863, despite Susan B. Anthony's
attempts to persuade these two women that they would better advance women's
rights if they would join forces.[7] All in all, mixing strategy with conviction, the
directors of these all-women's institutions put in place educational models that,
they believed, would produce the best practitioners possible and bring women
the recognition and prestige that was their due.

In this vein, one of Zakrzewska's first strategies was to ensure that the qualifications of the women who staffed her hospital could not be found wanting by
the profession's elite. Of the ten resident and attending physicians who worked
at the New England Hospital during its first twenty-five years, one graduated
from the University of Michigan, one from the Woman's Medical College of
Pennsylvania, and four from the University of Zurich. (The other four were
graduates of the New England Female Medical College.) All ten, moreover—
not just the four students who attended medical school in Zurich—spent at least
one year studying in Europe. Thus Lucy Sewall, who served as resident physician from 1863 to 1869, attending physician from 1869 to 1887, and advisory
physician from 1887 until her death three years later, spent a year studying
medicine in the Paris, Zurich, and London hospitals. And Helen Morton, who
joined Zakrzewska and Sewall in running the hospital for well over two decades,
spent four years in Europe, much of that time in Paris at La Maternité. Zakrzewska did not hesitate to draw attention to the European training of her
physicians in the hospital's annual reports.[8] She wanted to be sure that her
supporters understood her institution's embrace of modern scientific methods.

Zakrzewska also set out to distinguish her hospital from irregular institutions.
Thus she helped found the New England Hospital Medical Society to promote
regular women physicians and to distinguish them explicitly from "charlatans
of every description."[9] Indeed, almost immediately following its creation, the
members of the society petitioned the *Boston City Directory* to remove their names
from the heading "female physicians," which included everything from homeopathic physicians and Christian Scientists to midwives, nurses, and regular
physicians. Successful in their endeavor, the members of this society henceforth
appeared under a separate listing for their organization, hoping thereby to

make their elite standing clear. Zakrzewska's desire to distinguish her hospital from unorthodox institutions led her, moreover, to support a requirement in 1880 that all interns have the M.D. in hand before beginning their training and that this degree be from a regular medical school.[10]

In her promotion of medical orthodoxy, Zakrzewska also joined her peers in championing coeducational institutions. Indeed, she wrote optimistically of the day "when no separate institutions for women will be demanded, and when our Hospital will be only a charity for needy women who prefer women physicians to men, or where men and women may work together."[11] In fact, she was quite pleased when Massachusetts General Hospital decided in 1866 to permit her students to walk its wards on the days when Harvard medical students were not in attendance. She saw this as an indication that Harvard might soon follow suit and welcome women as well.

Still, Zakrzewska was not enthusiastic about coeducation at any price. Rather, like other pioneers of women's medical education, she wanted assurances that women would be educated in exactly the same way as men. Already in 1874, when the New England Female Medical College closed its doors and the question resurfaced whether Harvard would respond by accepting female students, Zakrzewska's reaction had been lukewarm. The specific proposal was to have women take the same entrance examinations as men and to have the same professors providing the instruction, but the women were to be educated in their own building, about two miles away from the main campus. "I did not favor such an arrangement," Zakrzewska explained years later, "but actually discouraged it, because it seemed to me disastrous to the whole spirit of woman's work in the profession." She feared in particular that such an arrangement would result in junior professors taking over the education of the female students, thereby perpetuating the notion that women were less qualified than men. Zakrzewska, along with several other women physicians, even offered Harvard fifty thousand dollars in 1881 if it would open its doors to women and grant them the same education as men. And in 1890, when a group of Baltimore women joined together to raise funds for the new medical school at the Johns Hopkins University on the condition that the school open its doors to women, Zakrzewska, whose opinion was specifically requested, urged them to police carefully exactly what the trustees meant by coeducation. In short, until the time that elite medical institutions in the United States would agree not to discriminate against their female students, Zakrzewska continued to favor schools, like the University of Zurich, that had proved their ability to treat all students alike. As she aged, she may have had increased doubts that that day would arrive any time soon, but she never abandoned her conviction that true coeducation would be superior to separate institutions.[12]

Zakrzewska's commitment to the standards of the elite medical profession were all part and parcel of her battle to advance women's rights. The same could be said of Ann Preston, Mary Putnam Jacobi, and many other regular women physicians.[13] An older scholarship lamented the loss of female solidarity that resulted as women became divided between orthodox and unorthodox practitioners.[14] Indeed, some contemporaries, such as Susan B. Anthony, regretted this as well. However, from Zakrzewska's perspective, the best way to advance the cause of women was to hold them up to what she considered to be the highest standards, and those were, in her opinion, the standards set by the best regular medical schools in the country and abroad. The advancement of women, not female solidarity, was the driving force in Zakrzewska's life.

• • •

In her promotion of medical orthodoxy and her embrace of coeducation Zakrzewska was thus far from alone among women physicians. Where she stood out was in her insistence that women did not practice medicine any differently than men. As we have seen, in none of her published work did she ever embrace language common among her peers that suggested women physicians had greater "sympathy" for their patients. In fact, in the hospital's fourth annual report in 1865, she even exhibited a marked concern that her previous emphasis on the homelike nature of the hospital had been misunderstood to mean that the hospital specialized foremost in providing care. Correcting that mistaken view, she now insisted that what mattered most was using science to save lives.[15]

Zakrzewska brought home this point by relaying two cases in which the medical staff had intervened directly in the birthing process. In the first, a woman in her ninth month of pregnancy had been found convulsing and unconscious in her home. She was transferred to the hospital, where "artificial delivery was immediately decided upon and commenced." Sixteen hours later "a living child was born," and thirteen days later mother and child were well enough to go home. In the second case, a woman with a "deformed pelvis," who had previously lost a child because of complications during delivery, was "kept under Hospital surveillance," so that when she became pregnant again, she could be helped to deliver the child prematurely, the assumption being that a smaller child would have an easier time passing through the birth canal.

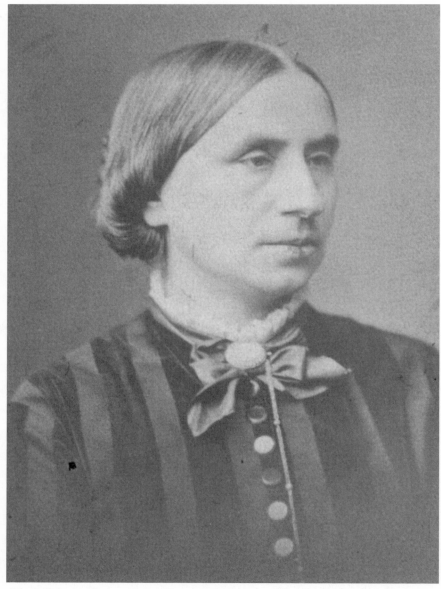

Marie Zakrzewska, ca. 1870s. (Courtesy Archives and Special Collections on Women
in Medicine and Homeopathy, Drexel University College of Medicine)

When the woman entered the hospital in the thirty-fifth week of her second pregnancy, Zakrzewska proudly wrote, "I induced labor at once, and three days afterwards a living, healthy child was laid by the side of its happy mother."[16] Zakrzewska had no doubt that because of these interventions her hospital had saved two lives, that of the woman in the first case and of the child in the second.

The medical staff at the New England Hospital, Zakrzewska was announcing, did much more than merely monitor the cases that came to them, offering gentle assistance. They were not practicing the kind of medicine Samuel Gregory had prescribed for women. Instead, the physicians intervened, when necessary, to ensure a healthy outcome. The powerful message in Zakrzewska's second anecdote is that she had been able to create an artificial situation (by inducing premature labor) that circumvented the natural limits of the woman's body. In other annual reports she repeated this focus on her staff's ability "to perform successfully the operative part of obstetrics."[17] The New England Hospital may have prided itself on the "necessary comforts" it offered women in need, but Zakrzewska wanted to make clear that the medicine they practiced was indistinguishable from that which was practiced at all-male institutions.

In this regard, a study conducted by Regina Morantz-Sanchez and Sue Zschoche comparing obstetrics practices at the New England Hospital and the Boston Lying-In Hospital is particularly telling. They found no significant differences between the two hospitals in terms of the frequency of intervention (as measured by the use of anesthetics and forceps), thus challenging historians for whom forceps had come to symbolize the practices of a male medical profession deemed antagonistic toward the needs of their patients.[18] The only difference they found was in postpartum care: women at the New England received more drugs and remained for a longer period of confinement. Morantz-Sanchez and Zschoche suggest that this may have reflected the persistence of "traditional holistic orientations," in comparison with the Boston Lying-In, which was moving toward "a more modern, technocratic approach to their patients." Yet given that the patient population at the New England came from a higher socioeconomic bracket than those who attended the Boston Lying-In (see Chapter 9), it seems more likely that the differential treatment reflected the patients' greater ability to pay for the medicines and extended stay.[19]

In short, Zakrzewska, who was determined to prove that women practiced medicine no differently than men, appears to have been successful in implementing essentially the same practices one would have found at hospitals staffed solely by men. Of course, it would be helpful to know what went on at other all-

women's hospitals. Certainly the emphasis the Woman's Hospital of Philadelphia placed on surgery, coupled with the Woman's Medical College's construction in 1875 of laboratories for microscopy, pharmacy, and chemistry, suggests that the style of medicine taught there would also have differed little from
what one found at elite all-male institutions.[20] If that was the case, it would
suggest that actual practices had little to do with whether women emphasized
their unique contribution to medicine (as Ann Preston, Elizabeth Blackwell,
and the majority of women physicians contended) or denied that they practiced
medicine any differently than men (as Zakrzewska and Mary Putnam Jacobi
insisted). It would also suggest that Zakrzewska's criticism of sympathy and her
lauding of science distinguished her from her peers more rhetorically than in
practice. Unlike Mary Putnam Jacobi, who engaged in laboratory investigations and fought to be permitted to teach and practice vivisection, Zakrzewska
differed little from others of her generation, male or female, in her actual
approach to the practice of medicine.[21]

Nevertheless, in one area, the fact that the New England was staffed solely by
women may very well have made a difference, and that was in the hospital's
ability to control puerperal fever. This disease was, in the words of one of the
hospital's physicians, "the constant dread of all the physicians of maternity
hospitals. At times all the cases would do well, and then without discoverable
cause, fever would begin and spread among the patients with appalling rapidity
and fatal results." The New England had, however, comparatively little trouble
with this infection. Between 1862 and 1872, its reported death rate from puerperal fever was 2 percent; the following decade the rate dropped to 0.5 percent.[22] This stands in comparison with the Boston Lying-In Hospital, which
may have had some years with similarly low rates (in 1879, for example, its
mortality rate from puerperal fever was only 0.9 percent) but which had considerable difficulty sustaining sanitary conditions. Thus in 1880, its rate jumped up
to 3.9 percent, in 1881 to 4.8 percent, and in 1883 to 5.2 percent. The comparable numbers for the New England Hospital during those same years were 0.9,
0.9, and 0 percent.[23]

One historian has suggested that the New England's success in controlling
puerperal fever may have resulted from female physicians' greater commitment
to eradicating a life-threatening condition that afflicted women alone.[24] Such
claims, however, are extremely difficult to prove. Nevertheless, gender may have
mattered in a different way: the low rates may have reflected the unexpected
consequences of the discrimination women faced in this country. Denied clini-

cal opportunities at home, female medical students often studied abroad, where they received a far better introduction to the scientific management of infection than they would have received had they remained in the United States. This was certainly true, as we have seen, of the women who staffed the New England. Susan Dimock, resident physician from 1872 to 1875, even submitted a thesis on puerperal fever to the faculty at the University of Zurich as part of the requirements for the M.D.[25] It is reasonable to assume, therefore, that the staff carried this greater awareness with them as they managed their cases at the hospital.

In addition, the New England had a director who had begun her career as a midwife, when she had been taught to manage childbirth with the minimum of intervention and certainly without the use of instruments. Zakrzewska's mentor, Joseph Hermann Schmidt, had also, as we have already mentioned, probably introduced her to the ideas of Ignaz Semmelweis, who had argued that puerperal fever was spread by the infected hands and instruments of physicians and medical students. She thus learned about the utmost importance of maintaining sanitary conditions in the maternity wards. But she was also convinced that hygienic measures alone would not always prevent the spread of infection. For that, one needed small hospitals divided into even smaller wards, thus allowing one both to isolate the infected patient and occasionally to close an entire ward for thorough cleansing.[26]

Armed with this knowledge, Zakrzewska instituted a variety of practices all of which must have contributed to the New England's low mortality rate from puerperal fever. When the hospital was still in the inner city and occupying a single building, she separated the maternity and surgical cases, making sure that no infections spread from one room to another. Recognizing, moreover, that crowded conditions created the perfect environment for the spread of the disease, she broke up the maternity ward into several smaller rooms, separating the women according to their stages of delivery. Zakrzewska also at times ordered the closing of almost the entire hospital for a few months for "the purpose of purifying and repairing"; she instructed her staff to wash their hands after examining a woman in labor and to dip their fingers in oil; and she did what she could to isolate any suspicious cases.[27]

After the move to Roxbury, hygienic needs were met by keeping hospital rooms small. Thus the rooms in the medical ward had one to four beds and those in the surgical ward one to three beds. The maternity ward, now housed in a separate cottage, had rooms with no more than two beds and a separate delivery room. Zakrzewska, as we have seen, drew special attention to the way in which the new hospital met hygienic standards, emphasizing that the new institution permitted her to leave rooms vacant for the purposes of purification. This strategy permitted the resident physician in 1873 to brag that in the new hospital's first year "we have had the great happiness not to lose one patient, notwithstanding the prevalence in Boston and vicinity of puerperal fever, and notwithstanding the several very serious cases of *septicaemia, pyoemia* and *peritonitis*, which have occurred in the Maternity Ward."[28]

Anyone familiar with nineteenth-century hospitals would recognize that to some extent there was nothing novel about Zakrzewska's insights. The difficulty of controlling the spread of infectious diseases in hospitals had even led one physician to coin the term "hospitalism" in the mid-nineteenth century to describe the periodic outbreaks that seemed nearly impossible to control. The widespread explanation for these occurrences drew on miasmatic theory and postulated that the generally unhealthy air within hospitals, consisting of a combination of urban fumes and bodily emanations, led to such periodic eruptions—hence the near obsession among hospital directors in the nineteenth century with clean air, good ventilation, and ample sunlight. This also explains the standard practice of occasionally closing hospitals, or at least wards, in order to whitewash them and take care of repairs.[29]

From this perspective, one could simply say that Zakrzewska managed to implement hygienic practices whereas others remained in the realm of theory. But Zakrzewska's insistence that hands be washed, her division of maternity cases by stages of delivery, and her isolation of suspicious cases all suggest that she held a more complicated view of infection that did not attribute the spread of disease to the air alone. Indeed, in 1862, three years before Lister published his findings, Zakrzewska noted after contracting an infection that "when my finger became infected, it was apparently perfectly sound, yet there must have been some point of entrance for the infection which followed."[30] Her comment suggests her awareness and acceptance of a view of disease that enjoyed considerable popularity among German academic physicians in the 1840s. Rudolph Virchow, whose work Zakrzewska knew, and Jacob Henle, among others, had defined disease as the response of the body's normal physiological processes to abnormal conditions; according to this definition, the abnormal conditions could be "contagions" or "miasmas."[31] Acting on these beliefs allowed Zakrzewska to limit the spread of infection even before the application of antiseptic techniques.

According to Emma Call, who practiced medicine at the New England

Hospital in the 1870s and 1880s, there was little evidence of any such antiseptic techniques before 1877, when the hospital finally introduced the use of carbolic acid and disinfected, through antiseptic douches, before, during, and after labor. Yet even then, she contended, the meaning of the germ theory had not yet penetrated, for these douches were often left in the drawer by the patient's bed, "with innocent disregard of the colonies of bacteria which might be reposing there."[32] It should not, of course, be surprising if, in the 1860s and 1870s, Zakrzewska had not yet fully embraced the germ theory. Few Americans or, for that matter, Germans had. But, as we have just seen, those who questioned whether bacteria were the sole cause of infectious diseases did not necessarily reject the idea that infections could be stimulated by the entry of some kind of external agent into the body's system. Of importance here, this view provided Zakrzewska with sufficient motivation to adopt rigorous standards of hygiene. In her own words, "carelessness and want of thorough cleanliness is at the bottom of epidemics of puerperal fever."[33]

Zakrzewska had set out to create an institution as mainstream as Massachusetts General or any of the other highly esteemed hospitals at the time. She sought to achieve this by staffing her institution with the most highly educated women physicians she could identify, by ensuring that members of Boston's medical elite served as consultants on her staff, and by implementing the most advanced medical techniques available at the time. But the New England Hospital was not merely a way of showcasing the skills and successes of a small group of highly accomplished women; it was also a teaching hospital, committed to providing the next generation of women doctors with the clinical training denied them at most other hospitals in the United States.

· · ·

When the New England Hospital for Women and Children first opened its doors in 1862, it was only the third institution in the country where women could acquire clinical training at the bedside.[34] It was thus filling an important niche. Like the New York Infirmary for Women and Children, which had opened with twenty-four beds, and the Woman's Hospital of Philadelphia, which had twelve beds, the New England started small, with just ten beds at its disposal. But by 1865 it had expanded to forty beds, and by 1872 to fifty-five.[35] This paralleled both an increase in the number of interns—three a year between 1862 and 1876 and six a year thereafter—and an increase in the number of patients admitted to the hospital, climbing from 118 in 1863, to 244 in 1873 (the first full year in Roxbury), to 585 in 1893 (the year Zakrzewska retired). Although in absolute numbers this increase might still be considered small, this would not be true of the number of dispensary patients. Here, the hospital cared for 1,507 patients in 1863, 2,905 in 1873, and 3,859 in 1893.[36] Clearly, the interns and resident physicians had ample opportunities to observe a variety of disease conditions and to learn how best to translate medical knowledge into practice.

Interns in the first decades of the New England's existence consisted of a diverse group of women. Some already had medical degrees; others were in the midst of their studies; and still others had not even begun their formal education. Such diversity reflected, at least in part, the unregulated nature of the profession itself. At a time when medical licensing was nonexistent, it is not surprising to find great variation in the way people acquired their medical expertise. But more than likely Zakrzewska was also responding to the particular situation faced by women: since they were denied entry to most medical schools, she probably considered it unfair, at least initially, to restrict the clinical internships to those with a medical school affiliation.[37]

The clinical program was built on the assumption that engaging students in "the actual care of and attendance upon the sick" was far better than "traversing the wards of a hospital in the suite of a professor."[38] Thus the interns, who usually remained one year, accompanied physicians on their daily rounds; assumed responsibility for the patients' care during the day; and kept the hospital notebooks, recording all prescriptions and describing each visit with the patient (sometimes twice a day), including the patient's condition and the treatments administered. Interns also occasionally assisted in operations; they frequently attended women during their confinements; and they may have learned to perform "version," the manual turning of a baby in utero to assist in a difficult delivery. Eliza Mosher, who trained at the New England Hospital in 1869 before entering medical school, later recalled that the interns "were permitted to examine as carefully as we wished, all the confinement patients in the different stages of labor. During those months there were over fifty confinements in the hospital. We were expected to make a diagnosis of position and condition and watch every delivery."[39] She remembered finding the obstetrics classes she later attended at the University of Michigan to be a waste of her time.

Sarah J. McNutt, who interned at the New York Infirmary for Women and Children around 1880, had a similarly positive experience. She described visiting the wards daily, assisting in surgical operations, taking charge of more than fifty maternity cases and observing another hundred or so, and mixing medicines in the dispensary.[40] The point, of course, is not that interns at all-women's hospitals received better or more extensive training than did male interns at other institutions. Rather, what the New England Hospital, New York Infirmary, and Woman's Hospital of Philadelphia provided was an opportunity for women to compete for elite hospital internships, which were few and far between even for men.[41]

Whatever independent work the interns might have been permitted to carry out in the hospital wards, nothing compared to their experiences in the dispensary. It was here, in the words of one hospital doctor, that interns learned "practically what it is to be a physician."[42] Sophia Jex-Blake, who volunteered for three months in 1865, described her day as follows: she was up every morning by 6:30, ate her breakfast at 7:00, and began her rounds with the doctors, making up the medicines ordered by the physicians. By either 9:00 or 10:00, depending on the day of the week, she was in the dispensary, where she spent the rest of the morning, "making up prescriptions as fast as [Dr. Sewall] writes them (two of us generally have our hands full, but sometimes I am alone), and very often we have not got through our work when the dinner-bell rings at 1 p.m."[43] In subsequent years, interns assumed more responsibility, especially for patients too ill to make it to the clinic. Thus, interns assigned specifically to the dispensary (after 1875 there were two) lived on the premises in order to be available when word came that someone was ill. Similarly, it was the student's job to attend the sick person at home and determine whether a physician needed to be called. Although statistics from the 1860s and 1870s are lacking, by the 1880s each intern made roughly a thousand visits during the four months that she spent doing rotation in the dispensary. It is not clear whether the interns administered any medical treatments during these visits, but chances are they had authorization to treat minor cases and to take care of any follow-up the physician deemed necessary.[44]

By the early 1870s, moreover, interns were responsible for recording various physiological processes on a daily basis. These included the patients' pulse, respiration, and temperature. One student remembered the thermometers Susan Dimock had brought back from her studies in Europe: they were "nearly a foot in length, and were not self-registering, so that they could only be read *in situ*, a feat not easy to accomplish in a poor light. They were used chiefly in the axilla [in the armpit]."[45] Interns then prepared charts from this information, which they presented to the resident physician twice weekly. According to one historian, the New England was the first hospital in Boston to keep such charts on a regular basis.[46]

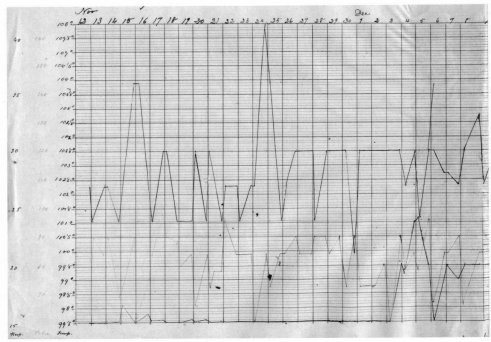

Record of a patient at the New England Hospital for Women and Children. (From the collection at the Boston Medical Library, Francis A. Countway Library of Medicine)

In the early 1870s, it also became more routine to conduct microscopic examinations of tumors and bodily discharges. And by the early 1880s a detailed analysis of the patient's urine was included in the standard physical examination, in which the amount, acidity, specific gravity, albumen, sugar, pus, blood corpuscles, and casts were all recorded.[47] That students performed these analyses themselves is clear from the experience of Kate Campbell Hurd-Mead, who interned at the hospital in 1888. "Those were the days," she later wrote, "of carbolic steam in the operating room, of instruments boiled and washed in corrosive sublimate solutions and scrupulously scoured by the internes, of all-night vigils with each abdominal case, besides crude bacteriological tests and sputum stainings in the cellar pharmacy where, with an old microscope and after a hard day's work, any interne not otherwise busy examined specimens of cancer or of urine, and made chemical investigations of any material sent to the laboratory."[48]

To the modern eye, none of this appears to be highly advanced science, but it was as advanced as one would find anywhere in the country at the time and considerably more sophisticated than in most hospitals. Of marked importance, considering complaints that would surface in the 1880s, the first generations of interns valued highly the kind of education they were receiving. "You don't know what an immense thing it is for us to have got free admission to the Woman's Hospital life here," wrote Jex-Blake in 1865.[49] Whether delivering babies, visiting the poor in their homes, or writing down directions for food and medicine, they appreciated both the novelty and the quality of their experiences.

Denied access to most medical institutions in the United States, the first generations of interns and staff physicians felt deep gratitude toward Zakrzewska and the New England Hospital for providing them an opportunity to study at the bedside. Filled with the excitement that comes when one is helping to chart a new path, the women who practiced medicine at the New England in its first years formed a close-knit group, often choosing to socialize together after a long day at the hospital. In her letters home to her mother, Jex-Blake described evenings spent at the theater, visiting ice cream shops, or simply spending time together in the hospital, singing songs, playing card games, and losing themselves in "roars of laughter."[50] Zakrzewska had set out to create a woman's hospital at the forefront of medical teaching and medical science, and judging by the standards of the regular medical profession—and the experiences of the first generations of interns—she had accomplished that and more. She had also fostered a shared sense of mission, which united staff and students in promoting "the *cause* of women-practitioners in medicine."[51]

* * *

The euphoria of the first years did not last. As early as 1876, some interns were already registering minor complaints. The situation was eventually resolved to everyone's satisfaction, but the tensions that surfaced set the stage for more serious problems later on. We know of this first encounter only from a text Zakrzewska prepared in anticipation of a meeting she arranged with the interns; a formal complaint was never submitted. But if Zakrzewska accurately represented the interns' concerns, then the central issue had to do with respect: the interns felt that the hospital staff's insistence on addressing them as Miss or Mrs., rather than Dr., belittled them before their patients. Zakrzewska, showing her usual impatience, turned the tables and accused the interns of being disrespectful themselves by failing to learn about "the motives and reasons for the existence of this Hospital."[52] Their needs, she implied, were petty compared with the greater mission of the institution. But she also found them silly. Interpreting their criticisms as an attack on her own pedagogical style, she insisted that she showed more respect toward them than any title ever could. In her eyes, her scrutiny of their clinical skills was designed to "teach them to form an opinion of their own"; moreover, she expected them to question her style of practice whenever they deemed it appropriate.[53] In other words, Zakrzewska imagined herself to be educating critical thinkers by fostering an open exchange of ideas. What she failed to understand was the power she wielded, unaware that students may have felt uncomfortable questioning her ways. Even turning their request for greater respect into a defense of her own pedagogical style may have made many uneasy. Certainly, the picture she painted of them as cowardly and self-centered, focused more on their own selfish desires than the needs of the hospital as a whole, would hardly have encouraged an open exchange.

More, however, was going on in this disagreement over the meaning of the title "Dr." Zakrzewska did not simply find it inessential; she also believed that the interns did not yet deserve it, even those who had already earned the M.D. No one, she insisted, yet knew enough to take responsibility for her own patients; only at that point would one earn the right to be called "Dr." "I, for my own self," she announced at this point, "would prefer never to be called 'Dr.' but rather 'Miss' or 'Madam' as so many of my patients like to address me. For me, it is far more agreeable to be considered first, a woman, and secondarily a 'Dr.' "[54]

This last line has received considerable attention from historians, who discern here a growing divide between a younger generation more committed to professionalism and an older generation for whom a commitment to female solidarity reigned supreme.[55] It is easy to see why Zakrzewska's comment would be interpreted in this light. She was announcing unequivocally that her identification as a woman was stronger than her identification as a physician, that she cared less about her professional identity than about the political work she was doing to help break down the barriers keeping women out of the medical profession or, for that matter, out of the public sphere at large. Indeed, later in the report, in a moment of exasperation, she wrote: "I only wish all women to have the right to do and to study what they like best."[56]

Yet to view this conflict as arising from different allegiances—female solidarity, on the one hand, and professionalism, on the other—obscures as much as it clarifies, largely because it makes little sense to cast Zakrzewska as someone who ever explicitly embraced a notion of "female solidarity." Indeed, it was right around the time of the skirmish with the interns that she petitioned the *Boston City Directory* to remove the names of the hospital's staff from the heading "female physicians." In addition, just one year after the initial trouble with the interns, Zakrzewska spoke before the New England Women's Club, expressing her concern that "the so hopefully sown good seeds are in danger of being suffocated by the still more thickly sown weeds."[57] Zakrzewska left little doubt that she intended her efforts to result eventually in the mowing down of these weeds.

It is, moreover, not at all clear that the interns would have disagreed with Zakrzewska in principle; where they seemed to differ was over the qualifications that entitled one to claim the honorific "Dr." Those students who had graduated from medical school believed they had already earned this privilege. Zakrzewska disagreed. That is why she viewed both graduates and undergraduates as receiving identical training during their internship year. It is also why she marked the point when interns were capable of assuming responsibility for their patients as the moment that "makes them really to be the 'Dr.' "[58]

In making this claim, Zakrzewska was staking out a position in a contemporary debate over the direction of medical education. Indeed, just a few doors down at Harvard University disagreements were surfacing between the university's president, Charles W. Eliot, who had issued educational reforms in 1871 that increased the time students spent in the laboratory, and some of the medical faculty. Oliver Wendell Holmes and Henry Jacob Bigelow, for example, both echoed the concerns John Ware had voiced almost twenty years earlier when they cast the curricular changes as a dangerous move toward the production of scientists rather than the education of practitioners.[59] Zakrzewska, as we will examine more closely in the next chapter, also viewed the recent move toward the laboratory with considerable ambivalence. It is in this context that one must understand her insistence that the knowledge imparted in medical schools did not translate into the clinical acumen students needed to diagnose and treat the ill. For that, she was telling her interns, they needed instruction at the bedside. Her interns, who may have felt buoyed by the educational reforms that were beginning to take place in medical schools around them, obviously disagreed. Still, this difference of opinion, which had more to do with how one evaluated both the nature and the impact of these educational reforms, is hardly indicative of a rift between those who embraced the new professionalism and those who remained critical.

In one way, though, a sharp division was emerging between the generations, and that was in the evaluation of the hospital's role in advancing women's medical education. At least, Zakrzewska reacted most strongly when her interns implied that medical students no longer viewed an internship at the New

England as desirable. Interpreting this as an indictment of the hospital's useful-ness, she responded by issuing her own threat, declaring her intent "to dispense with all students" if they believed they had ample opportunities for acquiring clinical training elsewhere. "Then," she elaborated, "the Hospital will change its character and stand as a charity carried on by women; and in this way, we shall perhaps effect as much towards convincing the medical profession of the ability of women physicians, and shall thus force them to open Harvard College to such women as desire entrance there. And after all, that is my object in life, to open the existing colleges to both men and women alike."[60]

Zakrzewska, whose tone was harsh and patronizing, clearly wanted to call the interns' bluff by expressing her readiness to close the teaching hospital. Her implication, of course, was that they were misreading the situation and would realize too late that they needed the hospital far more than it needed them. But Zakrzewska was also communicating her frustration that the interns did not share her vision of the hospital. Its purpose was not to serve their needs but rather to demonstrate the skills of women doctors in order to counter whatever prejudice still existed toward them. That they did not accept the central role of the New England Hospital in the movement to advance women's medical education rankled her to no end, and she responded by showing nostalgia for the shared sense of mission that had marked the first decade of the hospital's existence, when the interns were "earnest and anxious to learn, and worked hard."[61] Her message was clear, if simplistic: the current crop cared too much about titles and too little about advancing the cause of women.

How much of this report Zakrzewska shared with the students is unknown. Their reaction to her criticisms and complaints has also not been documented, but Zakrzewska did meet with the students, and a compromise was quickly reached. Admitting that "there seemed to be fault on both sides," Zakrzewska granted the interns the right to be referred to as "Dr." when they were working in the dispensary, where they had considerable contact with patients; in the hospital, however, they continued to go by "Miss" or "Mrs."[62] With this, the issue was laid to rest.

The ease with which the disagreement was resolved suggests that Zakrzew-ska, who had begun to take criticisms of the New England Hospital personally, may very well have been overreacting when she produced such a harsh response to the interns' concerns. It also suggests that whatever problems may have existed between her and the young interns in 1876 were still relatively minor. That was not the case when problems erupted in the early 1880s and again a decade later. Those tensions were never fully resolved and continued to trouble the institution well into the next century. Although some of the issues resembled those that had surfaced previously, the central bone of contention focused on the interns' demand that they be given greater responsibility for the care of patients. Zakrzewska responded again with lengthy reports, each more condescending and insulting than the last. Indeed, in 1883, after chastising the interns for not understanding their obligations, she told a particularly patronizing story about a nine-year-old patient who had severely burned his hand when he held on to a flatiron he had picked up, not dropping it for fear of waking up his sick sibling, whose care his mother had imparted to him. "My little patient," Zakrzewska wrote heavy-handedly, "may teach you a lesson on the fulfillment of responsibilities undertaken."[63]

Zakrzewska had little tolerance for the interns' request that they be granted primary responsibility for the care of patients. In fact, her evaluation of medical school education had not changed at all since the 1870s. She still contended that it provided poor preparation for the actual treatment of the sick, and she cautioned the interns not to let the self-respect they derived from the possession of a diploma "deteriorate into self-conceit. . . . The young doctor," she emphasized, "does not yet realise that to know a thing *'theoretically'* is far different from applying that thing *'practically.'* "[64]

In making these remarks, Zakrzewska seemed to be ignoring the sweeping reforms that had begun to change the face of medical education, at least among the nation's elite institutions. Several schools, most important among them the Woman's Medical College of Pennsylvania and the University of Michigan, where several of the interns had received their degrees, had long since lengthened the course of study, established a graded curriculum, and abandoned didactic teaching in favor of "practical" instruction. The graduates of these institutions had reason to believe that they brought with them more advanced skills than previous generations of interns. On the other hand, the reforms had more to do with laboratory instruction and less with clinical training. Indeed, even Harvard, when it decided in 1880 to add a fourth "clinical" year to the curriculum, did not make attendance mandatory. In a similar vein, the University of Michigan did not institute a required fourth-year clinical course until 1890.[65] Zakrzewska may very well have been thinking of this when she accused the interns of hubris.

However legitimate Zakrzewska's concerns may have been, her style of confrontation made compromise difficult. She had, in fact, painted herself into a corner; as a result, she went on the attack, insisting that the interns would be the losers in this battle. Forced to articulate why the interns should care, given that clinical internships at other hospitals were increasing at a slow but steady rate, Zakrzewska abandoned her lifelong defense of coeducational institutions, praising the New England for its exclusionary policies. "The main object of the Hospital," she impressed upon the interns,

> is to afford to young women . . . the opportunity to see *women* practising both as physicians and surgeons, that thereby they may acquire courage and self-reliance, which can never be so completely gained by seeing *men* acting as physicians and surgeons. Comparisons are often made between the opportunities offered to medical women now, and 25 years ago; but there is still very little opportunity for women to learn *from women.* The value of seeing *women* doing skilful medical work, cannot be over-estimated in its inspiring effect upon the young woman practitioner, and has a deeper influence than all the assurances of the college-Professor that women can be physicians and surgeons.[66]

Zakrzewska could no longer claim that the New England was necessary because most hospitals denied women clinical opportunities. At the time she was chastising the interns, about half a dozen previously all-male hospitals were offering internships to women, and more were to do so in the years to come. These included New York's Bellevue Hospital, Mount Sinai Hospital of New York, Cook County in Chicago, Philadelphia's Blockley Hospital, Boston's City Hospital, and Chicago's Wesley Memorial Hospital.[67] Zakrzewska thus shifted ground and presented the critical contribution of the New England Hospital as the chance it offered women to learn from other women rather than from men. Exactly what they would learn she never spelled out, but there is no evidence that she had come to embrace the popular view that women practiced a different kind of medicine. Instead, Zakrzewska seemed interested in the way female role models could empower younger women, stimulating self-confidence by demonstrating to women their ability to perform not different skills but rather the same skills as men. Notably, Emily Blackwell, director of the New York Infirmary and Medical College for Women, tempered her enthusiasm for co-education in a similar way. In 1900, the year her institution merged with Cornell University, she drew attention to the advantage that had accrued from the "presence of older and more experienced women in the Faculty," clearly lamenting that coeducational institutions would no longer offer such role models to their young female students.[68]

Zakrzewska's generation thus viewed with mixed feelings the end of the separate institutions they had founded, although one could argue that their position remained fundamentally pragmatic. After all, claiming that women now needed the New England because few other hospitals provided role models was not a different argument in kind than insisting that the hospital was necessary because women students lacked ample opportunities for clinical training elsewhere. The implication was that when other hospitals began placing women on their medical staffs, then and only then would an all-women's institution no longer be necessary. Still, to focus solely on the continuity in Zakrzewska's rhetoric would be to miss the ambivalence that had come to mark her attitude toward integration. She may not have embraced the notion of a distinct woman's sphere, but her attitude toward separatism had clearly softened, with the result that she now encountered resistance from the interns.

There is a definite irony here. The interns were merely questioning whether an all-women's institution provided the best education possible, something to which Zakrzewska herself (along with many of her peers) had previously answered no. That she now no longer held that view reflected in part her deepening suspicion that coeducational institutions were not always committed to *equal* education for women. Indeed, Emily Blackwell had watched Cornell refuse to hire the female faculty members who had staffed her college, an experience that would certainly lend credence to this view.[69] But Zakrzewska's change of heart also stemmed from her total immersion in the life of her hospital and her inability either to divorce herself from her creation or to articulate an alternative identity for the hospital, other than separatism, as all-women's institutions struggled to find a new sense of meaning and purpose. It was one thing to imagine that someday the New England Hospital would no longer exist; it was another thing entirely to hear suggestions that it may already have outlived its usefulness. In the end, Zakrzewska's caution proved prescient—women did not fare as well under coeducation as they had when all-women's institutions had flourished.[70] But however wise her position may have turned out to be, it was also fueled by a personal identification with the institution that made it difficult for her to contemplate a different path or, for that matter, to hear much criticism at all.

That personal identification appears, moreover, to have intensified over the years. Although that should hardly be surprising—one would expect a person's investment in his or her own creation to increase with time—more may have been going on here. Changes in Zakrzewska's personal life, foremost the shrinking of her family, may have led her to expect, and to need, a greater sense of allegiance from the individuals with whom she worked. The first member of Zakrzewska's family to pass away was her sister Minna, who succumbed to tuberculosis in 1877. Although they had not lived together for quite some time, Minna had stayed in Boston, and the two sisters had remained close. Even more devastating for Zakrzewska, however, was Heinzen's death in 1880. The day he let her know he was dying she described as "the hardest day of my emotional life."[71] She had been closer to no other man in her adult life and perhaps to no other person, with the possible exception of Sprague. We know too little about the exact nature of their friendship, but it is not difficult to imagine that Heinzen had been one of Zakrzewska's principal confidants as she struggled with the responsibilities and headaches of running a hospital. Despite his own hotheadedness, or perhaps because of it, he may have helped her to weather such controversies with more grace. But even if this was not the case, there can be little question that the two individuals had grown extremely close both intellectually and emotionally. Grieving his death, she may very well have thrown herself into her work with an even greater intensity than before.[72] Certainly it would have been normal for her to expect that the group of women who worked at the hospital would help to fill the void in her life.

Indeed, as Zakrzewska grappled with her interns' discontent, directed at least in part, she believed, toward herself, she turned more and more to the past and to a time when everyone in her hospital "assumed more of the condition of a family circle," united in their pursuit of the same goal.[73] As she made clear, it was a time when she had felt deeply appreciated. Even as late as 1875, just one year before the first troubles with the interns had manifested themselves, Zakrzewska had spoken proudly of the many graduates of her institution who "look towards Boston for their strength; strange to say, not so much towards the colleges from which they graduated, as towards the practical workers living and striving here in this Boston Hospital."[74] To some extent, she even viewed some of the interns as her children. This was true, at least, of Lucy Sewall, despite the fact that they were only nine years apart in age. In 1862, when Sewall was studying in Europe, Zakrzewska had written to her: "It is very strange how you have grown yourself into my heart. I never before have felt such strong attachment for a woman, that is, so 'tenderly' strong. I have always appreciated and loved women more intellectually. But you are my child."[75] To be sure, Zakrzewska did not develop such intense relationships with all her interns; indeed, the one with Sewall was probably unique. Nevertheless, judging from Sophia Jex-Blake's description of the early years at the New England, members of the staff did appear to have strong emotional attachments to one another, helping to foster a sense of family and belonging.

That deep bond seemed, however, to be eroding, and Zakrzewska, rather than engage in constructive ways of strengthening the young interns' commitment to the institution, widened the gap by chastising them. As she told them in 1891, "all the ladies present have served as Internes in this Hospital, and all had their grievances, and all had to endure annoyances of one kind or the other, as you have to endure; but just this training, which was borne with dignity and silence, has made them superior women, while everyone of the revolting sister-hood, have either remained on the lowest step of success, or fallen out of the profession entirely."[76] More than likely, Zakrzewska was not aware of the pun she made when referring to the "revolting sisterhood." Perhaps the interns had a good laugh when they read this phrase, but overall they would not have found her message humorous. Zakrzewska, hurt by their criticisms, had turned a discussion about the nature of clinical training into a statement about the character of the individuals involved. To be a superior physician, she stated in so many words, one must first engage in the arduous task of becoming a "superior woman."[77]

The young interns studying medicine in the early 1890s did not accept Zakr-zewska's assessment either of their own situation or of the importance of the institution. Submitting a statement to the medical staff in the fall of 1891, they voiced their anger that the staff refused to grant more responsibilities for patient care. "We have had abundant opportunities during our college years, to *see*," they complained; "we come here to *do*." But instead, they were "allowed to *do* absolutely nothing," forbidden from performing "even the simplest operations" or from handling any difficult maternity cases. They experienced this most significantly as a slight, feeling as though they were being treated "as mere children" who lacked any "professional standing." What they wanted was rec-ognition of the three or four years of medical school that they all possessed and of "the fact that we are now women; that many of us have occupied positions of responsibility;—that we have presumably reached the age of discretion." You may think, they argued, that you are doing us a favor by inviting us to spend a year here, but in fact you are reneging on your own promise "[t]o assist educated women in the practical study of medicine."[78]

This resentment was repeated and embellished two years later by Alice Hamilton, who interned briefly at the hospital. Voicing her complaints in private letters to her cousin Agnes, she did not exhibit any of the restraint the interns may have shown in an official communication. Hamilton, who eventually became an expert in industrial medicine and was the first woman to join the faculty at Harvard University (1919), did not hesitate in private to brand the New England Hospital a "narrow, petty, squabbly [sic], idiotic place." Accusing the staff of being narrowly focused on obstetrics and gynecology, she believed them to be "in a state of self-distrustful antagonism to all men doctors, . . . who escape discovering their own inferiority merely by avoiding their superiors." Adding insult to injury, instead of acknowledging that interns "could have an opinion of [their] own," they were "treated like a raw school-girl," even being chastised before their patients. All this was difficult for Hamilton to stomach. She had arrived in Boston excited about the prospect of spending an entire year developing her clinical skills; instead she found herself either "sitting around and reading text books" or filling her days with boring, menial tasks. Feeling as though she was wasting precious time, Hamilton resented the fact that "not a man medical graduate in the country . . . would accept so inferior a position as this." Although concerned that to quit would mean reneging on her promise to stay an entire year, Hamilton was so indignant that the staff had "not fulfilled their part of the contract," she ended up resigning her position before the year was out.[79]

The combination of the interns' complaints in 1891 and Hamilton's scathing remarks served as a devastating indictment of the New England's pedagogical policies and practices. While not every characterization need be taken seriously—Hamilton's accusation that the staff distrusted all male physicians would not, for example, have applied to Zakrzewska, who maintained close and respectful relations with Boston's elite male physicians her entire career—there can be little doubt that changes taking place outside the walls of the institution were taking a toll on the practices within. Not only had many schools adopted a four-year graded curriculum, but state legislatures had begun to grant physicians a limited monopoly over the practice of medicine. During the period in question, American society was endowing professions in general with increased power, and the medical profession was among the beneficiaries. Its new prestige had much to do with medicine's link to modern science, an approach to the acquisition of knowledge that many had come to believe would best allow one to make truth claims. Certainly everything from the germ theory to advancements in aseptic techniques was suggesting that scientific investigations were finally resulting in valuable knowledge about the nature of disease, even if therapeutic interventions were still a thing of the future. The resulting "culture of professionalism," as one historian has called it, placed great value on scientific objectivity and rationality, attributed both authority and honor to those who passed through the educational and licensing hoops, and encouraged individual autonomy, constrained only by the dictates of one's professional peers. Eventually, the medical profession, once a loosely knit conglomeration of highly diverse individual practitioners who frequently fought with one another as they struggled to achieve social standing, was transformed into a self-regulated group whose prestige, power, and autonomy reflected to a considerable extent the practitioners' possession of an esoteric and highly valued body of knowledge concerning health and disease.[80]

In the 1890s, when Zakrzewska was battling with the interns, the medical profession was still far from achieving this goal, but the world Zakrzewska had known seemed to be disappearing. Her own educational experiences had taken place at a time when the model of apprenticeship had still held sway. One need only think of the relationships she had with Joseph Hermann Schmidt in Berlin and John J. Delamater in Cleveland to appreciate the personal nature of her medical studies. This was, moreover, the model she had introduced to the New England Hospital, and for a while it had worked. Zakrzewska had assumed responsibility for her students' education, and they had accorded her the deference and respect that was her due. Feelings of gratitude to both Zakrzewska and the institution also dominated, given how few alternatives these young women had to acquire this kind of training elsewhere. Many also felt part of a greater mission and were excited by their own role in challenging social prescriptions against women's entry into the medical profession. The sense one often has when reading of the early years at the New England Hospital was that it did, in fact, resemble a happy family, aided no doubt by the relatively small size of the operation. The year Sophia Jex-Blake wrote her enthusiastic letters home, describing the ice cream socials and strong sense of camaraderie they all felt, only five physicians, three interns, three consultants, and twenty directors were associated with the hospital.[81]

By the early 1890s the situation was totally different. For one, the hospital was much larger, with sixteen physicians, six interns, fourteen consultants, and forty directors all involved in the life of the institution.[82] But most important, the interns made up a vastly different group than their predecessors: they were more highly and thoroughly educated; they had access to a wider variety of schools and hospitals; and they had more recent experiences in integrated settings. In addition, the increased social prestige being accorded physicians gave them a much greater sense of confidence and power. To be sure, women were still excluded from important aspects of this professionalization: medical schools still barred women from entry, and the vast majority of hospitals would not consider placing a woman on their staff.[83] Still, every year opportunities were increasing, and the interns felt inspired and empowered by these changes. It was difficult for them to arrive at the New England Hospital with the M.D. in hand, feeling as though they had earned a certain level of respect and honor, only to find themselves being treated as children. Undoubtedly they recognized that their training would occur under supervision, but it was an invisible hand, not a heavy hand, that they expected to guide their way. The hospital's failure to offer that was the source of their discontent and resentment. Zakrzewska may have viewed them as selfish, but to the interns, the New England was trapped in a model of stewardship that had long outlived its day. Worse yet, it was not providing the same quality of training they believed they could get elsewhere.

The generational tensions evident at the New England Hospital were by no means peculiar to this institution. Emily Blackwell also felt compelled to remind the 1899 graduating class of the New York Infirmary and Medical College not simply to work for their own advancement but to recognize "that the work of every woman physician, her character and influence, her success or failure, tells upon all, and helps or hinders those who work around her or come after her."[84] Indeed, historians who have studied late nineteenth-century women's organizations of all ilks have described the emergence of a "self-conscious professional culture" that seemed to have little in common with the professionalism of its predecessors.[85] The older form, referred to by some historians as "civic professionalism," was grounded in a sense of community. Professional responsibilities and civic duty were woven seamlessly together, one's place in the community defined by both.[86] The newer professionalism, in contrast, replaced the notion of a community with the image of a group of autonomous individuals joining together to protect their own interests. Even the women's rights movement showed signs of such tensions. Among the older generation (Zakrzewska's cohort), personal experiences of discrimination fueled a political critique that condemned the unjust concentration of power in the hands of white men. For the newer generation, the battle for women's rights was a battle for the rights of individuals to pursue their own interests.[87]

A similar dynamic was at play at the New England Hospital in the last decades of the century. The young interns, having so many more opportunities available to them, did not understand Zakrzewska's insistence that the time was not yet ripe to close down all-women's institutions. They certainly did not share her view that the fate of the women's movement for medical education depended upon the institution's ability to survive. This did not, however, mean that they were unaware of or indifferent to the plight of women physicians. Indeed, the interns' reminder to the medical staff that they were in fact "now women" and that the hospital was failing to fulfill its obligation to "assist educated women in the practical study of medicine" indicates that it was the thought of receiving a mediocre medical education *as women* that troubled them so much. Hamilton, we must remember, had been disturbed by the thought that she was being asked to tolerate a situation that "no man medical graduate in the country" would ever be expected to endure. Committed suffragist that she was, she understood only too well that her actions and experiences had consequences for the advancement of women at large.[88]

In response to this constant litany of complaints, Zakrzewska turned to the past, trying to convince the interns to see the New England as a "large family" that required them to place its needs before their own.[89] She even spoke passionately about the need for "a good deal of self-sacrifice" to bring to completion "one of the greatest historical reforms," thus embracing a language of self-sacrifice that she had so adamantly rejected in her youth because of her conviction that it kept women from implementing their own plans and satisfying their own interests.[90] But Zakrzewska's language, communitarian in spirit, no longer made sense to the younger generation. Thus, where she spoke of sacrifice, family, and stewardship, Hamilton spoke of contractual obligations. Both women were trying to characterize the relationship between two parties, but Zakrzewska assumed the primacy of the group and the existence of a clear hierarchy, where a "protector" assumed moral responsibility for those in her charge. Hamilton, on the other hand, assumed the primacy of the individual; in her view, relationships occurred between equal partners bound together by a written document ensuring that both parties would fulfill their obligations.[91]

There can be no question that the interns' embrace of the new professional ethos contributed to this clash of visions, but this clash was between different understandings of professionalism.[92] What must be emphasized, however, is that the interns never once mentioned science. Their complaints had nothing to do with the hospital's lack of laboratory facilities or with the medical ideas and theories of the staff. Hamilton may once have disparaged the diagnostic skills of one of the head physicians, but even that tirade focused more on the staff's refusal to let her treat her own patients than on the style of medicine being practiced.[93] This is not to say that the meaning and practice of scientific medicine had not changed by this time; they most certainly had. More to the point, as we will discuss in the next chapter, Zakrzewska struggled with some of these changes, criticizing bacteriology and a narrow definition of disease while identifying herself more closely with prevention and hygiene. It is likely that different understandings of medical science were in some subtle way contributing to the tensions that surfaced at the end of the century, but if that was the case, they were never clearly articulated. No, the battles that were fought focused almost solely on different styles of teaching and the distribution of power and responsibilities between interns and the physicians on the staff.

Matters did not improve in the following years; if anything, they worsened. And to add fuel to the fire, Zakrzewska ended up fighting contentious battles not only with the interns but with the board of directors as well. These kept her awake at night and led her on occasion to threaten to resign from the hospital's medical board.[94] On the surface, most of the disagreements had to do with the allocation of funds for the construction of new facilities, but beneath the surface another battle was taking place over who had ultimate authority to decide matters. In the first decades, when the directors had numbered twenty and the vast majority had been Zakrzewska's friends, her authority had rarely, if ever, been challenged.[95] Now, however, the number of directors had doubled, and most lacked any personal ties to her. There was a certain irony in this, given that most other American hospitals at the time were witnessing a handing over of power from the directors (or trustees) to the medical staff as medical care became more acute and less custodial.[96] Not so at the New England Hospital, and Zakrzewska, who had held the reins for so long, did not adjust to this shift in power any better than she had with the interns. With an absence of harmony (and a challenge to her authority) confronting her from both "above" and "below," the aging founder slowly withdrew from hospital affairs.

Zakrzewska had, in fact, already begun to redefine her relationship to the New England Hospital in 1887, when she was just a few years shy of her sixtieth birthday. On the occasion of the institution's twenty-fifth anniversary, she, Lucy Sewall, and Helen Morton had all stepped down as attending physicians. Although this had marked their withdrawal from the day-to-day management of the hospital, they had stepped immediately into another position created especially for them, that of advisory physician. This had allowed them to remain on the board of physicians, occasionally care for patients, and retain the authority to help run the hospital. Zakrzewska had operated in this capacity for another six years, but in 1893, the year not only of Alice Hamilton's internship but also of a particularly acrimonious battle with the directors, Zakrzewska "retired from professional work."[97] Although she never fully withdrew from the hospital, she severely curtailed her involvement with hospital matters, leaving to others the rewards and the headaches that go along with running an institution. As the years passed, she also found herself growing increasingly estranged from the world she had helped to create but had not anticipated. As she wrote seven months before her death, "The world becomes young daily, & new to me, into which newness I can hardly find myself."[98]

The hospital Zakrzewska left behind never regained its former glory as a teaching institution. The problems that had surfaced in the 1880s and 1890s continued to grow, and by the second decade of the twentieth century, the New England Hospital was having trouble filling its internships. By this time, moreover, students were complaining not only about the lack of clinical experience and professional standing but also about the hospital's indifference to the growing trends in medicine toward specialization and scientific research. With its focus on general medicine and its lack of laboratory facilities, the institution appeared old-fashioned and behind the times to many observers.[99] As its patient base also began to decline, the hospital struggled to find a niche for itself that would allow it to survive. Two questions, harkening back to its dual identity as a teaching hospital and an institution of charity, formed the core of the debates that ensued: should the New England Hospital abandon its identity as an all-women's institution and accept both male patients in its wards and male physicians on its staff? And should it forgo any attempt to become a research hospital and embrace instead its earlier heritage by promoting itself as a community hospital? In both cases, the answer ending up being yes. The first male patients entered the hospital in the interwar years; the first male physician (since Horatio Storer) joined the medical staff in 1950; and in 1969 the New England Hospital for Women and Children became the Dimock Community Center, catering to the poor and largely African American population that had moved into Roxbury in the postwar years.[100]

It is an interesting exercise to try to imagine how Zakrzewska would have responded to these changes. My guess is that she would have opposed gender integration, concerned that, despite the strides women had made by the 1960s, only a small percentage of the medical profession was made up of women, with the majority grouped in less prestigious specialties such as obstetrics and pediatrics. This would, I believe, have troubled her deeply, and chances are good that she would have insisted that an all-women's hospital, where women could develop surgical skills among others, remained an absolute necessity.

As far as the transformation to a community hospital was concerned, my guess is that Zakrzewska would probably have signed on. Most likely this would not have reflected a renewed commitment to charity—at the end of her tenure at the New England, Zakrzewska had announced her lack of interest in the institution's charitable work[101]—but rather a belief that research institutions did not provide the best environment for training physicians. In the early twenty-first century, we have come to believe that research hospitals provide both the best care and the best educational setting, but Zakrzewska may not have been so quick to agree. Her understanding of science translated into a commitment to careful bedside investigations, advanced diagnostic techniques, hygienic practices, and, increasingly in the 1880s and 1890s, surgery. But to the extent that the twentieth-century hospital became increasingly defined by a research ethic that at times placed the acquisition of medical knowledge before improvements in medical care, the New England Hospital was only tangentially a part.[102] Zakrzewska never saw herself as educating female scientists who conducted research in the laboratory or even, for that matter, at the bedside. In this regard, she could not have differed more from her colleague Mary Putnam Jacobi. Rather, her entire goal had been to educate good practitioners. Something regarded as "scientific thinking" or "scientific rationalism" had been an integral part of that, but scientific investigations had not been. Thus, as other hospitals strengthened their ties to medical schools and integrated themselves more directly into the emerging scientific complex of university/laboratory/hospital, Zakrzewska showed little interest in pursuing that path.[103] Indeed, as the century wore on, she joined the critics of bacteriology and even some branches of surgery. Zakrzewska may never have abandoned her commitment to science, rationality, and materialism, but she did hold on to an understanding of these categories that seemed increasingly out of place as the new century dawned.

The World Changes

The last decade of Zakrzewska's life was one of increasing disillusionment with the direction the medical world was taking. The battles with the interns at the New England Hospital had been only one manifestation of this. In a number of public and private writings in the late 1880s and 1890s, Zakrzewska criticized the increased use of instruments in the birthing process, bacteriology, vaccination, gynecologic surgery, and the narrowing of the definition of disease to the pathophysiological changes of the body. In their stead, she promoted prevention, hygiene, and therapeutic restraint, thus linking herself with an older style of medical practice that had assumed the primacy of the doctor-patient relationship, the notion of stewardship, and an expansive notion of science that was closer to a worldview than a specific method for acquiring knowledge.[1] In some ways, Zakrzewska had come a long way from the public pronouncements she had made in her youth when she had paraded the instrumental savvy of the New England Hospital's physicians and appeared more inclined to view the body in strictly biological terms. Yet in other ways, much had stayed the same, for Zakrzewska's criticisms of modern medicine stemmed largely from her inability to reconcile recent changes with the understanding of science and morality she had developed around midcentury and nurtured ever since.

Zakrzewska was not alone in her complaints. The last third of the nineteenth century was marked by contentious battles over the path modern medicine should pursue. Elizabeth Blackwell, certainly at one extreme, blamed laboratory medicine, especially vivisection, for blunting the medical student's sense of morality. Other critics of the laboratory, more moderate in their views, worried nevertheless about the denigration of the clinic and thus the kind of knowledge acquired at the bedside. The targets of their criticisms were, for the most part, young disciples of the rapidly proliferating German laboratories, who imagined a day when the specialized scientific knowledge produced in the laboratory would be capable of driving therapeutic practices.[2]

Zakrzewska, as we will see, occupied a somewhat anomalous position, in part because of her roots in German medicine, but there is no question that she, like many of her generational peers, questioned both the scientific and the moral legitimacy of the direction in which modern medicine was moving. True to her lifelong beliefs, however, she did not frame these tensions in gendered terms, although others certainly did. Indeed, one of the strategies of those enamored of the German laboratories was to discredit earlier approaches by gendering them feminine, implying that only the work that went on in the laboratory could wear the mantle of masculinity.[3] Elizabeth Blackwell, too, gendered·these competing medical approaches, but instead of lauding such masculine endeavors, she held them responsible for injuring medical students' ability to sympathize with the suffering of their patients.[4] Zakrzewska shied away from such gendered stereotypes, preferring to attribute different viewpoints to a generational divide. Nevertheless, through her promotion of prevention, hygiene, and therapeutic restraint and her rejection of bacteriology, she ended up aligning herself more closely with Blackwell and others who maintained that women practiced a different style of medicine. This alliance was strengthened, moreover, as she came to view women's bodies as sacred and childbirth as a central event in a woman's life. Zakrzewska never stopped promoting the virtues of science and rationality, and she never abandoned her belief in materialism, but the meanings she ascribed to these terms brought her, by the end of the century, closer to those who believed in a woman's distinct sphere of influence than she had ever been in her life.[5]

· · ·

One of the first public venues in which Zakrzewska criticized modern medicine was an article she published in 1889 in the *Boston Medical and Surgical Journal*. "Report of One Hundred and Eighty-Seven Cases of Midwifery in Private Practice" was the first and only article Zakrzewska ever published in a medical journal.[6] It was, as Zakrzewska announced, intended to counter the image young practitioners were receiving of obstetrics as a highly complex field of study that required the use of instruments. At the time she wrote this article, Zakrzewska's voice was one among many calling attention to the dangers of what was often referred to as "meddlesome midwifery." Although such cautions were not new—for at least the previous sixty years medical journals had

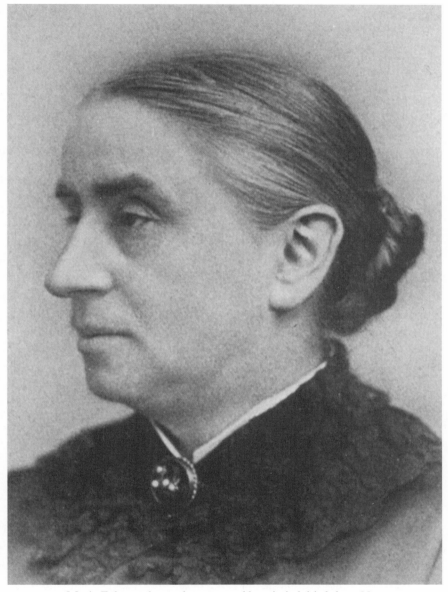

Marie Zakrzewska, perhaps around her sixtieth birthday, 1889.
(Courtesy Archives and Special Collections on Women in Medicine and Homeopathy,
Drexel University College of Medicine)

been carrying articles admonishing physicians to show restraint when attending women in labor—the proliferation of different types of forceps, the increased availability of anesthetics, and the greater percentage of laboring women who chose to have physicians in attendance rather than midwives had all so accelerated the tendency on the part of practitioners to intervene in the birthing process that the number and frequency of concerned voices had also grown. Thus, when Zakrzewska chose in 1889 to publish her views on childbirth, she was joining a large group of male and female physicians who had come to disparage not so much the use of instruments and drugs as their overuse.[7]

"I present here the summary report of these 187 cases in my private practice," Zakrzewska wrote, "recorded in the succession in which they occurred at the beginning of my obstetrical career." These cases were intended to demonstrate that childbirth was "the most natural process in a woman's life" and did not, therefore, require that a physician bring along "a well-equipped bag, containing instruments, disinfectants, drugs, etc." when attending a woman in labor. On the contrary, she insisted, since it is the woman, not the physician, who "brings the child into the world," the latter should play an active role only in the event of a complication. Otherwise, he or she had no reason to intervene until the baby crowned. At that point, the physician's job was to support the perineum to prevent tearing and then to wait again for the delivery of the placenta. Those who interfered by putting their hand in the uterus often caused inflammation and fevers. "Only in cases of haemorrhage or appearance of abnormal pains," Zakrzewska wrote, "do I interfere with nature."[8]

In Zakrzewska's estimation most of the complications that arose during and after delivery occurred because of the unwillingness of physicians "to wait quietly for the natural process to take its course." Instead, anxious to hurry labor along, they used forceps to deliver the child and then forcibly removed the placenta, both of which practices often required physicians to intervene further and sew up the tears they had caused. These, Zakrzewska remarked, are the "sorts of 'scientific' measures" that physicians employed "to bring a woman through."[9]

This was certainly quite a different picture than the one Zakrzewska had presented in the 1860s, when she had emphasized the instrumental skills of the physicians who trained at the New England Hospital. Now, however, faced by changes in medical practices of which she disapproved, Zakrzewska used language that not only sounded similar to that embraced by advocates of gender differences in medical practice but also harkened back to her earlier nemesis

Samuel Gregory. Indeed, someone who read in this article about the tears and ruptures caused by physicians, who "performed all sorts of 'scientific' measures" rather than allowing nature to take its course, might have thought that he or she had mistakenly picked up a copy of *Man-Midwifery Exposed and Corrected*. In portraying herself as someone who viewed childbirth as a natural process, promoted restraint rather than intervention, and heralded patience as one of the physician's most important attributes, Zakrzewska seemed almost to be modeling herself on Gregory's ideal female physician.[10]

She certainly seemed to be drawing considerable inspiration from her years as a midwife. Tellingly, Zakrzewska's first lengthy story in this article dealt with the time she spent both studying and then teaching midwifery at the Charité. Modeling this story closely upon that of Ignaz Semmelweis, she explained that the Charité midwives were instructed to let "nature do the work," with the result that they rarely used forceps and rarely had childbed fever in their wards. In contrast, when the male students received their instruction, "every third case was made a forceps-case, by untimely rupturing the membranes, or by other meddlesome interference with nature." Zakrzewska also had particularly harsh words for Dr. Credé, Joseph Hermann Schmidt's successor, who instructed the male students in the active removal of the placenta. The outcome, she claimed, was the persistence of "fevers, purulent ophthalmia, and peritonitis."[11]

Clearly, Zakrzewska's outlook on obstetric practices had changed—or perhaps all one can say is that she had chosen to give a different face to the style of practice she wished to promote publicly. Caution is necessary because we lack documents that would allow us to determine whether she had in fact always practiced restraint. There are also reasons to question the complete accuracy of the story she told about the Charité, not the least of which is its uncanny resemblance to the well-known account of Semmelweis.[12] Zakrzewska also failed to mention that midwives were forbidden by state law to use forceps. Hence, the differences in their education may very well have been as much legally as ideologically determined. Moreover, had she so clearly preached against the teaching methods of her superior, chances are that would have been mentioned in the archival records that discussed the conditions of her dismissal, and no such reference was ever made. But whether Zakrzewska offered an accurate appraisal of her earlier pedagogical style or not, what is significant is her decision, in 1889, to portray herself as someone who had always been a proponent of a noninterventionist approach to childbirth.

Still, before we erase any distinctions between Zakrzewska and Gregory, we must keep two caveats in mind: first, a careful reading of her story indicates that she was not in fact attributing any differences in practice to gender. Unlike Gregory, or a good number of women physicians for that matter, she was not claiming that women had less of a tendency to intervene or that male physicians had a greater tendency toward "meddlesome interference." Rather, in her story about the Charité, her message was that the male students had been taught incorrectly and that she had corrected this when she assumed the position of head midwife. At that time, so she claims, she adopted a different teaching method, instructing the male students in "the mechanism of normal labor, showing them when and how to assist nature in case of an abnormal deviation, using for this purpose the manikin, instead of the living woman." Furthermore, she added, she actively discouraged the male students from using the Credé method for removing the placenta. She was, in fact, so successful at altering the way her male students practiced medicine that "not one single time, were we removed to the isolating building during that summer."[13]

Second, unlike Gregory, Zakrzewska did not link her advocacy of restraint and nonintervention to a critique of science. On the contrary, this article, like all her other previous writings, argued for the virtues of proceeding scientifically. Indeed, she presented obstetrics not as an art but rather as the branch of medicine that most approached a science because of the near certainty with which one could make diagnoses and prognoses. Even her attack on the " 'scientific' measures" of some physicians was meant to rescue "science" from the hands of those who misappropriated the term. Her complaint was that what they labeled as scientific was actually grounded in a fallacious understanding of the birthing process.

Thus Zakrzewska had neither abandoned nor even modified her commitment to science. Still, in 1889 the meaning of science she promoted looked backward, not forward, grounded in anecdotes that were intended to demonstrate her "rational" approach to practice. For example, although she added statistical information to support her claim that childbirth was a natural process, her method more closely resembled the style of counting popularized by the early nineteenth-century French clinician Pierre Louis than the sophisticated statistical techniques that had taken hold by the end of the century.[14] Indeed, when Zakrzewska finally turned to the 187 midwifery cases in her private practice (on page 3 of a four-page article) she did little more than inundate the reader with as much information as possible. Thus, she recorded the ages of the mothers, the number of children born and their weight, the number of miscarriages and premature births, the length of labor, the time at which membranes ruptured, the number of normal births compared with the number requiring forceps, and so on. Nowhere did Zakrzewska offer any interpretation of this data. In fact, rather than conclude by calculating her infant and maternal mortality rates, her rates of complication, or even her rates of intervention, she ended with the description of a case involving a woman who gave birth to a stillborn after suffering from both typhoid fever and pneumonia during her pregnancy but who recovered within six weeks. The anecdote, not the numbers, was to Zakrzewska the more powerful form of persuasion.[15]

The centrality of the anecdote and, indeed, her older style of practice were even more evident in an article Zakrzewska published four years later in the *Woman's Journal*, the official publication of the American Woman Suffrage Association. Here, Zakrzewska told the story of a farmer's wife who came to her seeking medical advice. Despite the woman's glazed eyes, a pale complexion, and complaints of "sleeplessness, utter lack of appetite, backache, depression of spirits, etc.," a thorough examination revealed no evidence of disease. Zakrzewska did not, however, tell the woman that there was nothing she could do. Rather, suspecting exhaustion, she recommended "six months of rest." However, when the woman returned ten days later looking even more haggard, Zakrzewska realized she had misjudged the situation and needed to hear the woman's entire story. It turned out that earlier in the year the woman's husband had invested all the family's savings in the purchase of a Jersey cow, which had recently fallen ill. As a result, they were paying a hired man to tend the cow, which meant that they had to let the charwoman go who had been helping the wife with her housework. "The case looked so sad and hopeless," Zakrzewska commented, "that I sat silently thinking for a moment, when suddenly a bright thought sprang into my mind, and I said, 'Why don't *you* nurse that cow and let the charwoman do your work in house, kitchen and dairy?' " The farmer's wife at first dismissed such an idea, but Zakrzewska explained how "with my vivid power of imagination, I overthrew all of her objections one after another, until her conversation became really animated, and the plan appeared so plausible to both of us that the good woman went out of the office with no stronger tonic than hope and courage can bestow."[16]

The story ends with the return to Zakrzewska's office months later of "a plump, sunburnt, cheerful-faced woman." The farmer's wife, who had succeeded in persuading her husband to go along with Zakrzewska's plan, had spent every day since she had last visited Zakrzewska out in the field, helping feed the cow, even reading to it, while the two of them grew healthy together. The cow had even offered a return on its investment: it had given birth to a heifer, which her husband had already been able to sell for half the price he had paid for the cow. For Zakrzewska, this was clearly a success story, an example of hygiene and education in practice.

Putting aside for a moment the gendered meanings of a story in which a woman derives her health from nursing a cow, we can see that Zakrzewska was clearly criticizing an image of the modern physician, who would have terminated the clinical encounter after determining that the woman showed no physical signs of sickness. For Zakrzewska, in contrast, that piece of information marked the beginning of their relationship. The ideal physician she depicted took the time to learn about the circumstances surrounding her patient's experience of ill health; this is what allowed her to tailor her therapeutic advice to the specific situation at hand. Her diagnostic skills stemmed, moreover, not from the possession of a body of specialized knowledge, the command of the latest materia medica, or the handling of new instruments but rather from clear thinking, good judgment, and a "vivid power of imagination." Indeed, for Zakrzewska these traits allowed her to act rationally, dissecting the situation in order to determine both the true cause of the woman's ailments and a therapeutic regimen that would restore her to health.

Published in 1893, this article also represented a veiled attack on modern laboratory science. Indeed, two years earlier, Zakrzewska had written to Elizabeth Blackwell, complaining about the "Scientific Craze" that was leading her colleagues to talk about little else than "vaccination and inoculation." In her eyes, the eagerness with which physicians were embracing Pasteur's and Koch's discoveries was decidedly unscientific, "the same unproven '*Science*'(?) the same quackery" as could be attributed to Hahnemann, the founder of homeopathy. In contrast, she explained, she was never inclined to rely too heavily on medicines, usually giving them "as placebos in infinitessimal [*sic*] forms" and thus earning a reputation among her patients for "hardly any medicine but teaching people how to keep well without it. . . . I can assure you," she added, "it is far harder, requiring more thought and more endurance and more patience to practise hygiene than what is called medicine."[17] Certainly in Zakrzewska's mind, the way she brought the farmer's wife back to health was as clear a proof as she needed.

Therapeutic restraint, hygiene, skepticism toward instrumentation and bacteriology, anecdotal evidence—taken together, they all suggest the sizable gap that was growing between Zakrzewska's understanding of medical science and the focus on laboratory experiments, clinical studies, diagnostic instruments, and surgical acumen that were becoming the mark of modern medicine. Nor was Zakrzewska's a lone voice. In the late nineteenth century, medical researchers, clinical specialists, and practicing physicians were all engaged in contentious battles over the path modern medicine should pursue, much of their disagreement centering on competing definitions of science.[18] One of the more heated debates was between those who fought to ground medical practice in the knowledge produced at the bedside and those who favored the laboratory. Zakrzewska may not have chosen this particular language to frame her concerns, but her skepticism toward modern medical techniques cannot be understood apart from the issues that surfaced in this debate.

The debate between the clinic and the laboratory took place to some extent across a generational divide. On the one side were those physicians, older now, who had studied in Paris in the antebellum period and who had returned home lauding empirical studies at the bedside and denigrating the vacuous theories that they claimed were driving medical practices at the time. Whether in the clinic, the consulting room, or the patients' home, the physician's task, they insisted, was to collect as much information as possible about the particulars of the case before recommending a specific therapeutic regimen.[19] Now, however, they were being challenged by a younger generation of physicians who were more inspired by recent developments in the German laboratories and who sought universal laws that would explain the disease phenomenon. Ultimately, these German-trained physicians believed, such laboratory-based investigations would generate the specialized knowledge that would determine appropriate therapeutic measures. As John Harley Warner's sensitive study of the Paris-trained generation has illuminated, these battles were only in part about method. Because they marked disagreements over the very nature of the knowledge driving therapeutic practices, at their core were questions of professional authority, professional identity, and moral integrity.[20]

Zakrzewska, who struggled with many of the same issues, occupied a somewhat anomalous position. As we have seen, she shared with her generational peers a view of disease as embedded in the social environment, and she lauded the clinic as the most important site in the education of young physicians. Nevertheless, she shared none of the Paris-trained physicians' praise of empiricism. In her opinion, it left the physician without any rational foundation upon which to ground her or his therapeutic practices. This reflected, as I have been arguing, her own European training, which took place neither in Paris in the antebellum period nor in the German laboratories and clinics in the postbellum period but rather in Germany in the 1840s and 1850s, when a younger generation of physicians were making loud their demands for the implementation of what they termed "rational medicine." Conceived of as an antidote to the clinical empiricism that they believed had come to dominate medical theory and practice, they insisted that medicine would become a science only when the laboratory and the clinic joined together to study disease and to derive universal laws that would guide practice. This understanding of medical science, I have been arguing throughout this book, had a profound effect on how Zakrzewska shaped her own professional identity.

Thus one of the developments that so disturbed Zakrzewska at the end of the century was the severing of the laboratory's ties to the clinic, and thus to practice, not laboratory medicine per se.[21] This was at the heart of her criticism of bacteriology, and in this regard she may have had the most in common with other Germans of her generation who also viewed with dismay the narrowed focus on bacterial origins and isolated cells and organs that had come to mark German laboratory research. Thus Abraham Jacobi, a leading figure in American pediatrics who studied medicine in Germany before immigrating to the United States in 1853 (the same year Zakrzewska arrived), complained of the "bacteriomania" that had captured the imagination of his colleagues. And Rudolf Virchow, whose views on scientific medicine had so shaped Zakrzewska's own, criticized his colleagues' obsession with bacteriology, not so much denying that bacteria were responsible for the transmission of certain infectious diseases as rejecting both the notion that most diseases could be so explained and the idea that nothing else contributed to the diseased state.[22] Zakrzewska may have gone one step further and doubted that bacteriologists had actually found the cause of disease, but more important, she considered unscientific the frenzy among her colleagues to vaccinate and inoculate indiscriminately, as though all disease could now be reduced to the havoc caused by a bacterial infection. It was the leap being made from the laboratory to the doctor's office that she found troubling, not what was taking place within the laboratory itself.

· · ·

Zakrzewska may not have criticized laboratory work, but she also neither practiced nor promoted it. In terms of her own style of practice, and indeed of her professional identity, she positioned herself squarely at the bedside and in the consulting room, helping her patients to understand the link between their physical well-being and the social circumstances of their lives. Zakrzewska continued to emphasize the importance of proceeding scientifically—indeed, she never missed an opportunity to lay claim to the mantle of science—but her model was not the physician in the laboratory armed with test tubes and instruments but rather the steward and problem solver, who sought clues in the specifics of his or her patients' lives, relying on sound judgment, rational thought, and experience to devise the best therapeutic approach.

How much Zakrzewska had changed since the 1850s and 1860s, when she had promoted microscopy and thermometry, positioned at the vanguard of those arguing for the importance of grounding medical practice in the knowledge produced in both the laboratory and the clinic. Among women physicians she had certainly been one of the loudest and most public advocates of such an approach. Now, however, at the end of the century, her work was a far cry even from that of some of her contemporaries, like Mary Putnam Jacobi and Mary Dixon Jones, who were integrating modern laboratory techniques into their clinical practice, conducting microscopic and pathological investigations of the tumors and exudates they excised from their patients.[23] Zakrzewska may not have criticized their work, but she also did not identify with it.

Zakrzewska had come to embrace a style of practice that was, as several scholars have argued, becoming increasingly feminized.[24] This association did not, however, trouble her. On the contrary, she now seemed intrigued by the overlap between her own approach and those of her friends, like Elizabeth Blackwell, who had long insisted that women practiced medicine differently than men. "I sympathize with you on so many points, if not on all," Zakrzewska wrote Blackwell in 1891 after reading her friend's paper on hygiene, "but I feel grateful whenever I see your writings and try to spread its truths." It is not unreasonable to assume that Zakrzewska was rejecting Blackwell's explicit embrace of gender differences; at the same time, however, she shared her friend's insistence that medical practice and medical ideology be understood in moral terms. "You have the advantage over me that you talk and write in a strain of religious belief which will be understood by the many, while I can simply set forth the moral questions of moral righteousness as is expressed in the 'golden rule,'" Zakrzewska continued.[25] Ever skeptical of religious doctrine, Zakrzewska nevertheless shared with Blackwell—and, indeed, many others of their generation—a conviction that questions of justice were part and parcel of any discussion about health and disease. Indeed, her growing disillusionment with modern medicine may have reflected, more than anything

else, her sense that questions of "moral righteousness" were no longer as prominent as they had once been.

· · ·

As Zakrzewska's thoughts on medical practice changed, so too did her perception of the female body. There was already a hint of this in the 1889 obstetrics
article when she coupled her emphasis on childbirth as a natural process with a
reference to a woman's "first babe" as the "great event of her life." Even the
story she told in the *Woman's Journal* suggests a view of women's bodies as
intimately connected to nature. This is evident in the bizarre way she blurred
the line separating the wife and the cow, describing their blossoming friendship
as they helped each other grow fat (pregnant in the case of the cow), healthy, and
happy. The strongest indication, however, of Zakrzewska's altered view of wom-
en's bodies came in the 1891 letter she wrote to Blackwell, in which she followed
her criticism of bacteriology with an attack on gynecologic surgery. Zakrzewska
knew well Blackwell's own opinion of ovariotomies as "permanent mutilation."
Without mincing words, she let her friend know that she shared this position,
lamenting the "lack of sanctity for their own body growing up in girls and
women" that was sending women to the hospital "on the slightest cause" in
order to "urge upon us operations."[26]

At the time Zakrzewska wrote this letter, a spirited debate was under way in
the medical literature over the use of surgical solutions to cure women's health
problems. Women physicians were no strangers to this debate. Thus Blackwell,
with her total rejection of any kind of gynecologic surgery, represented one
position. In contrast, Mary Dixon Jones, one year older than Zakrzewska and
an 1875 graduate of the Woman's Medical College of Pennsylvania, made a
career for herself specializing in ovariotomies. Regina Morantz-Sanchez's rivet-
ing account of two late nineteenth-century trials against Dixon Jones—one for
manslaughter and the other for libel—reveals the difficulties encountered by
women who demonstrated too great an eagerness to cut and too much enthusiasm for their own self-promotion.[27] Although Dixon Jones's detractors were
many, she had her supporters as well, among whom Mary Putnam Jacobi could
be found. Less controversial than Dixon Jones but no less committed to using
the knife, Jacobi directly accused Blackwell of refusing to consider the lifesaving
nature of such operations. Besides, she fumed, "there is not such special sanctity
about the ovary!"[28]

Zakrzewska had once shared Dixon Jones's and Jacobi's views of women's bodies, but that was no longer the case. She may never have gone so far as to embrace Blackwell's notion of the "spiritual power of maternity," which supposedly taught "the subordination of self to the welfare of others," but she was clearly moving away from her highly mechanistic view of women's bodies and her absolute denial of difference.[29] Why she made this move is unclear, although the parallel between her embrace of a style of medical practice that was becoming gendered female and the sacredness with which she now viewed the female body would indicate a sharp turn toward the language of difference that had long characterized Blackwell's views.[30] Zakrzewska continued to reject any idea that her practices or her views represented a peculiarly female style, but there is no denying that in the last decade or so of her life the values and practices that were becoming feminized held far more appeal for her than those that were assuming the mantle of masculinity.

Zakrzewska's altered view of women's bodies had, however, personal roots as well and was tied to a number of changes right around her sixtieth birthday. As we have already noted, she had significantly reduced her involvement in the day-to-day affairs of her hospital in 1887 when she had resigned her position as attending physician. Pulling back from an institution that had been both her creation and a home away from home had already brought some sadness; the loss of two very dear friends just a few years later made things even more difficult. The first to pass away was her close friend Mary Booth, who was only fifty-eight when she died on 5 March 1889. They had remained close through the years and had shared, in Zakrzewska's words, an "intimacy [that] was only broken by death." Then, less than a year later, Lucy Sewall passed away at the age of fifty-two. The year, she wrote to Severance on the day of Sewall's death, had been a "sad" and "a cruel one," and she "felt almost tired of life" herself.[31]

These changes in Zakrzewska's life led her to think more about both her own mortality and the meaning of her life's work. There can be no doubt that she derived considerable satisfaction from the hospital she had founded and the work she had done to further the cause of women physicians, but on several occasions she implied that this was not enough. Indeed, in a particularly moving letter she wrote to Caroline Severance in 1889, she spoke of her regret that she had not brought any children into her life. Commenting on Severance's son's decision to remain a bachelor, she wrote: "I am sorry for him, because I know he will feel the penalty for doing so, just as keenly as I do, now that I completed my 60th year and have no young life, which belongs to me. . . . Now with mature thought, I see that life is selfish when the dread of sorrow prevents us to fulfil our natural mission, and whatever this sorrow may be, it is never as great, as not to be tentimes balanced by the joy, which precedes such grief & anxiety."[32]

In the midst of this contemplation and sadness, Zakrzewska found herself drawn to the German biologist and philosopher Ernst Haeckel, who had recently written of his view of the material world as both fundamentally mechanical and capable of generating soul-like properties.[33] Haeckel, who set out both to deny the existence of "immaterial forces" and to avoid a "soulless materialism," was arguing at the time that the first life forms, or Monera, had generated spontaneously from inorganic matter, emerging from that process endowed with the property of irritability. This property eventually evolved, moreover, into consciousness and the human soul. "I am a monist," Zakrzewska wrote Severance. "The whole universe is one great power or material & evolves the spirit."[34]

Zakrzewska appears to have found some comfort in Haeckel's ideas about the material world. She knew she could not, nor did she wish to, believe in an afterlife. She had no desire, she once explained, to join her friends once again "in a form, which is either by virtue of surroundings or an advanced development, so altered for the better or the worse, that they have become estranged to my comprehension or feeling."[35] But perhaps Haeckel's belief that matter could give rise to emergent properties, thus leaving room for something akin to a spiritual element, satisfied a need she had for something to persist after she died. That such thoughts were on Zakrzewska's mind is suggested by a comment she made to Elizabeth Blackwell a few years before her death: "I fully agree with you," she wrote, "and beleive [sic] that the spirit cannot die, is indestructible and lives forever, altho individual consciousness is lost in Nirvana."[36]

I am suggesting that Haeckel's blurring of the boundary between the natural and the spiritual not only offered Zakrzewska comfort but also contributed to her vision of the body as material but nevertheless sacred. At the very least, it offered her a language and a philosophical foundation, distinct from the religious doctrines she continued to hold suspect, in which to ground her increased reverence toward the human form. Still, this picture is too neat because, among the many emotions Zakrzewska expressed at this time of her life, she also showed considerable anger toward the younger generation. As we have seen, she did not hesitate to accuse the interns in her hospital of extreme selfishness, putting their own needs before the interests of women physicians as a whole. But her truly vituperative words she saved for the young women who sought ovariotomies in her hospital. In the letter she wrote to Blackwell in 1891, she accused these women of "indulgence in luxurious living, dislike to work and of self abnegation. . . . Yes," she added, "they rather die, than bring up a family of children and work and practise self-denials."[37]

Zakrzewska was clearly struggling to make sense of choices she had made when she was younger, including her decision to remain childless. Although it would be a mistake to imagine her dwelling on this sense of loss, at a time in her life when she perhaps felt overwhelmed by the loss of very dear friends and unmoored by her gradual retreat from the hospital she had created and nurtured, she directed her pain and anger at women who were choosing not to bring into the world the young lives she now lamented not having had herself. Some might be tempted to ascribe Zakrzewska's change of view to an elusive "maternal instinct" that finally surfaced toward the end of her life, but I choose to see this shift as evidence of the constraints under which women lived at the time and the difficulty of being an atheist and childless in a society that accepted neither. Disturbed by the changes taking place around her, Zakrzewska ended up embracing some of the very conventions she had once so vehemently opposed.

· · ·

Zakrzewska's ideas on gender, science, materialism, and medicine had changed considerably since her early adulthood. When she first began formulating her views in the 1850s and 1860s, she was trying to counter beliefs that women were physically and intellectually incapable of practicing medicine or that by their nature they were inclined to practice a gentler, more humane kind of medicine. She liked neither because, in her estimation, they both confined women's sphere of influence: the former by identifying women with the private sphere of the home, denying them access to positions of power in the public arena, the latter by relegating them to what she perceived to be a subordinate place in the medical hierarchy. In challenging these beliefs, Zakrzewska redefined woman, science, and the relationship between the two. She did this by minimizing the biological differences between men's and women's bodies; by promoting and performing women's ability to engage in rational thought; and by insisting upon an intimate connection between science and morality. Zakrzewska, who was convinced "that all [religious] belief weakens the moral sense," maintained, as did other German radicals, that only the embrace of a secular and materialist world could bring about a just and humane society.[38] It did this, they believed, by keeping one focused on fighting the social and economic forces responsible for the production of human misery and by promoting science education, which they cast as the best tool for encouraging the kind of critical thinking required for a democracy to succeed. Zakrzewska, who was determined that women both participate in and benefit from this social transformation, focused her attention on dismantling any notion that women and science stood in opposition to each other.

In her promotion of science in the early decades of her career, Zakrzewska had sounded to some extent like other women physicians who had also emphasized the importance of grounding medical practice in scientific knowledge of the human body. However, where she had stood out was in the political meaning she ascribed to science as a tool of emancipation. This reflected, as I have been arguing throughout this biography, her "position" as a German woman with particularly strong ties to German political radicals. Thus where the vast majority of her peers had sought to bridge "sympathy and science," viewing sympathy as a peculiarly feminine trait that would mitigate against the potential harshness of science, Zakrzewska had seen no reason for science to be monitored. On the contrary, she had viewed it as moral in and of itself. If anything needed monitoring, in her eyes, it was religion.

Significantly, the only other woman physician I am aware of who came close to sharing Zakrzewska's views on science was also influenced by European radical politics. Mary Putnam Jacobi had already turned her back on her Baptist upbringing as a young woman, but it was her experience in Paris, which overlapped with the Paris Commune, that led her to develop an alternative moral framework grounded in Comtian positivism. Jacobi thus came to favor scientific knowledge over metaphysics, the material world over that which cannot be seen, and the cherishing of humanity over the worshiping of a divine being. Like Zakrzewska, then, Jacobi came to see science as more than a tool for acquiring knowledge about the body; it also stood for a particular view of social progress grounded in a materialist, and explicitly antireligious, worldview.[39]

Zakrzewska never abandoned these convictions, yet by the last decade of her life, she viewed things differently. Make no mistake, she remained a materialist, an atheist, and a staunch advocate of both science and women's rights. But she now endowed matter with some sentience, she softened her diatribes against religion, and she viewed the narrow focus on the laboratory as unscientific. She also became an advocate of separate women's institutions just at the time when women's integration into the medical profession—as judged by their increased representation in medical schools and medical societies, their success in securing hospital internships, and their publications in elite medical journals—seemed most secured. To be sure, Zakrzewska's modification of her earlier emphasis on gender integration marked to a great extent her belief that women had not yet been guaranteed true equality. (She turned out, moreover, to be correct.) But her motivations were also more complex. She proved unable, for one, to view her own creation critically, but she also perceived her all-female institution as a necessary tool for guiding younger physicians to a deeper understanding of their professional responsibilities. Some of these responsibilities centered on their obligations to their patients, but Zakrzewska also focused on their obligations to other women physicians and to the "cause" as a whole. Thus where once she had sought to redefine "woman" in order to break down the doors preventing women from claiming their place in the public sphere, she now watched with concern as the kind of moral discourse she had come to take for granted vanished and the values she had fought for no longer seemed to matter to the young.

Zakrzewska was not alone among her generational peers in her distress. We have already mentioned the dismay Paris-trained physicians experienced as their professional authority, identity, and integrity were challenged by a younger generation more excited by the German laboratory sciences. There have also been several excellent studies of the struggles women in particular faced at the turn of the century as they sought to sustain their profession's earlier interest in integrating personal, civic, and professional responsibilities in the face of a new ethos that valued allegiance to one's profession over one's community ties.[40] Zakrzewska's sense of loss must be recognized as part of this growing disillusionment. She may have promoted science and rational medicine louder than some, been more critical of empiricism than others, and scorned any notion that woman's nature was more sympathetic than man's, but she felt no less acutely the attacks being made on an older style of medical practice that had valued judgment as much as science, the doctor-patient relationship as much as laboratory and clinical techniques, and the social context of disease as much as the pathophysiology of the disease itself. For all her differences—and Zakrzewska's materialism and atheism did continue to distinguish her from many of her peers—her complaints about the loss of a moral framework for guiding a physician's actions echoed loudly the concerns of others who were troubled by the way the medical world they had known and shaped was being radically transformed.

On top of it all, Zakrzewska missed the sense of community she had nurtured in her hospital and the feelings she had had of being admired and respected by her students. She missed a sense of allegiance, but what she lamented most was the loss of a sense of mission. This had bound her not only to the first generations of interns, many of whom had felt part of a larger movement to challenge cultural and institutional barriers to women's emancipation, but also to the wider community of Boston social reformers for whom the hospital had been but one part of a large program of social and political reform. The year before her retirement, Zakrzewska gave an address at the opening of the Sewall Maternity House at the New England Hospital. Her talk was filled with memories of the past: of Henry Ingersoll Bowditch's willingness to face "social ostracism" by supporting the cause of women's medical education; of the "spirit of justice" that led the Reverend James Freeman Clarke to support their cause; of Abby W. May, Lucy Goddard, and other "noble women" without whose work and financial support the New England Hospital would never have survived.[41] This was the community in which Zakrzewska's professional identity had taken form. With most of them now deceased, she no longer felt as though the institution was her own. This made her sad, to be sure, and she worried at times that the accomplishments of her generation would not be properly memorialized, but she also realized that her time had passed. "The world changes," she wrote a friend, "& with it, opinions & I am not at all desirous to have it stand still or do & go my way, others must lead & take the responsibility & I am only too glad to leave it in hands who want to have its strings."[42] Besides, she added at her retirement, "I want a few play days; and then I will go out of this life with that feeling of joy which ends a sensible existence."[43]

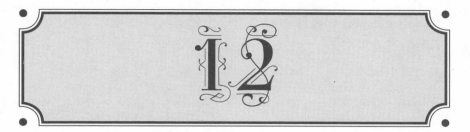

I Wish to Have My Own Way
in Taking Leave

Following her retirement in 1893, Zakrzewska engaged in activities that had long held her interest but for which she had had too little time. High on her list were two organizations, the Roxbury Women's Suffrage League and the New England Women's Club.[1] In both cases, she became almost immediately involved in historical projects—researching the first women's rights conventions for the league and the origin of women's associations for the club—but what she enjoyed most of all were the afternoon teas, lectures, and discussion groups, when she could spend time with old friends like Julia Ward Howe, Ednah Dow Cheney, Anna H. Clarke, Lucy Goddard, and Mary Livermore. Always on the lookout for opportunities to distinguish her generation from the younger one, she insisted that the club's get-togethers had nothing to do with the fashionable "*socials*" of the day, "where one goes once or twice during the whole season, shakes hands with the hosts, says some nothings, meets friends and foes and says more nothings, shakes many hands without knowing why, and takes some refreshment in thimble cups." In sharp contrast, she maintained, the members of the club made up "an association of friends," who met regularly and spent their afternoons listening to and discussing "well expressed thoughts."[2] But whether their conversations were truly more meaningful or not, Zakrzewska enjoyed the opportunity to visit with old friends.

Zakrzewska's retirement also meant that she now had more leisure time to share with her companion, Julia Sprague. By this point their family had, in Sprague's words, become "small, only we two." They had recently moved to a small house in Jamaica Plains, not far from their old Roxbury residence. (This

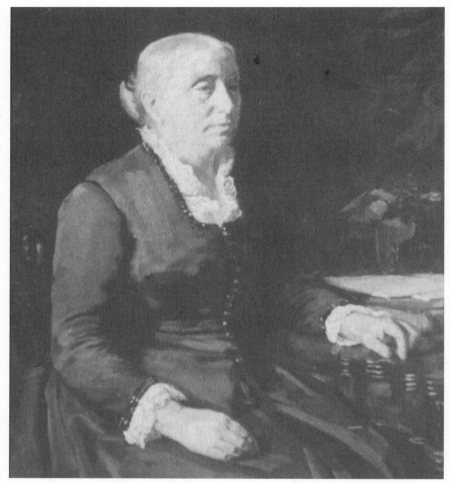

Marie Zakrzewska, ca. the turn of the century. (Courtesy Archives and
Special Collections on Women in Medicine and Homeopathy,
Drexel University College of Medicine)

was, in fact, the second move in less than ten years—they had left Cedar Street
and moved to Boston sometime in the mid-1880s.) As Zakrzewska explained,
scaling down to a smallish residence allowed her to "use the little spare money
to build me a little seashore home retreat." She and Sprague had spent the
summer of 1889 in York Harbor, Maine, and had found it restful for "both body
& mind." Remaining class conscious to the end, Zakrzewska described how

they had selected a spot far away from both "the fashionable" and "the un-fashionable plain people" and built a small cottage that they occupied every summer between 1 July and 15 September. As late as 1899, Sprague was still commenting upon "the perfect rest we have . . . in the beauty of land- and waterscape" every time they traveled to their summer abode.[3]

When Zakrzewska and Sprague were not spending their afternoons at the club or vacationing in York Harbor, they were often traveling. In the winter of 1895, as a surprise present to Sprague on the occasion of her seventieth birthday, Zakrzewska announced that they would be spending the holidays in England. Her hope was that Sprague would find that the "climate suits" her, as she had not been feeling well of late.[4] It also gave Zakrzewska an opportunity to visit once again with Elizabeth Blackwell. The two women had had their rocky moments from time to time, stemming most likely from the tensions that had developed while they were both still working in New York. But Zakrzewska had developed considerable admiration and affection for Blackwell over the years, and she looked forward to sharing memories of the beginning of the women's medical movement and their thoughts on what the future might hold.[5] By all accounts, the visit went well; Zakrzewska and Sprague spent almost three weeks of their three-month sojourn with Blackwell and her daughter, Kitty, attending teas, socializing with other friends, and enjoying the Christmas holiday to-gether. It was to be their last visit. Zakrzewska never returned to Europe; nor did she expect to. Although she was not yet experiencing serious health problems, she was feeling the effects of age. As Sprague wrote Kitty the year after they returned, "I know her, better of course than any one else," and know how much she has always hated letting anyone see her when she was unwell. Now, however, "she has had to find out that she also is mortal and must yield to mortal's fate."[6]

The last long excursion the two women made together was in 1901, one year before Zakrzewska's death. This time they spent ten weeks on the West Coast, visiting Caroline Severance and other friends. Zakrzewska, whose health had deteriorated by this point, thought the trip might provide a distraction from her ills. As she described it, she had begun to have "some confusion of mind" years earlier, which had turned into "noises" in her head by December 1900.[7] Since Sprague was also not well, Zakrzewska hoped the trip would restore both of them to some degree. Zakrzewska did, in fact, appear to be buoyed by this trip. Sprague described in a letter to Severance, one day after they left their friend to head up the coast, how Zakrzewska had forgotten "while at the beach in Mon-terey, that she was not 'sweet 16,' climbed about on the rocks, slipped about on the anemones and sea-weed, etc., and went to bed last night as lame as if she were 70, and today groans with a headache, but as it is improving now, she rouses to say, 'give her my love, and tell her I wish I had half a dozen of her oranges now.' "[8]

Whatever benefits Zakrzewska may have enjoyed from her trip did not last. "I had the benefit of a change," she wrote Blackwell, "but no improvement in the condition of my troublesome head." Most upsetting to her was that she could no longer engage in any mental activities. She found reading too difficult, and even when Sprague read aloud to her in order to keep her abreast of current events, she could barely remember what she had heard the following day. Distressed by her limitations, she felt as though she were "killing the time day after day until the time of everlasting rest will come."[9]

"Everlasting rest" would arrive within the year. Early in 1902, Zakrzewska had a series of angina attacks that, combined with her headaches, made her life "a burden."[10] Still, she held on for several more months, much of that time in pain. Although she continued to walk to the market and ride the cable car every day with Sprague, she could no longer tolerate visits from friends and had reached a point where she needed opium at night in order to get any rest. Unable to engage in any enjoyable activity at all, she shared with Sprague her desire that her life come to an end.[11] That happened on the morning of 16 May 1902, after a restless night. The physician who attended Zakrzewska in the last months of her illness listed "Arterial Schlerosis," "Valvular disease of the heart," and "Apoplexy" as the causes of death. More than likely Zakrzewska suffered a heart attack brought on by hardening of the arteries. This may explain the noises she had been hearing for the previous few years: they may have resulted from an aneurysm caused by the arteriosclerosis.[12]

"Your letter had a little strengthening remark in it," Sprague wrote to Severance a few months after Zakrzewska passed away, "which some day will be of use to me, I hope. No, I ought to be thankful in not having to look on, and 'see her mind farther eclipsed than it was.' "[13] But after forty years together, Sprague was having difficulty adjusting. They had done everything together, from building a home life to traveling, to caring for each other in times of need. "I am living a life so different that I do not know myself," she confided several months later to Kitty Blackwell. "But you will comprehend the difference in my two lives. The void is great, but I am trying to be strong, and what helps me is the knowledge that she understood her disease and wanted to die."[14]

Sprague lived on several more years, supported by her inheritance from Zakrzewska's estate. Realizing that Sprague had become too feeble to care for a home herself, Zakrzewska had placed the Jamaica Plains property in trust for her friend's benefit: Sprague was to have the income, whether the home be sold or rented. Zakrzewska also gave the York Harbor property as a life estate to the trustee's wife, Mrs. Dary, "except," as Sprague explained, "one room, my room which is mine for life, with its contents." Mrs. Dary, Sprague explained, "knew what it meant, that the Dr. wanted her to take care of me, and she wants to do so."[15]

Slowly Sprague adjusted to her loss, feeling blessed that they had had "a rare companionship." What she continued to struggle with, though, especially as she grew increasingly feeble herself, was Zakrzewska's denial of immortality. "I have found myself wondering," she wrote to Severance, "how she could pass on through life, and out of it, as she did, differing from most of those around her, and pass out of sensible living, believing as she did to the last, that *that was all*. Yet she *did go*, and not until she was in another sphere, did she change from what you knew her."[16]

Zakrzewska did pass on without ever accepting the idea of an afterlife, but her denial of immortality did not mean that she was willing to depart this earth without making sure that something more than her friends' memories of her lived on. What she could also leave were her own words, a statement of what her life had meant to her and how she wished to be remembered. Thus, in what may be considered the ultimate assertion of one's independence, Zakrzewska had penned her own eulogy three months before her death, with the request that it be delivered at her funeral.

. . .

On 15 May 1902, three days after Zakrzewska passed away, her friends and acquaintances gathered together one last time to hear her words recited by Emma Merrill Butler, a member of the New England Hospital's board of directors:

> During my whole lifetime, I have had my own way as much as any human being can have it without entirely neglecting social rules or trespassing upon the comfort of others more than is necessary for self-preservation.
>
> And now, upon this occasion, I wish to have my own way in taking leave of those who shall come for the last time to pay such respect as custom, inclination and friendship shall prompt, asking them to accept the assurance that I am sorry to pass from them, this time never to return again.
>
> While these words are being read to you, I shall be sleeping a peaceful, well-deserved sleep—a sleep from which I shall never arise. My body will go

back to that earthly rest whence it came. My soul will live among you, even among those who will come after you.

I am not speaking of fame, nor do I think that my name, difficult though it be, will be remembered. Yet the idea for which I have worked, the seeds which I have tried to sow here and there, must live and spread and bear fruit. And after all, what matters it who prepared the way wherein we walk? We only know that great and good men and women have always lived and worked for an idea which favored progress. And so I have honestly tried to live out my nature—not actuated by an ambition to be somebody or to be remembered especially, but because I could not help it.

The pressure which in head and heart compelled me to see and think ahead, compelled me to love to work for the benefit of womankind in general, irrespective of country or of race. By this, I do not wish to assert that I thought of all women before I thought of myself. Oh, no! It was just as much in me to provide liberally for my tastes, for my wishes, for my needs. I had about as many egotistical wants to be supplied as has the average of womankind.

To look out for self and for those necessary to my happiness, I always considered not only a pleasure but a duty. I despised the weakness of characters who could not say "No" at any time, and thus gave away and sacrificed all their strength of body and mind, as well as their money, with that soft sentimentality which finds assurance in the belief that others will take care of them as they have taken care of others. . . .

And now, in closing, I wish to say farewell to all those who thought of me as a friend, to all those who were kind to me, assuring them all that the deep conviction that there can be no further life is an immense rest and peace to me. I desire no hereafter. I was born; I lived; I used my life to the best of my ability for the uplifting of my fellow creatures; and I enjoyed it daily in a thousand ways. I had many a pang, many a joy, every day of my life; and I am satisfied now to fall victim to the laws of nature, never to rise again, never to see and know again what I have seen and known in my life.

As deeply sorry as I always have been when a friend left me, just so deeply sorry shall I be to leave those whom I loved. Yet I know that I must submit to the inevitable, and submit I do—as cheerfully as a fatal illness will allow. I have already gone in spirit, and now I am going in body. All that I leave behind is my memory in the hearts of the few who always remember those whom they have loved. Farewell.[17]

Rejecting all religious beliefs that an individual's soul lives on after his or her body dies, Zakrzewska nevertheless wanted to make sure that her words would survive her and perhaps shape the memories her friends would take with them when they left her graveside. This was Zakrzewska's last performance, and she used the opportunity to emphasize once again her fierce independence, her sense of duty, and her total lack of any sentimentality. As in her autobiographical sketch, which she had penned forty years earlier, Zakrzewska linked religion and sentimentality and placed them in opposition to materialism and progress. She may not have mentioned science explicitly, but it was nevertheless present in her repeated references to nature. Indeed, as an indication of how Zakrzewska's thoughts had developed since her early adulthood, her eulogy can almost be read as a manifesto for Darwinian evolution and its power to bring about social progress. Certainly influenced by Ernst Haeckel's own reading of Darwin, Zakrzewska left her friends with an image of herself as driven by self-interest and a desire for "self-preservation" to "work for the benefit of womankind." Progress did not require sacrifices; her work for others did not come at her own expense. The laws of nature do not work that way. No, in pursuing what was best for herself she had played her part in creating a better world for others as well.

Zakrzewska clearly wished to go out of this world taking a stand on how one could live a moral life—one committed to social progress—without necessarily embracing any religious beliefs. She knew that this was something many of her American friends, including Sprague, had difficulty understanding, and she tried one last time to reassure them that, rather than being troubled by the absence of a deity, she derived comfort from knowing that she was a part of nature, driven by the same laws that govern the material world and that lead inevitably to social progress.

But perhaps more than anything else, Zakrzewska wished to leave her friends with a final image of herself as strong and resourceful, a type that was an alternative to the stereotypical picture of women as submissive and unable to refuse a request that they sacrifice their own needs for the good of others. She had fought for this alternative image all her adult life, promoting it in her autobiographical sketch and living it to the fullest extent possible. Sprague had once described how Zakrzewska "disliked being thought bodily weak or ailing"; how she was "mortified by any such condition" and went to great pains to hide any signs of physical or mental fatigue, even during her final illness.[18] As Zakrzewska herself shared with her friend Ednah Cheney just a few years before her death: "I am still proud enough as a woman not to serve as an example of woman's frailty, which will lead to a sad ending in life."[19]

Zakrzewska's closest friends may have seen another side of her—the woman who felt exhausted by all the responsibilities she had taken on, who felt immeasurable grief at the loss of loved ones, who regretted some decisions she had made, or who even let go of herself enough to skip around on the rocks on the beach—but it was a side of herself that she kept tightly under wraps. Even Sprague's letters suggest that she and Zakrzewska had come to know each other more by simply going through life together rather than by discussing their feelings in any great depth.[20] Zakrzewska was an immensely private person, one who left no diary and relatively few letters that would allow one to learn more about her personal reflections. The letters that survived in Caroline Severance's papers were an exception. Another cache of letters that Zakrzewska had written to Cheney might have been just as enlightening, but Sprague deemed them too revealing for public consumption.[21] In what she must have considered one of her last acts of love, she destroyed the letters that Zakrzewska certainly would not have wanted anyone to see.

· · ·

Zakrzewska had no wish to have her personal life paraded before others; rather, she wished her name to be identified with an idea, both during her lifetime and afterward. That idea was justice, particularly in the name of women.[22] She had cast her net wide, trying to work in general "for the benefit of womankind," but her greatest contribution was to those women who wished to enter the medical profession. Among the first generation of women to graduate from medical school and founder of one of the first hospitals where women could receive clinical training, she had fought hard to guarantee that women would receive the best training possible. For Zakrzewska, that meant learning not only diagnostic techniques, such as microscopy and thermometry, but, more important, the use of reason, critical judgment, and rational deductions in determining the best therapeutic regimen. This approach, vague to be sure, nevertheless captures most closely what Zakrzewska meant by the term "science": rather than a specific method, it referred to an entire way of thinking, one that, very much in Enlightenment fashion, was expected to dispel prejudice, poverty, and disease, helping to bring about a world in which justice and humanity would reign.

That was not, however, the direction medicine followed. By the time of Zakrzewska's death in 1902, a rather different understanding of scientific medicine had taken hold. Instead of a worldview, science referred more specifically to the methods associated with strict scientific protocols. The results of this approach—the discovery of ever more disease-causing microbes; the production of the first vaccines and therapeutic treatments, such as diphtheria antitoxin; and the development of new diagnostic tools, such as X-rays—hailed a new day in which specific medicines would target specific diseases, but they also functioned to further divorce disease from its social context. These developments were, moreover, accompanied by a change in the site of medical practice—more and more medicine was practiced in the hospital rather than in the home—and by changes in medical training. Higher entrance requirements, longer periods of study, more attention to the basic and clinical sciences, and, ultimately, the expectation that students would pursue postgraduate internships all marked the increased standardization of medical training and the growing prestige of a style of medical practice that circulated around the laboratory and the clinic. Indeed, just eight years after Zakrzewska's death, Abraham Flexner published his famous muckraking report that, taking the Johns Hopkins Medical School as its ideal, cemented in place an educational model that privileged the physician-as-researcher over the physician-as-practitioner; this model led ultimately to the demise of medical schools that had as their primary goal the training of physicians who would treat the everyday health problems of their local communities.[23]

Most of these changes were made in the name of science, but the meaning ascribed to the term only loosely overlapped with what Zakrzewska had so loudly proclaimed. When, for example, educational reformers referred to modern science as a way of developing a critical habit of mind, then it had some resemblance to Zakrzewska's notion, although the political meaning she had ascribed to science was lost. When, however, the claim was made that scientific thinking could only, or even best, be learned in the laboratory, especially when it was linked with a style of medical practice that ignored the wider context of disease, then it had little to do with the scientific approach that Zakrzewska had promoted her entire life.

Zakrzewska had voiced her displeasure with many of these changes before her death. She had, however, only vaguely understood the effect these changes would have in particular on women physicians. Even before Flexner published his report, all-female medical colleges had begun closing their doors, unable to raise the funds necessary to implement such reforms as the building and furnishing of teaching clinics and laboratories. At first some women viewed the increase in coeducational institutions as a clear sign of progress, but this optimism turned out to be short lived. Whereas women made up 5 percent of the medical student body in 1899, three years after Zakrzewska's death they had dropped to 3.5 percent and then to an all-time low of 2.9 percent in 1910. This drop marked a decline in absolute numbers as well, from 1,063 students in 1899 to 573 eleven years later.[24]

As historians of women and medicine have revealed, the reasons for this decline were varied and complex. Overt discrimination, such as the implementation of sex-based quotas, certainly played a role. The loss of female role models —coeducational institutions, unlike the all-female medical schools, rarely hired female educators—also contributed to an atmosphere that could be inhospitable to women. Another factor that worked to lower the numbers of women studying medicine was the greater investment of time and money that an elite medical education now demanded. For some this meant that their families were now reluctant or unable to finance their careers; for others, the four years of study following graduation from college meant a greater commitment and sacrifice than they were willing to make. In fact, the medical profession simply lost its appeal for some. Whether this reflected the increasingly masculine image of the scientist-physician, the greater difficulty women experienced trying to balance family and career, or the gradual severing of modern medicine from any kind of social reform agenda, the result was that in addition to the structural impediments to women's pursuit of medicine, a growing number of women no longer seem to have been as drawn to medicine as their predecessors once were.[25] Zakrzewska would most assuredly have watched all this with great sadness, disturbed both by medicine's embrace of a research ethic that often lost sight of the people it was trying to serve and by women's gradual exclusion from the elite echelons of the profession. I am not sure, though, that she would have been totally surprised. Her skeptical attitude toward coeducational institutions in the last decade of her life had reflected her deep suspicion that the United States was not yet ready to grant women full equality with men. She was right.

· · ·

In the twentieth century, as women physicians continued to struggle to achieve fair representation, Zakrzewska's story would occasionally be told in the interest of advancing women's medical careers. Thus in 1924, Agnes Vietor, previously an assistant surgeon at the New England Hospital, published *A Woman's Quest: The Life of Marie E. Zakrzewska, M.D.* This 514-page biography, written largely from materials Zakrzewska had given to Vietor, served a particular purpose for the author. At the time, a good medical education had come to include a year's internship following graduation from medical school, yet women faced a new wave of discrimination when they applied to fill these posts. Vietor thus used Zakrzewska's biography to argue for the injustice of keeping the doors to hospital and clinical internships closed to women. "[T]he battle which she [Zakrzewska] faced and fought is not ended," Vietor told her readers. "It remains for all lovers of justice to sustain the impulsion which carried her on and so to continue the fight till the truth of her watchword, 'Science has no sex,' is acknowledged. Then, and only then, will her life's work be fulfilled."[26]

Vietor, who fully embraced the role hospitals had come to play as "great centers of laboratory and clinical investigation and research," worried little that Zakrzewska, at the end of her life, had viewed such a development critically. What Zakrzewska symbolized to her was not a particular medical style but rather a quest to prove that women had the same ability as men to think scientifically and should, therefore, be granted opportunities "on equal terms with men."[27] It was Zakrzewska's insistence that "science has no sex" to which she drew most attention because she continued to believe that the greatest obstacle before her remained the notion that gender differences existed in men's and women's scientific abilities. To Vietor, Zakrzewska's life was "one more document testifying to the Humanity of Woman," a humanity that was "neither male nor female; it is both."[28]

When World War II broke out, Zakrzewska's name was once again used in the service of advancing women's cause, this time as part of a battle to give women physicians, in Dr. Emily Dunning Barringer's words, "complete equality as to rank and professional status within the Medical Reserve Corps of the Army." Barringer, president of the American Medical Women's Association in 1942, had been spending much of her time in Washington trying to convince Congress to pass legislation that would allow women to receive these commissions.[29] Whether it was her idea to feature Zakrzewska in an installment of the Du Pont Corporation's series "Cavalcade of America" is unclear, but she clearly played a role.[30] At the end of the broadcast, Barringer gave an impassioned speech defending women's right "to stand shoulder to shoulder with their male colleagues."[31]

"That They Might Live," which aired on 19 October 1942, opens at the Charité, where Zakrzewska, portrayed as a physician rather than as a midwife, has just successfully completed "a very delicate operation."[32] Her mentor, "Dr. Joseph," informs her immediately that, despite objections from those who are vehemently opposed to women doctors, he plans to hand over to her the directorship of the hospital when he steps down. That, of course, does not happen. As soon as Doctor Joseph passes away, Zakrzewska is derided as the "daughter of a Polish mid-wife" and dismissed. From this moment until the end of the episode, which concludes in America with the founding of the New England Hospital, Zakrzewska is cast as a symbol of "progress" in battle with those who represent "the age of darkness." Armed with microscopes, test tubes, thermometers, a strong sense of justice, and compassion for the poor, she conquers misery, ignorance, and prejudice.

Although in different ways, both Vietor and Barringer embraced the link Zakrzewska had made between science, progress, and morality. Their goal was to ensure that women be allowed to participate in the scientific work that would promote not only their own careers but also a better world in which to live. When Zakrzewska was rediscovered in the 1970s, however, the link between science and morality had been subjected to a devastating critique. The disillusionment with an idea that had inspired Enlightenment thinkers and nineteenth-century radicals alike had grown in the immediate World War II period as intellectuals considered with horror both Germany's use of science and technology to mastermind the Holocaust and the coming together of great scientific intellects to produce the ultimate weapon of destruction, the atom bomb. Within a few decades, feminists had added to this critique an analysis of the way professional communities used science to erect institutional barriers and to define constrictive social roles that made it difficult for women to enter the public sphere. It is hardly surprising that science itself would come to be seen by many as antithetical to the advancement of women's goals, a position from which it was impossible to make sense of Zakrzewska's own convictions. Small wonder a confusing picture of her emerged, one that, in the end, showed her at best to be embracing a masculine discourse for strategic purposes, determined that women achieve equality in a man's world.

The first wave of feminist scholarship is responsible for exposing many of the deep-seated cultural, political, and institutional barriers that functioned to deny women power. Over the past few decades, however, a number of feminist scholars have been questioning the very binary oppositions that had once shaped this work. Thus, instead of continuing to contrast public and private, masculinity and femininity, professionalism and feminism, heterosexuality and homosexuality, morality and science, they now employ concepts such as "situatedness" and "positionality" to draw our attention to how such binary oppositions function to erase the great multiplicity of positions that fit uncomfortably on one side or the other of the dyad.[33] In terms of the scholarship on women and science, some of the most exciting new work asks no longer whether women have a different style when they practice medicine. Instead, it focuses on whether a feminist perspective, defined as the embodiment of a commitment to gender equality, can make a difference in how science is practiced. This approach has several advantages: it encourages us to look at the questions that are deemed important as much as the methodological styles that are employed; it allows for a multiplicity of styles in the practice of science but does not assume that these styles stem from the sex of the practitioner; and since both men and women can be feminists, it views a scientist's political orientation as more important than his or her sex.[34]

Zakrzewska's story brings home the power of these feminist insights, for although she lived in a society very much structured by a discourse of binary opposites, she found cracks and fissures that allowed her to position herself differently than many of her peers. She did not, like the majority of her colleagues, justify women's entry into the medical profession by embracing a picture of women as more nurturing and compassionate. Instead, she set out to redefine women by emphasizing their rational capabilities, thus claiming science for women and using it as a weapon against the arguments put forth to keep them from claiming their rightful place in the public sphere. Most significant, Zakrzewska insisted that science, morality, and social progress went hand in hand. Inspired by German radical thought, she viewed science as a political weapon in the battle against all forms of inhumanity, but especially against sexual discrimination. In the end, Zakrzewska's project faltered. She proved unable to fully disassociate science from gender and to link it with a vision of freedom. But the debate that animated Zakrzewska and others in the nineteenth century has not yet been put to rest, bringing home the importance of continuing Zakrzewska's battle to prove that "science has no sex."

NOTES

AR Annual Report of the New-England Hospital for Women and Children. Boston: Prentiss and Deland, 1863–1902.

Countway Boston Medical Library in the Francis A. Countway Library of Medicine, Boston, Massachusetts.

Dall Papers Caroline Healey Dall Papers, Massachusetts Historical Society, Boston, Massachusetts.

GStA PK Geheimes Staatsarchiv Preussischer Kulturbesitz, Files of the Ministry of Culture, Berlin, Germany.

HL Huntington Library, San Marino, California.

LBC Labadie Collection, Ann Arbor, Michigan.

LC Library of Congress, Washington, D.C.

NEHWC New England Hospital for Women and Children.

PBL Potsdam-Brandenburgisches Landeshauptarchiv, Potsdam, Germany.

PI Marie E. Zakrzewska. *A Practical Illustration of "Woman's Right to Labor"; or, A Letter from Marie E. Zakrzewska, M.D.* Edited by Caroline H. Dall. Boston: Walker, Wise, and Co., 1860.

Severance Papers Caroline Maria Seymour Severance Papers, Huntington Library, San Marino, California.

SL Schlesinger Library, Radcliffe, Cambridge, Massachusetts.

SS Sophia Smith Collection, Smith College, Northampton, Massachusetts.

UA der HUB Universitätsarchiv der Humboldt Universität zu Berlin, Berlin, Germany.

WQ Agnes Vietor, ed. *A Woman's Quest: The Life of Marie E. Zakrzewska, M.D.* 1924. New York: Arno Press, 1972.

Zakrzewski file Martin Ludwig Zakrzewski's personnel file, Rep. 76 I, Sekt. 31, Lit. Z, Nr. 2, Geheimes Staatsarchiv Preussischer Kulturbesitz, Files of the Ministry of Culture, Berlin, Germany.

INTRODUCTION

1. "That They Might Live," Archives and Special Collections on Women in Medicine and Homeopathy, Drexel University College of Medicine, Philadelphia, Pa. On "The Cavalcade of America," see Grams, *History of the Cavalcade of America*; Grams, "Cavalcade of America"; and Riley, Lucas, and Pettit, "Cavalcade of America."

2. For earlier works on Zakrzewska, see *WQ*; Walsh, *"Doctors Wanted"*; Drachman, *Hospital with a Heart*; Morantz-Sanchez, *Sympathy and Science* (unless noted otherwise, all citations of this work are to the 1985 edition); and Abram, *"Send Us a Lady Physician."* While the medical school Zakrzewska attended was popularly known as Cleveland Medical College, its official name at the time was the Medical Department of Western Reserve College. In 1967 Western Reserve University joined with the Case Institute of Technology to form Case Western Reserve University.

3. The first quotation is from Mary Putnam Jacobi, "Women in Medicine," 166. The second is from Mary A. Smith, who interned at the New England Hospital in 1874; cited in *Fiftieth Anniversary of the New England Hospital*, 14.

4. Cited in *WQ*, 459.

5. [Zakrzewska] Eine "Aerztinn," "Weibliche Aerzte." On nineteenth-century women physicians' use of satire, see Wells, *Out of the Dead House*, 92–99.

6. See Abram, *"Send Us a Lady Physician"*; Blake, "Women and Medicine in Ante-Bellum America"; Cayleff, *Wash and Be Healed*; Drachman, *Hospital with a Heart*; Moldow, *Women Doctors in Gilded-Age Washington*; Morantz, Pomerleau, and Fenichel, *In Her Own Words*; Morantz-Sanchez, *Sympathy and Science*; Shryock, "Women in American Medicine"; and Walsh, *"Doctors Wanted."* For more recent studies, see, among others, Bittel, "Science of Women's Rights"; Bonner, *To the Ends of the Earth*; Kirschmann, *Vital Force*; Morantz-Sanchez, *Conduct Unbecoming a Woman*; More, *Restoring the Balance*; Peitzman, *New and Untried Course*; Schoepflin, *Christian Science on Trial*; and Silver-Isenstadt, *Shameless*. See also the new preface in the 2000 republication of Morantz-Sanchez, *Sympathy and Science*, ix–xxxi.

7. Morantz-Sanchez, *Sympathy and Science*.

8. Zakrzewska, *Introductory Lecture*; Morantz, " 'Connecting Link.' "

9. On mid-nineteenth-century American physicians' attitudes toward German medicine, see Warner, *Therapeutic Perspective*, esp. chaps. 3 and 6, and the very moving final chapter of Warner, *Against the Spirit of System*, 330–64.

10. Ackerknecht, "Beiträge zur Geschichte der Medizinalreform." I discuss this program in detail in Tuchman, *Science, Medicine, and the State*.

11. On the German radical community in America, see Levine, *Spirit of 1848*; Nadel, *Little Germany*; Brancaforte, *German Forty-Eighters*, esp. the article by Hamerow, "Two Worlds of the Forty-Eighters"; and McCormick, *Germans in America*.

12. Cited in Wells, *Out of the Dead House*, 77–78. For a brief discussion of the place of religion, orthodox or unorthodox, in the lives of nineteenth-century women physicians in the United States, see Morantz-Sanchez, *Sympathy and Science*, 102–6, 187–88. The only other well-known nineteenth-century female physician who came close to sharing Zakrzewska's views

on scientific materialism was Mary Putnam Jacobi. See Bittel, "Science of Women's Rights"; Harvey, "*La Visite*"; and Harvey, "Medicine and Politics."

13. On religion and American radicals, see, for example, Perry, *Radical Abolitionism*; Lerner, *Grimké Sisters from South Carolina*; and Grodzins, *American Heretic*.

14. Some classic examples of this interpretative framework are Wood, " 'Fashionable Diseases' "; Ehrenreich and English, *For Her Own Good*; and Drachman, *Hospital with a Heart*. While Drachman presented a more complex picture than the other two, she nevertheless subscribed to this dichotomy.

15. Compare Drachman, *Hospital with a Heart*, 39, 150–53; Walsh, *"Doctors Wanted,"* 58–59, 86; and Morantz-Sanchez, *Sympathy and Science*, 63, 133–34, 177.

16. Morantz-Sanchez, *Sympathy and Science*, 200.

17. In *Sympathy and Science*, Morantz-Sanchez did much to challenge this dichotomy by representing the great diversity of positions women physicians held in the past. Nevertheless, the chapter in which she compared Elizabeth Blackwell and Mary Putnam Jacobi, although intended to represent two ends of a spectrum, had a tendency to reify this dichotomy. Morantz-Sanchez's own realization of this led her to write a subsequent piece, "Feminist Theory and Historical Practice," in which she cast Blackwell as someone who, while critical of modern laboratory methods and especially vivisection, nevertheless valued knowledge derived from scientific methods of investigation as long as it was combined with knowledge acquired through such qualities as sympathy and compassion. See also More, *Restoring the Balance*.

18. Leavitt, " 'Worrying Profession.' "

19. Morantz-Sanchez, *Conduct Unbecoming a Woman*; Bittel, "Science of Women's Rights."

20. See, for example, Alcoff, "Cultural Feminism versus Poststructuralism," and the various essays in Nicholson, *Second Wave*.

21. Alcoff, "Cultural Feminism versus Poststructuralism." See also Fraser, "Structuralism or Pragmatics?," 391; Keller, "Developmental Biology as a Feminist Cause?," 17; and Haraway, "Situated Knowledges."

22. Butler, *Gender Trouble*, esp. 134–41.

23. *WQ*, 359.

24. Bonner, *To the Ends of the Earth*, 32–48.

25. On the idealized feminine type, see Welter, "Cult of True Womanhood." On the rhetoric of domesticity, see Sklar, *Catherine Beecher*, and Evans, *Born for Liberty*, 101. For a provocative analysis of the transgressive gender performances of nineteenth-century American women physicians, see Wells, *Out of the Dead House*.

26. *WQ*, 268.

27. Zakrzewska to Paulina Pope, 28 October 1901, NEHWC Collection, box 1, SS. On Heinzen, see Wittke, *Against the Current*.

28. *WQ*, 296–97. I have been unable to find much biographical information on Sprague. Most of what I know I have culled from her own correspondence and the occasional reference to her in histories of the New England Women's Club.

29. Sprague wrote these letters between 1886 and 1911. They are all housed in the Caroline

Maria Seymour Severance Papers at the Huntington Library in San Marino, California. I am grateful to Virginia Elwood-Akers, who is writing a biography of Caroline Severance, for informing me of these letters and for arranging to have them copied and sent to me.

30. On women's relationships in the nineteenth century, see Smith-Rosenberg, "Female World of Love and Ritual"; Sahli, "Smashing"; Rupp, " 'Imagine My Surprise' "; and Faderman, *Surpassing the Love of Men*. On Boston marriages in particular, see di Leonardo, "Warrior Virgins and Boston Marriages," and Freedman, *Maternal Justice*, esp. 107, 178, 242.

31. On the New England Hospital for Women and Children, see Drachman, *Hospital with a Heart*. This study, now twenty years old, looks at this hospital as both a medical institution and an example of the all-women's institutions founded in the nineteenth century to provide a public space for women excluded from all-male schools and clubs. I build on Drachman's work in my chapters on the New England Hospital, although I place greater emphasis on a third context for understanding the hospital: as one of many charitable institutions founded in the second half of the nineteenth century to deal with the rapidly increasing number of poor. I also do not always share her assessment of the reasons for the hospital's decline.

32. On social welfare in the nineteenth-century United States, see Boyer, *Urban Masses*; Gordon, *Pitied but Not Entitled*; Katz, *In the Shadow of the Poorhouse*; Kunzel, *Fallen Women, Problem Girls*; Rosenberg, *Care of Strangers*; and Vogel, *Invention of the Modern Hospital*, 9–19.

33. On the policies at other hospitals, see Kass, *Midwifery and Medicine*, 103; Vogel, *Invention of the Modern Hospital*, 35; and Quiroga, *Poor Mothers and Babies*, 63–64. On Zakrzewska's defense of unwed mothers, see, for example, Zakrzewska, "Report of the Attending Physician," *AR*, 1868, 9–21.

34. See Rosenberg, "Inward Vision and Outward Glance"; Rosenberg, *Care of Strangers*; and Starr, *Social Transformation of American Medicine*.

35. Walsh, *"Doctors Wanted,"* 76–105. Chapter 3 of this book, which deals solely with the New England Hospital, is entitled "Feminist Showplace."

36. Ibid., 76. On the founding of all women's institutions in the nineteenth-century United States, see Freedman, "Separatism as Strategy."

37. Morantz-Sanchez, *Sympathy and Science*, 66–89.

38. Ibid., 73–74; More, *Restoring the Balance*, esp. 16–23, 45–56; Wells, *Out of the Dead House*, 126–28.

39. Kirschmann, *Vital Force*, 1–6; Rogers, "American Homeopathy Confronts Scientific Medicine" and *Alternative Path*, 1–9; and Warner, "Orthodoxy and Otherness."

40. Ludmerer, *Learning to Heal*.

41. See Drachman, *Hospital with a Heart*, 127; Walsh, *"Doctors Wanted,"* 83–84; More, " 'Empathy' Enters the Profession of Medicine," 25.

42. On the multiple meanings of science within the nineteenth-century American medical community, see the work of John Harley Warner, especially "Ideals of Science and Their Discontents" and *Against the Spirit of System*.

43. Rosenberg, *Care of Strangers*; Rothstein, *American Physicians in the Nineteenth Century*; Starr, *Social Transformation of American Medicine*; and Ludmerer, *Learning to Heal*.

44. Morantz-Sanchez, *Sympathy and Science*; More, *Restoring the Balance*; and Walsh, *"Doctors Wanted."*

45. The literature is quite large. For some examples, see Abir-Am and Outram, *Uneasy Careers and Intimate Lives*; Kohlstedt, "Women in the History of Science"; Kohlstedt and Longino, "Women, Gender, and Science Questions"; Rossiter, *Women Scientists in America: Struggles and Strategies* and *Women Scientists in America: Before Affirmative Action*; and Schiebinger, *Mind Has No Sex?*

46. See, for example, Benjamin, *Science and Sensibility*; Jordanova, *Sexual Visions*; Keller, *Reflections on Gender and Science* and "Gender and Science"; and Schiebinger, *Nature's Body* and *Has Feminism Changed Science?*

CHAPTER ONE

1. Marie's last name is the feminine form of the family name and thus is different from her father's. Personal information on the Zakrzewski family is drawn largely from the Zakrzewski file in the Prussian archives. For useful definitions of the German bourgeoisie, see Blackbourn and Evans, *German Bourgeoisie*, xiv. See also Conze and Kocka, *Bildungsbürgertum im 19. Jahrhundert*, and Habermas, *Frauen und Männer*.

2. Sheehan, *German History*, 432.

3. This comment was from the writer Heinrich Laube; cited in ibid., 513. On the place of the *Bildungsbürgertum* in Prussian state reforms, see ibid., 291–310; Blackbourn, "German Bourgeoisie"; and Koselleck, *Preussen zwischen Reform und Revolution*.

4. Zakrzewski to the state minister, 13 July 1841, Zakrzewski file, 89.

5. The quotations are from J. Meyer, *Das grosse Conversations-Lexicon* (1848), cited in Hausen, "Family and Role Division," 54. See also Frevert, *Women in German History*, and Habermas, *Frauen und Männer*.

6. On the Prussian government's desire to attract "cultivated women [gebildete Frauen]" to midwifery, see the correspondence between the mayor of Berlin and the Ministry of Interior, 19 September 1817, 29 April 1818, and 12 June 1818, Zakrzewski file, 7–10, 48–52, 53–56.

7. *Marie Elizabeth Zakrzewska: A Memoir*, 7. This story is repeated in *WQ*, 483 n. 1. On the importance of reading such stories as legends and not simply factual accounts, see Davis, *Fiction in the Archives*, and White, *Content of the Form*.

8. Klaus Zernack, professor emeritus of history at the Free University in Berlin, pers. comm. Martin Ludwig claimed that his father had come to Prussia in 1787, yet the second partitioning of Poland, when Russia claimed Polish territory, occurred in 1793. See Zakrzewski to the state minister, 11 June 1842, Zakrzewski file, 105–6.

9. Davies, *God's Playground*, 1:369. On the Polish nobility, see ibid., 201–55, 321–72, 511–46.

10. Smith, *German Nationalism and Religious Conflict* and *Protestants, Catholics, and Jews*.

11. The information on Zakrzewska's grandfather is from the following letters: Zakrzewski to the king, 24 November 1839, and Zakrzewski to the state minister, 11 June 1842, Zakrzewski file, 28–29, 105–6.

12. La Vopa, *Prussian Schoolteachers*, 38.

13. Ibid., 53. On the reform of the elementary school system, see ibid., 17–77. For a brief

discussion of Prussian educational reform, see Sheehan, *German History*, 513–16, and Nipperdey, *Deutsche Geschichte*, 451–82.

14. La Vopa, *Prussian Schoolteachers*, 32; Koselleck, *Preussen zwischen Reform und Revolution*, 78–115. The list of who counted as an *Eximierte* is from Frevert, *Women in German History*, 32.

15. Sheehan, *German History*, 291–310; Rosenberg, *Bureaucracy, Aristocracy, and Autocracy*, 207.

16. Martin Ludwig never tired of pointing out that his father's struggles to support the family had made it impossible for him to attend good schools or the university. See, for example, Zakrzewski to the king, 24 November 1839, Zakrzewski file, 28–29.

17. Martin Ludwig mentioned that not only had his father tutored him privately but the services of a local preacher had been engaged for this purpose as well. See Zakrzewski to the king, 24 November 1839, and Zakrzewski to the state minister, 7 May 1840, Zakrzewski file, 28–29, 49–50. On the internship system, see Sheehan, *German History*, 519–20.

18. This information is culled from the following sources: a military attest of Zakrzewski's service, dated 18 July 1837; Zakrzewski to the state minister, 20 November 1838, 29 June 1839, and 13 July 1841; and Zakrzewski to the king, 24 November 1839, all in Zakrzewski file, 17, 7–8, 16, 89–94, 28–29.

19. *PI*, 32.

20. Zakrzewski to the state minister, 13 July 1841, Zakrzewski file, 89–94; quotation on 89. See also his letters to the state minister on 13 October 1837 and 29 June 1839, in ibid., 2, 16–17.

21. Zakrzewski to the state minister, 20 November 1838 and 25 August 1839, in ibid., 7–8, 20–22.

22. Sophie was probably born in 1830, Anna in 1833, and Herman in 1834. The stillbirth probably occurred in 1832. I have made these determinations based on information culled from the following: *PI*, 19, 22, 93, 127; Zakrzewski to the state minister, 5 October 1843 and 25 October 1856, Zakrzewski file, 122–23, 333–34.

23. Zakrzewski to the state minister, 13 July 1841, Zakrzewski file, 89–94. Although the letter is dated 1841, Zakrzewski is referring to his situation at the time he first requested a civilian position in 1831.

Although exact figures are difficult to come by, a salary of thirty taler per month (or the equivalent of 1,080 marks a year) probably placed the Zakrzewski family in the top 10–20 percent of the population as far as earning power was concerned. Even as late as 1849, a beginning government clerk did not earn much more. These judgments are based on a series of tables collected in Fischer, Krengel, and Wietog, *Sozialgeschichtliches Arbeitsbuch I*. See esp. the tables on 122–25, 153, and 161–65. In addition, Levine (*Spirit of 1848*, 19) cites a nineteenth-century source that claimed one needed at least 400 gulden (or 225 taler) to achieve personal independence.

24. *Marie Elizabeth Zakrzewska: A Memoir*, 8. This story is repeated in *WQ*, 484 n. 1.

25. Fraser, *Gypsies*; Hancock, introduction to *The Gypsies of Eastern Europe*, ed. Crow and Kolsti, and "Gypsy History in Germany and Neighboring Lands."

26. Zakrzewski to Adalbert von Ladenberg, minister of culture, 30 October 1849, Zakrzewski file, 185–86. Zakrzewska discusses her experiences visiting her grandfather at the almshouse in *PI*, 26–31.

27. Frevert, *Women in German History.*

28. Zakrzewski to the state minister, 13 July 1841, Zakrzewski file, 89–94.

29. Zakrzewski to the state minister, 25 October 1856, in ibid., 333–34. See also *PI*, 148.

30. Zakrzewski mentions Ladenberg's help in a letter to the state minister, 13 October 1837, Zakrzewski file, 2. See also *PI*, 33. On Ladenberg's various positions in the Prussian government, see Lüdicke, *Die Preußischen Kultusminister*, Beilage II. On Caroline Fredericke's repeated attempts to gain entry to the school of midwifery, see Zakrzewski to the state minister, 13 July 1841, Zakrzewski file, 89–94.

31. For information on the general course of instruction at the midwifery school, see Augustin, *Die Königlich Preußische Medicinalverfassung*, 526–33. See also Sudhoff, "Aus der Geschichte des Charite-Krankenhauses zu Berlin," and Diepgen and Heischkel, *Die Medizin an der Berliner Charité.* The special arrangements for the midwifery pupils from Berlin are spelled out in Schmidt, "Die geburtshülflich-klinischen Institute," 503.

32. Caroline Fredericke is listed as a licensed practitioner in *Verzeichneß der approbirten und praktisirenden Hebammen*, PBL, Rep. 30 Berlin, C-Polizei Präsidium, Tit. 50, Nr. 2234, p. 109.

33. Zakrzewski to the state minister, 16 October 1846, Zakrzewski file, 145.

34. Zakrzewski to the state minister, 13 July 1841, in ibid., 89–94.

35. The material on this turf battle is extensive and can be found in GStA PK, Rep. 76 Va, Sekt. 2, Tit. X, Nr. 8, Bd. V, pp. 135–256. See also Tuchman, "'True Assistant to the Obstetrician.'" For Caroline Fredericke's particular role in this battle, see the Ministry of Culture to the midwives Freyer, Zakrzewski, and Genossin, 14 January 1842, which mentions the complaint they registered on 4 December 1841, in PBL, Rep. 30 Berlin, C-Polizei Präsidium, Tit. 50, Nr. 2232, pp. 51–52, and Eichhorn to the midwives Freyer, Zakrzewski (spelled Zackrzewski in the original), and Zimmerman geb. Meinicke, 3 December 1847, which mentions the complaint they registered on 12 July 1845, in GStA PK, Rep. 76 Va, Sekt. 2, Tit. X, Nr. 8, Bd. VI, p. 84. For the deliveries Caroline Fredericke Zakrzewski carried out through Busch's polyclinic, see the lists Busch submitted to Eichhorn on 27 July 1850, 8 February 1851, 29 September 1851, 26 January 1852, 21 September 1852, 15 January 1853, and 30 August 1853, all in ibid., 193–203, 216–26, 235–43, 248–56, 272–79, 372–75, 383–86.

36. *PI*, 55–56.

37. See Chapter 10 of this book.

38. Zakrzewski to the state minister, 20 November 1838, Zakrzewski file, 7–8. See also the War Ministry's explanation of why he lost his pension, in its letter to Altenstein, 2 May 1840, in ibid., 44–45. For Zakrzewski's various positions and promotions, see Zakrzewski to the state minister, 13 October 1837; Felgentreff to the state minister, 29 June 1838; State Ministry to the General Registrar (General = Kasse), 7 July 1838, all in ibid., 2, 4, 5. On the status of nineteenth-century German civil servants, see Sheehan, *German History*, 504–23.

39. Zakrzewski to the state minister, 13 July 1841, Zakrzewski file, 89–94.

40. Zakrzewski to the state minister, 5 October 1842, in ibid, 116–17. On Zakrzewski's promotion, see the state minister to Zakrzewski, 12 August 1841, in ibid., 95. On the scripted nature of many archival documents, see Davis, *Fiction in the Archives.*

41. On Rosalie's birth, see Zakrzewski to the state minister, 27 October 1844 and 25 October 1856, Zakrzewski file, 132, 333–34. On the birth of their seventh child, see Zakrzew-

ski to the state minister, 9 February 1847, in ibid., 148. On Caroline Fredericke's dropsy, see Zakrzewski to the state minister, 5 April 1847, in ibid., 150–51. On the nineteenth-century German middle class and the ideology of separate spheres, see Hausen, "Family and Role Division."

42. Zakrzewski to the state minister, 16 October 1846, Zakrzewski file, 145.

43. In 1838, Zakrzewski mentioned that his two older daughters were in school and that it was costing him 2.25 taler per month. See Zakrzewski to the state minister, 20 November 1838, in ibid., 7–8. For other discussions of his children's schooling, see his letters to the state minister on 5 October 1843 and 5 April 1847, in ibid., 122–23, 150–51. On girls' seminaries, see Albisetti, *Schooling German Girls and Women*.

44. La Vopa, *Prussian Schoolteachers*, 25–51; Schöler, *Geschichte des naturwissenschaftlichen Unterrichts*; Sheehan, *German History*, 513–16; Tuchman, *Science, Medicine, and the State*, 44–49.

45. Herman Zakrzewski began attending the *höhere Bürgerschule* run by Marggraff on Sophien-Kirchgasse in October 1843. See Zakrzewski to the state minister, 5 October 1843, Zakrzewski file, 122–23. Herman ended up becoming an engineer. See *PI*, 127.

46. *PI*, 39. On the content of the curriculum in the girls' seminaries, see Albisetti, *Schooling German Girls and Women*.

47. Zakrzewski to the state minister, 5 October 1843, Zakrzewski file, 122–23.

48. See *PI*, 25. Zakrzewski mentions his daughters' confirmations in his letters to the state minister on 19 January 1845, 3 September 1848, and 28 December 1848, all in Zakrzewski file, 135–36, 174–75, 176.

49. Zakrzewski to the state minister, 9 February 1847, in ibid., 148.

50. Zakrzewski's worst bout of illness had been in the summer of 1840, when he had landed in the Charité hospital for almost two months, convinced that his own death was imminent. See Zakrzewski to the state minister on 5 May 1840, 7 May 1840, and 11 May 1840, in ibid., 46, 49–50, 52. On his other bouts of illness, see Zakrzewski to the state minister, 25 August 1839 and 25 May 1848; Felgentreff to the state minister, 6 November 1843 and 17 December 1843; and Wiegner to the state minister, 3 July 1851, in ibid., 20–22, 161–62, 125, 130, 202.

51. Hachtmann, *Berlin 1848*; Sheehan, *German History*, 656–729; Siemann, *Gesellschaft im Aufbruch*.

52. Hachtmann, *Berlin 1848*; Sheehan, *German History*, 665–69.

53. "Extract," no date, Zakrzewski file, 188. On the *Bürgerwehr*, see Hachtmann, *Berlin 1848*, 234–59.

54. Fricke, *Lexikon zur Parteiengeschichte*; Paschen, *Demokratische Vereine und Preußischer Staat*; Sheehan, *German History*, 656–710.

55. Sheehan, *German History*, 704–18.

56. "Extract," no date, Zakrzewski file, 188. See also Adalbert von Ladenberg, minister of culture, to Karl Ludwig von Hinckeldey, president of the police, 21 March 1850; Hinckeldey to Ladenberg, 6 June 1850; and Undersecretary of State Hermann Lehnert to Ladenberg, 19 June 1850, all in ibid., 189, 192–93, 194–95.

57. Zakrzewski to Ladenberg, 19 June 1850, in ibid., 196–99. For the letter in which he at first denied everything, see Lehnert to Ladenberg, 19 June 1850, in ibid., 194–95.

58. Lüdicke, *Die Preußischen Kultusminister*, Beilage II.

59. Sheehan, *German History*, 656–729.

60. Lehnert, "to Zakrzewski's file," 29 June 1850, Zakrzewski file, 200–201. Zakrzewski "read, approved, and signed" this letter. The formality of the exchange suggests that this may have been a pattern adopted as the police pursued its investigations of middle-class individuals and members of the civil service, most of whom were exonerated. The vast majority of people killed during the street battles or later investigated were, in contrast, from less privileged segments of the population. See Sheehan, *German History*, 708.

61. *PI*, 39.

62. Ibid., 32–33.

63. Military attest, 18 July 1837, Zakrzewski file, 17.

64. Zakrzewska mentioned this in a letter to Paulina Pope, 28 October 1901, NEHWC Collection, box 1, SS. I am grateful to Regina Morantz-Sanchez for sending me a copy of this letter. A brief excerpt from this letter is cited in *WQ*, 297.

65. Zakrzewska to the state minister, 5 April 1847, Zakrzewski file, 150–51. For his oath, see 7 October 1841, in ibid., 99.

66. I develop this in greater detail in Chapter 6 of this book.

67. *PI*, 33–35.

68. Wells, *Out of the Dead House*, 3–4.

69. *PI*, 42.

70. It was unusual for nineteenth-century women to write autobiographical sketches in which they presented themselves as being in control of their lives. See Heilbrun, *Writing a Woman's Life*.

71. *PI*, 44.

72. Zakrzewski mentions his adopted son in two letters to the state minister, 30 October 1849 and 16 April 1855, Zakrzewski file, 185–86, 310–11. Zakrzewska also mentions her brother in *PI*, 147.

73. *PI*, 39, 52.

74. Ibid., 86. See also her comment on 72.

75. Zakrzewska to Caroline Severance, 8 September 1889, in Severance Papers.

76. *PI*, 36.

77. Ibid., 44–46.

78. Bonner, *To the Ends of the Earth*, chap. 5.

CHAPTER TWO

1. Zakrzewska discusses this experience in *PI*, 53–61.

2. Schmidt, *Lehrbuch der Geburtskunde*, 2; Credé, *Die Preußischen Hebammen*, 9. Zakrzewska states the reasons for her rejection in *PI*, 57–58.

3. *PI*, 58, 60. I have not been able to find any corroborating evidence that Schmidt did, in fact, take Zakrzewska's case to the king.

4. See Fassbender, *Geschichte der Geburtshilfe*, 256–57, and Donnison, *Midwives and Medical Men*, 54.

5. Schmidt, *Die Reform der Medizinalverfassung Preußens*, 26–29. On the various changes that led to the emergence of a powerful medical profession, see Fischer, *Geschichte des deutschen Gesundheitswesens*; Huerkamp, *Der Aufstieg der Ärzte*; McClelland, *German Experience of Professionalization*; and Tuchman, *Science, Medicine, and the State*.

6. Biographical information on Schmidt can be found in Fraatz, *Der Paderborner Kreisarzt*. See also Hirsch, *Biographisches Lexikon*, 95–97.

7. Johann Nepomuk Rust et al., "Vorbericht zur ersten Aufgabe," in Schmidt, *Lehrbuch der Geburtskunde*, p. VIII.

8. Schmidt, *Die Reform der Medicinalverfassung Preußens*. On Schmidt's call to Berlin, see Fraatz, *Der Paderborner Kreisarzt*, 48, and Dudenhausen, Stürzbecher, and Engel, *Die Hebamme im Spiegel*, 15.

9. Physicians were licensed to practice medicine and surgery; surgeons of the first class were also licensed to practice both, but they could practice internal medicine only if they lived in a district where no physician had established himself. Surgeons of the second class were licensed only to perform minor surgeries and to assist their superiors. See Huerkamp, *Der Aufstieg der Ärzte*, 45–50.

10. Schmidt, *Die Reform der Medizinalverfassung Preußens*, 16. On the midcentury medical reforms in Prussia and elsewhere, see Huerkamp, *Der Aufstieg der Ärzte*; Sczibilanski, "Von der Prüfungs- und Vorprüfungsordnung"; and Tuchman, *Science, Medicine, and the State*, chap. 8. For a general analysis of professionalization strategies, see Larson, *Rise of Professionalism*, especially the introduction.

11. Zakrzewska, "Sind Hebammenschulen wünschenswerth?" I discuss this in greater detail in Chapter 4.

12. *PI*, 57–64.

13. For a more detailed analysis of this debate, see Tuchman, " 'True Assistant to the Obstetrician.' "

14. Schmidt, *Lehrbuch der Geburtskunde*, 1.

15. See "Erörterungen der bisherigen Verhältnisse," 53–54; the minister of culture to the police president, 16 March 1852, PBL, Rep. 30 Berlin, C-Polizei Präsidium, Tit. 50, Nr. 2236, p. 87; and *PI*, 80.

16. Mayer to Eichhorn, 20 December 1847, GStA PK, Rep. 76 VIIIA, Nr. 896. This file was not paginated. However, the comment appears on the fourth page of Mayer's document. See also "Erörterungen der bisherigen Verhältnisse," 50.

17. Schmidt to Undersecretary of State Hermann Lehnert, 16 January 1848, GStA PK, Rep. 76 VIIIA, Nr. 896, 9.

18. I return to this point in Chapter 4.

19. Borst, "Training and Practice of Midwives" and *Catching Babies*; Leavitt, *Brought to Bed*; Smith, "Medicine, Midwifery, and the State"; Ulrich, *Midwife's Tale*. On the relationship between the state and the licensing of midwives in states and countries throughout Europe, see Lindemann, *Health and Healing*, 194; Loetz, *Vom Kranken zum Patienten*, 144–49, 182–90; Marland, *Art of Midwifery* and *Midwives, Society and Childbirth*; and Wilson, *Making of Man-Midwifery*.

20. On the sense of professionalism among German-trained midwives who immigrated to the United States, see Borst, "Training and Practice of Midwives."

21. Cited in Gregory, "Kant, Schelling, and the Administration of Science," 26.

22. When the previous director of the Charité's midwifery institute died in 1848, his position was divided between Ernst Horn, who assumed the directorship of the institute and the responsibility for providing practical instruction, and Schmidt, who took over the theoretical instruction. One year later, however, the government reunited the various responsibilities and handed them over to Schmidt. See Ladenberg to the Charité director, 18 August 1848, and Ladenberg to the Charité director, 24 September 1849, both in UA der HUB, Charité Direktion, Nr. 192, unpaginated.

23. For a discussion of physicians' interest in bridging theory and practice and how the meanings of those terms changed over time, see Tuchman, *Science, Medicine, and the State*.

24. Schmidt, *Lehrbuch der Geburtskunde*.

25. The dissections are mentioned in Schmidt to Ladenberg, 19 March 1849 and 15 April 1850, both in GStA PK, Rep. 76 VIIIA, Nr. 1004, 75, 94.

26. Schmidt, "Die geburtshülflich-klinischen Institute," 485–523, esp. 498.

27. Ibid., 502; Schmidt to Ladenberg, 15 April 1850, GStA PK, Rep. 76 VIIIA, 93. Schmidt mentions the breech birth in a letter to von Raumer, minister of culture, 21 March 1851, in ibid., 145–46. It is possible that this pupil was Zakrzewska. She would not yet have graduated, and she was his prize pupil. Schmidt does not, however, mention the pupil's name.

28. On the problem of puerperal fever in the nineteenth century, see Carter, "Puerperal Fever"; Leavitt, *Brought to Bed*; Loudon, *Childbed Fever*; and Wertz and Wertz, *Lying-in*.

29. Schmidt, "Die geburtshülflich-klinischen Institute," 499–501.

30. Walsh, *"Doctors Wanted,"* 92–95; and Chapter 10 of this book.

31. Schmidt, "Die geburtshülflich-klinischen Institute," 506.

32. Ibid., 505–6.

33. Ibid., 507.

34. Ibid., 506. On the relationship between physicians and patients in the nineteenth-century hospital, see, for example, Waddington, "Role of the Hospital," and Rosenberg, *Care of Strangers*.

35. Cited in *PI*, 12.

36. Ginzberg, *Women and the Work of Benevolence*.

37. Atwater, "Touching the Patient"; Ludmerer, *Learning to Heal*, chap. 1; Rosenberg, *Care of Strangers*, 193–209; Warner, *Against the Spirit of System*, 28–29.

38. Schmidt, "Die geburtshülflich-klinischen Institute," 498.

39. See Schmidt to Ladenberg, 15 April 1850, GStA PK, Rep. 76 VIIIA, Nr. 1004, 93; Schmidt, "Die geburtshülflich-klinischen Institute," 503–4; and "Instruction für die, in der mit dem Königlichen Charité-Krankenhause verbundenen Hebammen-Lehranstalt auszubildenen Hebammenschulerinnen," 12 October 1846, UA der HUB, Nr. 802, 81–83.

40. Schmidt to the Charité directors, 3 March 1850, UA der HUB, Nr. 200, 103.

41. *PI*, 59, 62.

42. Schmidt to the Charité directors, 3 March 1850, UA der HUB, Nr. 200, 104.

43. Schmidt to Esse (Charité director), 23 November 1849, in ibid., Nr. 802, 170–72.

44. Schmidt to the Charité directors, 20 March 1850, in ibid., Nr. 200, 116–23.

45. Schmidt to the Charité directors, 3 March 1850, in ibid., 106–7.

46. Schmidt to the Charité directors, 20 March 1850, in ibid., 122–23.

47. See Catherina Bernhardina Schmidt to the Charité directors, 31 March 1850, and the Charité directors to Joseph Hermann Schmidt, 4 April 1850, both in ibid., 126, 127–28. See also Zakrzewska's discussion of this in *PI*, 78–79.

48. *PI*, 60.

49. Zakrzewska claimed that he was so weak at times that he had "to lecture in a reclining position." Ibid., 48.

50. Ibid., 64.

51. Ibid., 65. Zakrzewska's excellent performance at her exams is also mentioned in Schmidt to von Raumer, minister of culture, 29 March 1852, GStA PK, Rep. 76 VIIIA, Nr. 1004, 152. Of the thirty-five pupils who were examined, eleven received "excellent"; eleven, "very good"; and thirteen, "good." This was the first year Schmidt listed each of the midwives by name, along with their grades and the extent of their clinical practice. Accordingly, Zakrzewska received an "excellent," delivered thirty-six babies herself, and assisted in another seventy deliveries.

52. Charité directors to the minister of culture, von Raumer, 2 February 1852; Lehnert to Esse, 11 February 1852; and Schmidt to the Charité directors, 21 March 1852, all in UA der HUB, Nr. 200, 144–45, 146, 149.

53. This series of events was described and recorded during a meeting of Esse, Horn, and Lehnert, on 8 May 1852, in ibid., 156–59.

54. Zakrzewska to Schmidt, 16 April 1852, in ibid., 153–54.

55. Report on meeting of Esse, Horn, and Lehnert, 8 May 1852, in ibid., Nr. 200, 156–59.

56. Esse and Horn to Schmidt, 10 May 1852, in ibid., 160–61.

57. *PI*, 75–79. See Schmidt's obituary on 22 May 1852, in GStA PK, Rep. 76 I, Sekt. 31, Litt. S, Nr. 55, 129–32.

58. Zakrzewska describes these responsibilities in *PI*, 81–82. In 1889, in an article she published on the midwifery cases she had attended in private practice during her career, she also mentioned briefly the work she performed as head midwife at the Charité. See Zakrzewska, "Report of One Hundred and Eighty-Seven Cases."

59. "Dienst-Instruction für die Charité-Hebammen," 6 March 1827, Charité Direction, UA der HUB, Nr. 199, 147–53.

60. *PI*, 85. See also "Erörterungen der bisherigen Verhältnisse," 55, and the minister of culture to the police president, 16 March 1852, PBL, Rep. 30 Berlin, C-Polizei Präsidium, Tit. 50, Nr. 2236, 87.

61. "Dienst-Instruction für die Charité-Hebammen," 152–53. Zakrzewska's problems with Horn are mentioned as well in a letter Martin Zakrzewski wrote, requesting that his daughter be allowed to immigrate to America. See Zakrzewski to the state minister, von Raumer, 29 January 1853, Zakrzewski file, 305–6.

62. *WQ,* 67.

63. Barney, *Passage of the Republic*, 177; Nadel, *Little Germany*, 1–26, 173 n. 1.

64. *PI*, 88.

65. Ibid., 92.

CHAPTER THREE

1. *PI*, 92. See also "Biographical. Sketches of the Life and Work of the Pioneer Women in Medicine." This article (which was part of a series) was written in the third person, suggesting that Zakrzewska was not herself the author. Although it had some new information, by and large the series drew on Zakrzewska's 1860 autobiographical sketch.

2. *PI*, 94–95.

3. Ibid., 96–97.

4. Ibid., 97.

5. Nadel, *Little Germany*, 1–26, 173 n. 1.

6. On *Kleindeutschland*, see ibid. Zakrzewska recounts their experiences upon arriving in New York in *PI*, 98–99.

7. Theodor Griesinger, a contemporary, claimed that at the time one could get a "parlor with two windows and . . . a windowless bedroom" for about four dollars a month. If one wanted "a pleasant apartment with three windows and two bedrooms," one would need to spend eight to ten dollars; cited in Nadel, *Little Germany*, 36. Zakrzewska mentioned her apartment and furniture in *PI*, 105–7.

8. Stansell, *City of Women*, chaps. 6–9. Stansell provides a good description of the system of outwork on 109. The estimate of the amount of money needed to support oneself is cited on 111. See also Nadel, *Little Germany*, 75–78.

9. Stansell, *City of Women*, 179.

10. *PI*, 106, 112.

11. Ibid., 114, 125–26.

12. Ibid., 105–6; *WQ*, 113–14; "Biographical. Sketches of the Life and Work of the Pioneer Women in Medicine," 136. On the apprenticeship system, see Haller, *American Medicine in Transition*, 192–97; Warner, *Against the Spirit of System*, 17–31. That Zakrzewska could simply open a midwifery practice stemmed from the fact that midwives, like all other medical practitioners at the time, were not yet subjected to state laws. See Borst, "Training and Practice of Midwives."

13. Cited in Bonner, *To the Ends of the Earth*, 6. On Blackwell's experience at Geneva Medical College, see also Morantz-Sanchez, *Sympathy and Science*, 47–49.

14. Kirschmann, *Vital Force*, chaps. 2 and 3; Morantz-Sanchez, *Sympathy and Science*, chap. 4; More, *Restoring the Balance*, 17–23; and Walsh, *"Doctors Wanted,"* 35–75.

15. Kirschmann, *Vital Force*, 4; Rogers, "Women and Sectarian Medicine."

16. The quotation is from the AMA's 1847 Code of Ethics, cited in Baker, "American Medical Ethics Revolution," 42. In this essay, Baker offers an important revisionist interpretation of this code.

17. Rogers, "American Homeopathy Confronts Scientific Medicine"; Rothstein, *American Physicians in the Nineteenth Century*, 177–246.

18. Cayleff, *Wash and Be Healed*; Donegan, *"Hydropathic Highway to Health"*; Gevitz, *Other Healers*; Kaufman, *Homeopathy in America.*

19. Rothstein, *American Physicians in the Nineteenth Century*, 170–73; Warner, "Orthodoxy and Otherness."

20. William Lloyd Garrison II once commented that Zakrzewska "held firmly to the conviction . . . that homeopathy has no claim to science"; cited in *WQ,* 459, no date.

21. Bittel, "Science of Women's Rights"; Kirschmann, *Vital Force*, 61–62; Morantz-Sanchez, *Sympathy and Science*, 73–74; Peitzman, *New and Untried Course*, 45–55; Wells, *Out of the Dead House*, 57–79.

22. On Dixon-Jones, see Morantz-Sanchez, *Conduct Unbecoming a Woman*; on Dolley, see More, *Restoring the Balance*, 45–56.

23. For biographical information on Blackwell, see Sahli, *Elizabeth Blackwell.*

24. *PI*, 130.

25. Elizabeth to Emily Blackwell, 12 May 1854, reprinted in Blackwell, *Pioneer Work*, 201. An excerpt from this letter is cited in *WQ,* 109.

26. Sahli, *Elizabeth Blackwell*, 124, 129; L'Esperance, "Influence of the New York Infirmary."

27. *PI*, 131.

28. For a detailed account of Cleveland Medical College in the 1850s and its policy toward women, see Goldstein, "Roses Bloomed in Winter."

29. *WQ,* 142, 147, 170, 177; *PI*, 113, 136.

30. Goldstein, "Roses Bloomed in Winter," 115.

31. Zakrzewska must have chosen not to repeat the experience she had had in New York, for she could just as easily have buried herself in Cleveland's German-speaking population, which was by no means small at this time. See Miller and Wheeler, *Cleveland*, 52–55.

32. *PI*, 121, 139–42; *WQ,* 162.

33. On Severance, see Jensen, "Severance," and Ruddy, *Mother of Clubs.*

34. *WQ,* 134, 151.

35. Ibid., 153. On the turmoil caused by the Fugitive Slave Law and the Kansas-Nebraska Act, see Stewart, *Holy Warriors.* On differences between the antislavery movements in the Northeast and the Midwest, see Gamble, "Moral Suasion in the West."

36. *WQ,* 138. On the Severances' role in founding the Independent Christian Church, see Jensen, "Severance."

37. Williams, "Unitarianism and Universalism."

38. Jensen, "Severance." On Mayo, see Robertson, "Mayo, Amory Dwight," and Robinson, *Massachusetts in the Woman Suffrage Movement*, 28. Mayo was a strong supporter as well of women's rights. See Mayo to Mrs. Paulina W. Davis, 24 August 1853, reprinted in Stanton, Anthony, and Gage, *History of Woman Suffrage*, 1:851–52.

39. Severance to Mrs. Elizabeth Cady Stanton, no date, reprinted in Ruddy, *Mother of Clubs*, 13–14. On her election to the vice presidency of the national movement, see Stanton, Anthony, and Gage, *History of Woman Suffrage*, 1:548.

40. *WQ,* 134. Zakrzewska is referring to Paulina Wright Davis and to the Seneca Falls Convention in 1848. See also ibid., 137, in which she mentions again that she needed time to

come to understand "their demands for a larger sphere for women." On the early women's rights conventions, see Stanton, Anthony, and Gage, *History of Woman Suffrage*, 1:216.

41. We must also keep in mind that Zakrzewska first told this story at the end of the century. It may not, therefore, accurately reflect how she felt at the time. Casting herself as someone who had initially stood in opposition to the women's rights movement but had ultimately changed her mind may have been a way of reaching out to potential readers who were ambivalent about the women's rights movement of their day.

42. On Hunt, see her autobiography, Hunt, *Glances and Glimpses*, and Walsh, *"Doctors Wanted,"* 135–37. On the meeting between Hunt and Zakrzewska, see *PI*, 142.

43. Reprinted in Stanton, Anthony, and Gage, *History of Woman Suffrage*, 1:259–60. On the first National Woman's Rights Convention, see ibid., 215–16, and Robinson, *Massachusetts in the Woman Suffrage Movement*, 20–22, 215–17.

44. Hunt, *Glances and Glimpses*, 347.

45. *PI*, 149; *WQ,* 149–51. Zakrzewska later described the day she met Theodore Parker as "the greatest event of my three days' sojourn in Boston," largely because he introduced her to Garrison and Phillips. See *WQ,* 151. On the New England Woman's Rights Convention, see Robinson, *Massachusetts in the Woman Suffrage Movement*, 36–37, and Barry, *Susan B. Anthony*, 107.

46. Goldstein, "Roses Bloomed in Winter," 252–60; *PI*, 139–40; Jensen, "Severance."

47. *WQ,* 153–54.

48. Ibid., 155.

49. Ibid., 134–35.

50. Mary Roth Walsh tends to attach more importance to the "web of feminist friendship" in Zakrzewska's life, but I share Goldstein's sense that Zakrzewska's support network was much broader. See Walsh, "Feminist Showplace," and Goldstein, "Roses Bloomed in Winter," 22.

51. *WQ,* 145; *PI*, 140, 149. On the parallel between Zakrzewska's relationships with Schmidt and Delamater, see Goldstein, "Roses Bloomed in Winter," 214.

52. On Delamater's role in opening Cleveland Medical College's doors to women, see Goldstein, "Roses Bloomed in Winter," 125–30, 170. The six who matriculated and received their M.D.'s are Nancy Talbot Clark (1852), Emily Blackwell (1854), Marie Zakrzewska (1856), Sarah Chadwick (1856), Cordelia Agnes Greene (1856), and Elizabeth Griselle (1856). The other three are Eliza Brown, Mary Frame Thomas, and Eliza Lucinda Smith Thomas. See ibid., chap. 4.

53. Waite, *Western Reserve University*, 427.

54. Goldstein, "Roses Bloomed in Winter," 154.

55. Ibid., 107–247, 314–22.

56. Ibid., 142, 181, 183.

57. Waite, *Western Reserve University*, 431; Goldstein, "Roses Bloomed in Winter," 181–82, 262. I am grateful to Naomi Rogers for helping me to better understand the way regular physicians linked unorthodox medicine and women's entry into the regular profession. See also Kirschmann, *Vital Force*.

58. Waite, *Western Reserve University*, 514. On competition between the two institutions, see ibid., 431.

59. Kirschmann, *Vital Force*.

60. Ludmerer, *Learning to Heal*, chap. 1; Rosenberg, *Care of Strangers*; Rothstein, *American Physicians in the Nineteenth Century*, 85–121.

61. Cited in Rosenberg, *Care of Strangers*, 202.

62. Ludmerer, *Learning to Heal*, 12. For a less critical view of antebellum medical training, see Warner, *Against the Spirit of System*, 17–31. Nevertheless, Warner agrees that the quality of a medical student's training depended largely on either the skills of his preceptor or the nature of the training he received outside of formal educational requirements.

63. *WQ,* 121.

64. Ibid., 178.

65. *PI*, 140–41; *WQ,* 124–25. On Chadwick, see Goldstein, "Roses Bloomed in Winter," 215–25, 386–404.

66. *PI*, 141, 204–5; Goldstein, "Roses Bloomed in Winter," 267–69.

67. *PI*, 141–42.

68. Ibid., 147–48; *WQ,* 148. Caroline Zakrzewski died on 30 August 1855. See Martin Ludwig Zakrzewski to the state minister, 26 February 1856, Zakrzewski file, 320–21.

69. Zakrzewska mentions the birth of her nephew in *WQ,* 159.

70. *PI*, 148.

71. Ibid., 148–49, 154.

72. *WQ,* 152.

73. Mayer to Eichhorn, 20 December 1847, GStA PK, Rep. 76 VIIIA, Nr. 896. I discussed his views at greater length in Chapter 2.

74. Thus a physician had once commented that it was "as if the Almighty, in creating the female sex, had taken the uterus and built up a woman around it"; cited in Smith-Rosenberg and Rosenberg, "Female Animal," 113, and in Wood, " 'Fashionable Diseases,' " 223–24. See also Schiebinger, *Nature's Body*.

75. Zakrzewska, "Thesis. The Organ of Parturition," 1. I am grateful to the Archives of the Allen Memorial Medical Library at Case Western Reserve University for sending me a transcription of Zakrzewska's thesis. The transcription was prepared by Linda Lehmann Goldstein.

76. Ibid., 5.

77. Ibid.

78. Ibid., 9.

79. Ibid., 5. On the notion of the "type," see Lenoir, *Strategy of Life*.

80. Zakrzewska, "Thesis. The Organ of Parturition," 13, 9. On German nature philosophy, see Lenoir, *Strategy of Life*.

81. Emily Blackwell wrote "A Thesis on Certain Principles of Practical Medicine," and Cordelia Greene wrote "A Thesis on Prolapsus Uteri, and Other Malpositions of the Abdominal and Pelvic Viscera." See Goldstein, "Roses Bloomed in Winter," 260–314.

82. For a provocative interpretation of nineteenth-century women physicians' medical writings as strategies for establishing a place and a voice for themselves in a hostile profession,

see Wells, *Out of the Dead House*. Although Wells does not examine Zakrzewska's medical thesis, she does begin her book with Zakrzewska's story about getting locked in the dead house (hence the title of the book).

83. Zakrzewska, "Thesis. The Organ of Parturition," 2.

84. The physician was the famous seventeenth-century Dutch physician Jan Swammerdam. See ibid., 14.

85. *WQ*, 163.

86. Ibid., 165.

87. Ibid., 168.

CHAPTER FOUR

1. *WQ*, 177–78; Zakrzewski to the state minister, 26 February 1856, 25 October 1856, and 19 November 1856, all in Zakrzewski file, 320–21, 333–34, 331. Zakrzewski never took the trip, presumably because Anna and Sophie, who had not been well during the summer of 1856, both recovered.

2. *WQ*, 179–80. See also *PI*, 153.

3. *WQ*, 181–82. Zakrzewska's youngest sister, Rosalia, also eventually joined them. See Sahli, *Elizabeth Blackwell*, 128.

4. *Appeal in Behalf of the Medical Education of Women*, 5–6. I am grateful to Richard Wolfe, former rare book librarian of the Countway, for making a copy of this available to me. Although the pamphlet was published anonymously, there can be no question that it reflected the work of both Blackwell and Zakrzewska. More than likely, though, given Zakrzewska's trouble with the English language, Blackwell was the one who sat down and wrote it. Zakrzewska discussed the content of this pamphlet in *WQ*, 191.

5. Morantz-Sanchez, *Sympathy and Science*, 72–76.

6. *WQ*, 180, 206.

7. Gordon, "Voluntary Motherhood"; Mohr, *Abortion in America*; Reagan, *When Abortion Was a Crime*.

8. *Appeal in Behalf of the Medical Education of Women*, 6.

9. Ibid. Once women graduated from medical school, they had another option. Many European clinics and hospitals opened their doors to graduates for brief periods, even while European medical schools remained closed to them. See Bonner, *To the Ends of the Earth*, 25.

10. Rosenberg, *Care of Strangers*; Warner, "Selective Transport of Medical Knowledge" and *Against the Spirit of System*.

11. To get around this problem, private programs were often established in which medical faculty who had access to hospital wards would complement formal school requirements by providing clinical lectures for a fee. It is unclear, though, whether students enjoyed any hands-on experience through these extracurricular courses of instruction. Indeed, the very language of the advertisements suggests that students observed clinical cases and anatomical dissections rather than being guided to develop their own practical skills. See Warner, *Against the Spirit of System*, 28–29.

12. *Appeal in Behalf of the Medical Education of Women*, 8–9.

13. Ibid., 6–7.

14. See, for example, Bonner, *American Doctors and German Universities*; Ludmerer, *Learning to Heal*; Rosenberg, *Care of Strangers*; Shryock, *Development of Modern Medicine*; and Warner, *Therapeutic Perspective*. Two exceptions to this are Bonner, *To the Ends of the Earth*, and Warner, *Against the Spirit of System*.

15. *Appeal in Behalf of the Medical Education of Women*, 10.

16. Warner, *Against the Spirit of System*.

17. *WQ*, 198–202.

18. Ibid., 227, 230.

19. On Booth, see ibid., 184–85; Zakrzewska, "Mary L. Booth"; and "Mary Louis Booth."

20. William Lloyd Garrison to Wendell Phillips Garrison, 9 March 1857, Garrison Family Collection, Biography, box 84, SS. See also *WQ*, 185–86, 194.

21. William Lloyd Garrison to his wife, Helen, 13 May 1857, in Merrill and Ruchames, *Letters of William Lloyd Garrison*, 4:438–39. On the opening of the hospital, see *PI*, 158–59; *WQ*, 209–11; and Sahli, *Elizabeth Blackwell*, 134–35.

22. Zakrzewska to Harriot Hunt, 14 May 1857, Dall Papers, box 2, folder 15. This is, to my knowledge, the only time Zakrzewska ever gave the slightest hint of a belief in God. By the end of the decade she had become an atheist.

23. Elizabeth to Emily Blackwell, 12 May 1854, reprinted in Blackwell, *Pioneer Work*, 201; Hunt, *Glances and Glimpses*, 347. Both have already been discussed in Chapter 3.

24. Zakrzewska to Paulina Pope, 28 October 1901, NEHWC Collection, box 1, SS.

25. Blackwell, "New York Infirmary." See also *PI*, 159–60; *WQ*, 211–14; and Blackwell, *Pioneer Work*, 207–11.

26. For a discussion of these criticisms, see Rosenberg, *Care of Strangers*, 200–209, and Warner, *Against the Spirit of System*, 53, 98–99.

27. *Appeal in Behalf of the Medical Education of Women*, 7–10. See also *WQ*, 212–13.

28. Zakrzewska to Paulina Pope, 28 October 1901, NEHWC Collection, box 1, SS.

29. *PI*, 159–60; *WQ*, 182, 211–27; L'Esperance, "Influence of the New York Infirmary"; Morantz-Sanchez, *Sympathy and Science*, 75. For another example of male physicians lending support to an all-female institution, see Peitzman, *New and Untried Course*.

30. On the German radical community in America, see Brancaforte, *German Forty-Eighters*; Hamerow, "Two Worlds of the Forty-Eighters," 19–35; Levine, *Spirit of 1848*; McCormick, *Germans in America*; and Nadel, *Little Germany*. For an important study that also analyzes the impact of German radical politics on nineteenth-century American medicine, see Viner, "Healthy Children for a New World."

31. Wittke, *Against the Current*.

32. Zakrzewska mentioned this in her letter to Paulina Pope, 28 October 1901, NEHWC Collection, box 1, SS. See also *WQ*, 297, and Wittke, *Against the Current*.

33. "Boston 'Pionier.' " See also Wittke, *Against the Current*, 110.

34. Originally written on 13 July 1852, Greeley's comments were reprinted in "Die teutsche Organisation," 2. Cited in Wittke, *Against the Current*, 90.

35. Wittke, *Against the Current*, 145.

36. Zakrzewska to Paulina Pope, 28 October 1901, NEHWC Collection, box 1, SS.

37. On Heinzen's decision to move to Boston, see Heinzen, "Verlegung des 'Pionier' nach Boston," 1. On the negotiations surrounding Zakrzewska's move to Boston, see Waite, *History of the New England Female Medical College*, 43; *WQ*, 236–38; and "History of the New-England Hospital for Women and Children," *AR*, 1876, 5.

38. [Zakrzewska] Eine "Aerztinn," "Weibliche Aerzte"; Zakrzewska, "Sind Hebammen-schulen wünschenswerth?" Note that Zakrzewska published "Weibliche Aerzte" anony-mously, signing it Eine "Aerztinn" rather than with her own name. It is doubtful that she did this to protect herself. The German radical community was too small for there to be any doubt as to who had penned the article. No other German female physician had such close ties to Heinzen; the views expressed in this article match those Zakrzewska expressed else-where; and the writer's biting wit is reminiscent of Zakrzewska's sense of humor. A more likely explanation is that she wished to imply that the views expressed therein reflected those of the typical female physician, rather than hers alone.

39. For an analysis of biological arguments against women's entry into the public sphere, see Morantz-Sanchez, "'Connecting Link'"; Smith-Rosenberg and Rosenberg, "Female Animal"; and Schiebinger, *Mind Has No Sex?*

40. [Zakrzewska] Eine "Aerztinn," "Weibliche Aerzte."

41. Ibid. On nineteenth-century women physicians' use of satire in their battle to gain entry into the medical profession, see Wells, *Out of the Dead House*, 92–99.

42. [Zakrzewska] Eine "Aerztinn," "Weibliche Aerzte." On the concerns physicians voiced about the potential of dissection to brutalize medical students, male and female alike, see Warner, *Against the Spirit of System*, 264–65.

43. [Zakrzewska] Eine "Aerztinn," "Weibliche Aerzte."

44. Ibid.

45. Ibid.

46. Morantz-Sanchez, "Feminist Theory and Historical Practice." See also Morantz-Sanchez, *Sympathy and Science*, chap. 7.

47. On Preston, see Wells, *Out of the Dead House*, 57–79, and Peitzman, *New and Untried Course*, 45–55.

48. Wells, *Out of the Dead House*, 122–45.

49. Ibid., 146–92; Bittel, "Science of Women's Rights."

50. I am grateful to the participants in the National Library of Medicine's symposium "Women Physicians, Women's Politics, and Women's Health: Emerging Narratives," espe-cially Carla Bittel, Regina Morantz-Sanchez, Ellen Singer More, and Susan Wells, for en-couraging me to explore the connections between Zakrzewska's performances and those of some of her contemporaries. This symposium took place 9–11 March 2005.

51. Morantz-Sanchez, *Sympathy and Science*.

52. See Tuchman, "'Only in a Republic.'" See also Chapter 5 of this book. Interestingly, Jacobi's positive assessment of science stemmed as well from her embrace of a brand of European radicalism. See Bittel, "Science of Women's Rights."

53. The extent to which Zakrzewska may, at this point in her life, have been influenced by women's rights advocates like Susan B. Anthony and Elizabeth Cady Stanton is unclear. On

Anthony's and Stanton's embrace of rationality over sentimentality and their denial of sexual differences, see Barry, *Susan B. Anthony*, 124–34, and Pellauer, *Toward a Tradition of Feminist Theology*.

54. Borst, *Catching Babies*; Kobrin, "American Midwife Controversy"; Litoff, *American Midwives*; Wertz and Wertz, *Lying-in*.

55. Zakrzewska mentioned this in Eine "Aerztinn," "Weibliche Aerzte."

56. On the large number of German-trained midwives in the United States, see Borst, *Catching Babies* and "Training and Practice of Midwives."

57. Zakrzewska, "Sind Hebammenschulen wünschenswerth?"

58. Ibid.

59. Ibid.

60. Zakrzewska to Paulina Pope, 28 October 1901, NEHWC Collection, box 1, SS.

61. *WQ,* 237.

62. Zakrzewska to Hunt, 14 May 1857, Dall Papers, box 2, folder 15.

63. Nadel, *Little Germany*, 136.

64. *WQ,* 230, 239. See also ibid., 235, and Zakrzewska, "Mary L. Booth," 105.

65. Heilbrun, *Writing a Woman's Life*, 108.

66. Faderman, *Surpassing the Love of Men*; Smith-Rosenberg, "Female World of Love and Ritual."

67. Zakrzewska, "Mary L. Booth," 106.

68. "Woman and the Press." Zakrzewska and Booth abandoned this plan because of the Civil War.

69. *PI*, 162.

70. Smith-Rosenberg, "Female World of Love and Ritual."

CHAPTER FIVE

1. Zakrzewska, "Ueber Hospitäler" (4 February 1863). On home ownership as a mark of middle-class respectability, see Ryan, *Cradle of the Middle Class*, 181–82.

2. Austin, *Voice to the Married*, 38, cited in Ryan, *Cradle of the Middle Class*, 147. See also Deutsch, *Women and the City*, 54–77, and Cott, *Public Vows*.

3. Zakrzewska made this comment in a eulogy she wrote for herself, which was published in C. W., "Dr. Zakrzewska's Funeral." The eulogy is reprinted in *WQ,* 474–78, quotation on 477. For the makeup of her household, see Zakrzewska to Paulina Pope, 28 October 1901, NEHWC Collection, box 1, SS, and Wittke, *Against the Current*, 22–23.

4. Hausen, "Family and Role Division," 51. Zakrzewska was not alone among women physicians in creating an alternative family. Ann Preston also shared her home off and on with others, including other unmarried women, a woman and her child, and a married couple. See Peitzman, *New and Untried Course*, 50.

5. Morantz-Sanchez, *Sympathy and Science*, 135. See also More, *Restoring the Balance*, 24.

6. *PI*, 119–20.

7. Cott, *Public Vows*.

8. The term "streetcar suburb" is from the title of Warner's book *Streetcar Suburbs*. On Roxbury, see ibid., 21–29, and Handlin, *Boston's Immigrants*, 99.

9. On the Tremont area and Roxbury Highlands, see Handlin, *Boston's Immigrants*, 86–116. On Zakrzewska's home and garden, see Zakrzewska to Paulina Pope, 28 October 1901, NEHWC Collection, box 1, SS; *Fiftieth Anniversary of the New England Hospital*, 48; and Zakrzewska to "Miss Baker," 15 May 1879, New England Hospital Collection, Miscellaneous, Countway.

10. *WQ*, 269. On 20 December 1859, Martin Zakrzewski's widow wrote to the Prussian ministry informing it that her husband had died that day. See Widow Zakrzewski to "Ew. Excellenz," 20 December 1859, Zakrzewski file, 343. Zakrzewska's claim in *WQ* (268) that she had heard of her father's death in November must, therefore, be mistaken.

11. "Wilhelmine J. Zakrzewska"; Zakrzewska to Paulina Pope, 28 October 1901, NEHWC Collection, box 1, SS. Although Zakrzewska never mentioned her dependent sisters by name, they could only have been Rosalia and Minna. See Zakrzewska to Lucy Sewall, 25 January 1863 and 7 May 1863, cited in *WQ*, 306, 311, and Zakrzewska to Paulina Pope, 28 October 1901.

12. Kitty Barry Blackwell, "Reminiscences," cited in Sahli, *Elizabeth Blackwell*, 178 n. 56.

13. Zakrzewska made this comment in a letter to Lucy Sewall, 7 May 1863, reprinted in *WQ*, 311. See also ibid., 296. I wish to thank Bob Doerr, the great-grandson of Zakrzewska's brother Herman, for sharing his knowledge with me of his family's genealogy. He informed me of Rosalia's marriage to John C. Steinebrey.

14. Zakrzewska to Paulina Pope, 28 October 1901, NEHWC Collection, box 1, SS. See also *WQ*, 297, where Vietor has cited from this letter after improving Zakrzewska's English.

15. See, for example, her letter to Heinzen, 5 February 1873, Karl Heinzen Papers, LBC. There are more than a dozen letters from Neymann to Heinzen in this collection, mostly from 1872 and 1873. See also Wittke, *Against the Current*, 131–34.

16. The quotation is from "Organisation der freisinnigen Teutschen," 6. On Zakrzewska's political activities, see, for example, *Der Pionier*, 9 September 1863, which lists her as a donor for the Feuerbach fund, and 24 January 1877, 5, which mentions her involvement in the Society for the Dissemination of Radical Principles.

17. Cited in *WQ*, 460.

18. Heinzen, *Die Helden des teutschen Kommunismus*, 17.

19. See, for example, Heinzen, "Ueber die 'Liebe,'" 34–35.

20. Zakrzewska to Paulina Pope, 28 October 1901, NEHWC Collection, box 1, SS.

21. Heinzen, "Was ist Humanität?," 310. See also Wittke, *Against the Current*, 84–94.

22. Wittke, *Against the Current*, 171–98; Gienapp, "Nativism and the Creation of a Republican Majority," 529–59; Levine, *Spirit of 1848*. On Heinzen's alienation of many of his friends because of his views on Lincoln, see Julia Sprague to George Schumm, 11 March 1909, George Schumm Papers, LBC. On Heinzen's views on the source of racial differences, see Heinzen, *Communism and Socialism*, 9.

23. Heinzen, *Die Helden des teutschen Kommunismus*, 3.

24. *PI*, 119.

25. Heinzen, *Communism and Socialism*, 4.

26. Ibid., 16–19. See also Heinzen, *Die Helden des teutschen Kommunismus*, 17–18. Wittke discusses Heinzen's views on communism in *Against the Current*, 229–49.

27. Heinzen, *Communism and Socialism*, 29, 34, 36, 38. The reference to "socialistic institutions" can be found on 34.

28. Heinzen, *What Is Real Democracy?*, 64.

29. Heinzen, "Wer and was ist, das Volk," 199.

30. Heinzen, *Separation of State and Church*, 1, 8.

31. Heinzen, *Communism and Socialism*, 43. See also Heinzen, "Zur Moral des Radikalismus," 9; "Was ist Humanität?," 274–312; "Weiberrecht und Liebe vor dem Richterstuhl der Moral," 237–48; "Ueber die 'Liebe,' " 31; and *Rights of Women and the Sexual Relations*, 136.

32. Heinzen, *Six Letters to a Pious Man*, 29.

33. On the kind of Christian humanism that motivated American radicals like William Lloyd Garrison to burn the Constitution in protest against the institution of slavery, see Perry, *Radical Abolitionism*.

34. Heinzen, *Six Letters to a Pious Man*, 25.

35. Ibid., 27–28.

36. Ibid., 61. Heinzen frequently used religious language to describe radical materialism, such as in an essay on the morality of radicalism, when he went through all ten commandments and rewrote them for radicals. See his "Zur Moral des Radikalismus," 5–27.

On the German scientific materialists, see Gregory, *Scientific Materialism in Nineteenth Century Germany*.

37. I develop this argument in greater detail in Tuchman, *Science, Medicine, and the State*.

38. In *Communism and Socialism*, Heinzen insisted that a just society had to guarantee equal rights for all individuals, "without distinction of descent, of rank, and of sex" (37).

39. Heinzen, "Die Ungenügsamkeit der 'Rechts'-Weiber," 409.

40. Heinzen, *Communism and Socialism*, 48. See also his *Rights of Women and the Sexual Relations*, 37. The relative novelty of this position in the German radical community is mentioned in Levine, *Spirit of 1848*, 102–3.

41. Zakrzewska's disputes with Garrison are mentioned by the latter's son, William Lloyd Garrison II, in a letter, no date, published in *WQ*, 459–60.

42. Zakrzewska to Lucy Sewall, 1862 (probably November or December), cited in *WQ*, 303, 316; C. W., "Dr. Zakrzewska's Funeral." Zakrzewska mentioned the tensions with friends over her lack of religious beliefs in a letter to Lucy Sewall, 25 January 1863, cited in *WQ*, 308.

43. Wittke, *Against the Current*, 137.

44. I have derived my sense of the relationship between Zakrzewska and Mrs. Heinzen from the following letters: Zakrzewska to Caroline Severance, 6 March 1881; Sprague to Caroline Severance, letter fragment from 1892; Sprague to Severance, 29 December 1898, all in Severance Papers. Also Zakrzewska to Miss Channing, 27 December 1892, NEHWC Collection, box 1, folder 10, SS, and Sprague to Perry, 20 February 1899, New England Women's Club Records, SL. Carl Wittke, Heizen's biographer, claims that the two women "remained the closest friends," but I have not found anything to support this assertion. See Wittke, *Against the Current*, 137.

45. Cited in Wittke, *Against the Current*, 135.

46. On the battle and its aftermath, see Wittke, *Against the Current*, 136–37, and Randers-Pehrson, *Adolf Douai*, 315–32.

47. Cott, *Public Vows*.

48. See Zakrzewska's letters to Lucy Sewall in 1863 in which she mentions the practice of boarding, cited in *WQ*, 309, 311. On the practice of boarding among the middle class, see Ryan, *Cradle of the Middle Class*.

49. I have calculated her age from a letter she wrote in 1905 to Severance in which she mentioned that her friends had thrown her a surprise party for her seventieth birthday ten years earlier. See Sprague to Severance, 9 November 1905, Severance Papers.

50. This is clear from an undated letter Sprague wrote to Heinzen sometime after she moved in. She assured him that "when I came back last August, it was expected that my stay here would be temporary; this is not to be my home; I am only remaining here awhile in preparation for a change to some place not yet fully decided upon." She also asked him not to mention to Zakrzewska "this 'want of harmony' between us. . . . I cannot leave her house without some pangs and the less the matter is discussed, the pleasanter will be my visits here in the future." Karl Heinzen Papers, LBC.

51. Zakrzewska to Sewall, 7 May 1863, cited in *WQ*, 311. The first mention of Sprague is in a letter Zakrzewska wrote to Sewall on 21 October 1862 (see ibid., 301). She mentions that on 12 November they will be celebrating Sprague's birthday.

52. On Sprague's career as a schoolteacher, see William Lloyd Garrison to Fanny Garrison Villard, 14 February 1877, reprinted in Merrill and Ruchames, *Letters of William Lloyd Garrison*, 6:455–57; Wittke, *Against the Current*, 102.

53. Sprague, *History of the New England Women's Club*.

54. Sprague to Kitty Barry, 28 December 1896, Blackwell Family Papers, LC.

55. Sprague to Caroline Severance, 8 July [1902?], Severance Papers.

56. Sprague to Kitty Barry, 28 December 1896, Blackwell Family Papers, LC. On women's relationships in the nineteenth century, see Smith-Rosenberg, "Female World of Love and Ritual"; Sahli, "Smashing"; Rupp, " 'Imagine My Surprise' "; Faderman, *Surpassing the Love of Men* and *Odd Girls and Twilight Lovers*; and di Leonardo, "Warrior Virgins and Boston Marriages."

57. Di Leonardo, "Warrior Virgins and Boston Marriages"; Freedman, *Maternal Justice*, esp. 107, 178, 242.

58. The information on these relationships is not extensive, but the fact of their companionship is unmistakable. On Dimock and Greene, see Cheney, *Memoir of Susan Dimock*, 8–9, 38, 39, 43, and Cheney, "Report," *AR*, 1875, 10. On Booth and Wright, see "Obituary. Mary L. Booth." On Sewall and Jex-Blake, see Todd, *Life of Sophia Jex-Blake*. See also Morantz-Sanchez, *Sympathy and Science*, 133. Although writing of a later period, Linda Gordon found that approximately one-fourth of the women active in reform work had female companions. See Gordon, *Pitied but Not Entitled*, 78–79.

59. See especially Smith-Rosenberg, "Female World of Love and Ritual," and di Leonardo, "Warrior Virgins and Boston Marriages."

60. Zakrzewska to Lucy Sewall, 28 December 1862, cited in *WQ*, 305–6.

61. Not surprisingly, the one time Zakrzewska voiced her opinion on divorce, which was during a debate with Horace Greeley, she sided with Susan B. Anthony and Elizabeth Cady Stanton, who created quite a storm at the 1860 Women's Rights Convention when they insisted that divorce be considered a woman's civil right. On Zakrzewska's debate with Greeley, see *WQ,* 204. On Anthony, Stanton, and the 1860 Woman's Rights Convention, see Barry, *Susan B. Anthony,* 137–45.

62. *WQ,* 297.

63. Sprague to Severance, 22 February, no year but sometime after 1902, Severance Papers. The particular correspondence Sprague was referring to was between Zakrzewska and Ednah Dow Cheney.

64. Sprague to Severance, 31 January 1893, Severance Papers.

65. In the early 1890s, when Sprague and Zakrzewska moved to a new home, Sprague wrote to Severance that for the first time "our family will be small, only we two." See Sprague to Severance, 9 August [1892?], Severance Papers.

66. *Der Pionier* included announcements about the New England Hospital about once or twice a year. See, for example, "Das Hospital für Frauen und Kinder," 6, and "Stadt Boston" (2 July 1872), 6. On Sprague's work as a matron, see *AR,* 1863, 7. On the family's support of the newspaper, see Wittke, *Against the Current,* 104, 113, 317; Heinzen to Schmemann, 10 March 1879, Karl Schmemann Papers, LBC; and Sprague to George Schumm, 11 March 1909 and 3 November 1909, George Schumm Papers, LBC. Sprague's translation of "Sechs Briefe an einen frommen Mann" is mentioned in *Der Pionier,* 5 March 1879, 1.

67. In her wonderful book *Women and the City,* Sarah Deutsch distinguishes between middle-class and working-class women's understandings of domesticity by suggesting that in contrast to the former, the latter "did not organize their lives around the concepts of 'public' and 'private' " (287). Zakrzewska's indifference to this organizing framework suggests, however, that what Deutsch describes as a class difference may have had more to do with whether women worked outside the home.

68. On Zakrzewska's friendship with William Lloyd Garrison II, see Chapter 4; on Heinzen and the elder Garrison, see Zakrzewska to Garrison, 7 December, no year, Garrison Family Collection, Correspondence, SS, and Wittke, *Against the Current,* 114. On Büchner's visit, see Ludwig Büchner to Heinzen, 6 October 1872, Karl Heinzen Papers, LBC.

69. Cited in *WQ,* 459.

70. The reminiscences are of Dr. Augusta Pope, which she shared during a speech she gave at the fiftieth anniversary of the New England Hospital. See *Fiftieth Anniversary of the New England Hospital,* 48. For other reminiscences of parties at what Zakrzewska playfully called her "Rock Garden," see *WQ,* 458–59.

71. The comparison between Washington and Heinzen is from a summary and translation that Sprague provided of a speech given by Clara Neymann, a German radical journalist. See "Address by Mrs. Clara Neymann," 441–42. Zakrzewska's comment is from a tribute to Samuel Sewall, printed in the appendix to Sprague, *History of the New England Women's Club,* 83. The fact that Zakrzewska's household continued to commemorate Heinzen's birthday is mentioned in Sprague to Perry, 20 February 1899, New England Women's Club Records, Julia A. Sprague, SL.

72. Zakrzewska to Sewall, 28 December 1862, cited in *WQ,* 305.

73. Zakrzewska to Pope, 28 October 1901, NEHWC Collection, box 1, SS.

74. Zakrzewska to Sewall, 29 November 1862, cited in *WQ,* 303.

CHAPTER SIX

1. Dall, *"Woman's Right to Labor."* On Dall, see Bowman, "Caroline Healey Dall," and Wach, "Boston Feminist."

2. Zakrzewska, "Ueber Hospitäler" (18 February 1863).

3. Cited in Barry, *Susan B. Anthony,* 115.

4. Dall, introduction to *PI,* 3. Dall wrote the first eighteen and the last two pages of *PI.*

5. Wagner-Martin, *Telling Women's Lives.*

6. See Wells's discussion of the feminist scholarship on autobiography in *Out of the Dead House,* 131. According to this scholarship, women had a greater tendency to follow a less linear, more episodic narrative structure when telling the stories of their lives.

7. *PI,* 46.

8. Dall, *"Woman's Right to Labor,"* 11–12.

9. Dall, introduction to *PI,* 4–5.

10. Ibid., 9, 13.

11. Ibid., 4–5, 15.

12. Dall discusses this in ibid., 16. In her concluding comments to the autobiographical sketch, Dall again emphasized how it was "free from all egotism" (164).

13. *PI,* 18. See also 161–62 and a letter Zakrzewska wrote to Dall on 1 December 1860, Dall Papers, box 3, folder 5. Notably, several of the book's reviewers addressed the appropriateness of publishing an autobiography, only to explain why Zakrzewska's sketch should not be seen as lacking in decorum. See the collection of reviews in Scrapbook #1, Dall Papers.

14. On the genre of women's autobiography, see Heilbrun, *Writing a Woman's Life,* esp. the introduction, 11–31; Jelinek, *Tradition of Women's Autobiography,* 90; and Wagner-Martin, *Telling Women's Lives.*

15. On Longshore, see Wells, *Out of the Dead House,* 131. On Dixon-Jones, see Morantz-Sanchez, *Conduct Unbecoming a Woman.*

16. Booth to Dall, 19 October 1860, Dall Papers, box 3, folder 4.

17. The stories from her early childhood appear in *PI,* 19–24. Quotations are from 19, 20, and 24.

18. Ibid., 24.

19. Ibid., 36–37.

20. Ibid., 26.

21. Cott, "Passionless"; Douglas, *Feminization of American Culture.*

22. Numbers and Schoepflin, "Ministries of Healing." For a different take on Zakrzewska's story of the night she spent with the corpse, see Wells, *Out of the Dead House,* 3–5.

23. *PI,* 35–36.

24. Ibid., 67.

25. *Boston Transcript*, Scrapbook #1, Dall Papers.

26. *PI*, 97.

27. Ibid., 119.

28. Ibid. On prostitution in New York City, see Stansell, *City of Women*, chaps. 6–9, and Nadel, *Little Germany*, 75–78. On antebellum melodramatic tales of seduction and abandonment, see Kunzel, *Fallen Women, Problem Girls*, chap. 1.

29. *PI*, 115–19.

30. Dall, conclusion to *PI*, 166–67.

31. Heinzen, *Rights of Women and the Sexual Relations*, 32.

32. Ibid., 36.

33. Ibid., 30, 38.

34. *WQ*, 156. See also Zakrzewska's comment that when she had first arrived in Boston the fear still existed "that the study of medicine would unsex girls." Ibid., 245.

35. *Portland Transcript*, *London Critic*, and *Monthly*, all in Scrapbook #1, Dall Papers.

36. *Boston Transcript*, *Christian Register*, *Christian Examiner*, all in ibid.

37. C. K. W., *Liberator*, *Portland Transcript*, *Christian Examiner*, all in ibid.

38. *London Critic*, *Boston Transcript*, *Boston Journal*, all in ibid.

39. *Boston Journal*, *Christian Inquirer*, *London Critic*; C. W. Curtis, *Harper's*, all in ibid.

40. *PI*, 153.

41. Ibid., 24, 69.

42. Ibid., 37.

43. Ibid., 46.

44. "Woman and the Press," 95; "Notizen," 6. The announcement was repeated in both newspapers every week throughout June and July.

45. The title of the announcement was the same in each journal: "Postponement of the Woman's Journal," *Liberator*, 43, and *Der Pionier*, 6.

46. Walker, Wise, & Co. to Mrs. C. H. Dall, 16 October 1861, in Dall Papers, box 5, folder 68. Dall and Booth also exchanged words about who was responsible for the financial failure. See Booth to Dall, 10 October 1861, in ibid., box 3, folder 8.

47. Zakrzewska to Dall, 13 February 1867, in ibid., box 4, folder 12.

CHAPTER SEVEN

1. Gregory penned these words in the college's *Tenth Annual Report*, published in 1859, cited in Gardner, "Midwife, Doctor, or Doctress?," 142. For other sources on the New England Female Medical College, see Waite, *History of the New England Female Medical College*; *WQ*, 243–87; and Walsh, *"Doctors Wanted,"* chap. 2.

2. Ludmerer, *Learning to Heal*, 11–12. The absence of clinical instruction in medical schools did not, however, mean that practical instruction was deemed unimportant. Rather, students were expected to acquire this knowledge on their own. See Warner, *Against the Spirit of System*, 26–29.

3. Waite, *History of the New England Female Medical College*, 11–44, 112–13; *First Annual Report*

of the Clinical Department of the New England Female Medical College, Boston, 1860, NEH Annual Reports, Blanche Ames Ames Papers, box 2a, folder 24a, 4, SL.

4. "Circular," reprinted (in English) in *Der Pionier*, 2 July 1859, 6.

5. Waite, *History of the New England Female Medical College*, 45–46; *WQ*, 243–44; *First Annual Report of the Clinical Department of the New England Female Medical College*, 61; "Annual Meeting of the 'Hospital for Women and Children,'" 182; "Bostoner Heilanstalt für Frauen und Kinder," 8.

6. Jacobi, "Women in Medicine," 166. See also Gardner, "Midwife, Doctor, or Doctress?," 177.

7. At the time Zakrzewska joined the faculty of the college, the requirements for a medical degree stated that one had to be twenty-one years old; have studied medicine three years, all of them under a licensed physician; have attended two courses of lectures, with at least one course at the college; have passed examinations in all subjects taught at the college; and have written a dissertation. See Waite, *History of the New England Female Medical College*, 30. For criticisms of the way Gregory has been portrayed in the stories told about his battles with Zakrzewska, see Gardner, "Midwife, Doctor, or Doctress?," 143, and Tuchman, "Situating Gender."

8. Zakrzewska, *Introductory Lecture*, 7. On nineteenth-century American medical education, see Ludmerer, *Learning to Heal*; Rosenberg, *Care of Strangers*; and Rothstein, *American Physicians in the Nineteenth Century*. For a comparative analysis of medical education in the United States, Great Britain, France, and Germany, see Bonner, *Becoming a Physician*.

9. Warner, *Therapeutic Perspective*, esp. chaps. 3 and 6, and *Against the Spirit of System*, esp. chap. 10.

10. Bleker, *Die naturhistorische Schule*; Tuchman, *Science, Medicine, and the State*. For Zakrzewska's comments about "empirics," see *WQ*, 165.

11. Wunderlich, "Einleitung," xvi. On German rational medicine, see Tuchman, *Science, Medicine, and the State*.

12. Ware, "Success in the Medical Profession," 518, 503.

13. Morantz-Sanchez, *Sympathy and Science*.

14. Ware, "Success in the Medical Profession," 520. Interestingly, Zakrzewska and Ware developed a warm friendship. After reading her autobiographical sketch, he expressed his admiration for her accomplishments. Nevertheless, he still declared "intolerable" the idea that any of his daughters would pursue a medical career. He thus chose to view Zakrzewska as an anomaly. See Ware's letter to Zakrzewska, 13 December 1860, cited in *WQ*, 255–56.

15. The quotation, which appears in *WQ*, 251, is not directly from Gregory. Rather, Zakrzewska is reporting hearsay, although she places this statement in quotation marks. See also ibid., 284. For a very good recent discussion of Gregory and the New England Female Medical College, see Gardner, "Midwife, Doctor, or Doctress?" Gregory's concerns about the microscope were voiced by others as well. See Warner, *Against the Spirit of System*, 342.

16. Zakrzewska to Samuel E. Sewall, no date but probably written in the summer of 1861, cited in *WQ*, 281–82.

17. Ibid., 272, 256 (reference to Bowditch and Cabot), 251.

18. Gardner, "Midwife, Doctor, or Doctress?," 143–44.

19. Gregory, *Man-Midwifery*, 45. See also Gregory, *Letter to Ladies*, 31–32.

20. Gregory, *Man-Midwifery*, 29. See also Gregory, *Letter to Ladies*, 33.

21. Gregory, *Man-Midwifery*, 32, 46. Realizing that he had made unnecessary enemies through such harsh comments, Gregory dropped all accusations of greed and depravity from later publications. See Gardner, "Midwife, Doctor, or Doctress?," 68–73.

22. Donegan, *Women and Men Midwives*; Leavitt, *Brought to Bed*; Wertz and Wertz, *Lying-in*.

23. Gregory, *Man-Midwifery*, 41–42.

24. Ibid., 35.

25. Ibid., 8. On the regulation of European midwives, see Marland, *Art of Midwifery* and *Midwives, Society and Childbirth*.

26. Gregory, *Letter to Ladies*, 22. Walsh also discusses the ambiguity in Gregory's attitudes toward women in *"Doctors Wanted,"* 36.

27. Gregory, *Letter to Ladies*, 16–19. Madame Marie Louise Lachapelle (1769–1821), author of the three-volume *Pratique des Accouchemens* (Paris, 1821–25), was one of the better-known French midwives. A German translation of the first volume was published as early as 1825, which means Zakrzewska may very well have read her work. Madame Marie Anne Victorine Boivin, a student of Lachapelle's and author of *Traité pratique des maladies de l'utérus et de ses annexes* (Paris, 1833), was awarded an honorary degree from the medical faculty of the University of Marburg in 1827. See Donnison, *Midwives and Medical Men*, 54, and Fassbender, *Geschichte der Geburtshilfe*, 256–57.

28. Gregory, *Letter to Ladies*, 37.

29. Gregory, "Female Physicians," 246, 247.

30. Zakrzewska, *Introductory Lecture*, 5–6.

31. Ibid., 24. See also her article "Ueber Hospitäler" (4 March 1863).

32. Ginzberg, *Women and the Work of Benevolence*. For an excellent analysis of the attack on the rhetoric of female benevolence, see Kunzel, *Fallen Women, Problem Girls*. On the tradition of female benevolence, see also Cott, *Bonds of Womanhood*; Deutsch, *Women and the City*; Ryan, *Women in Public* and *Cradle of the Middle Class*; Sklar, *Catherine Beecher*; Smith-Rosenberg, *Disorderly Conduct*; and Welter, "Cult of True Womanhood, 1820–1860."

33. More, " 'Empathy' Enters the Profession of Medicine."

34. For the strengths and weaknesses of earlier work on women and the professions, see Kunzel, *Fallen Women, Problem Girls*, 1–8.

35. On Blackwell, see Morantz-Sanchez, "Feminist Theory and Historical Practice"; on Dolley, see More, *Restoring the Balance*, 13–41; on Preston, see Peitzman, *New and Untried Course*, 45–55, and Wells, *Out of the Dead House*, 57–79; on Dixon-Jones, see Morantz-Sanchez, *Conduct Unbecoming a Woman*; on Jacobi, see Bittel, "Science of Women's Rights," and Morantz-Sanchez, *Sympathy and Science*, 184–202.

36. Zakrzewska, *Introductory Lecture*, 8–9. Ann Preston also shaped an introductory lecture she gave at the Female Medical College of Pennsylvania in 1855 around the theme of medical progress. See Wells, *Out of the Dead House*, 66.

37. Zakrzewska, *Introductory Lecture*, 14.

38. Cited in *WQ*, 175.

39. Cited in ibid., 251. This quotation is not directly from Gregory but is rather Zakrzew-

ska's rendition of what Sewall told her Gregory had said. There is, however, no reason to doubt that this quotation accurately reflects Gregory's sentiments. Gregory's comment is little different from that of other American physicians, who also spoke disparagingly of microscopes. See Warner, *Therapeutic Perspective*, 219.

40. Cited in *WQ*, 165. Ironically, one of the criticisms American physicians had of science was that it led physicians to adopt a "routine practice," by which they meant a fixed course of treatment rather than focusing on the peculiarities of the case before them. See Warner, *Therapeutic Perspective*, 218.

41. Cited in *WQ*, 281.

42. Ibid., 257, 276; Waite, *History of the New England Female Medical College*, 47; "Stadt Boston" (27 February 1862), 6, where it is mentioned that Zakrzewska had resigned her position.

43. Jacobi, "Women in Medicine," 146.

44. Peitzman, *New and Untried Course*, 2, 24, 38–44; Morantz-Sanchez, *Sympathy and Science*, 74–75, 77. Chicago's Woman's Hospital Medical College, which was founded in 1870 under the leadership of Mary Thompson, also required clinical instruction and dissection when it opened its doors. See Morantz-Sanchez, *Sympathy and Science*, 80.

45. *WQ*, 382. On the merger, see Gardner, "Midwife, Doctor, or Doctress?," 226–34, and Waite, *History of the New England Female Medical College*, 107–11.

CHAPTER EIGHT

The title of this chapter is taken from the title of a lecture Zakrzewska gave in January 1863, in which she laid out her vision of the hospital she had just helped to create.

1. On the Woman's Hospital of Philadelphia, see Peitzman, *New and Untried Course*, 24–26.

2. Zakrzewska, "Ueber Hospitäler" (4 March 1863).

3. Huggins, *Protestants against Poverty*, 93; Irving, *Safe Deliverance*; Vogel, *Invention of the Modern Hospital*, 9–19; Watson, *Charity Organization Movement*, 178, 197–201.

4. See Boyer, *Urban Masses*; Deutsch, *Women and the City*; Katz, *In the Shadow of the Poorhouse*; Kunzel, *Fallen Women, Problem Girls*; Rosenberg, *Care of Strangers*; and Vogel, *Invention of the Modern Hospital*.

5. See Katz, *In the Shadow of the Poorhouse*, 66, 70–75, and Boyer, *Urban Masses*, 86–94. On the blend of medical care and moral education at the New England Hospital, see Drachman, *Hospital with a Heart*, 60–64, 83–85.

6. "Lecture on Hospitals," 19.

7. Zakrzewska, "Ueber Hospitäler." Ironically, since she gave the lecture in English, it had to be translated into German for the readers of *Der Pionier*. The English translation here is my own.

8. Zakrzewska, "Ueber Hospitäler" (4 February 1863). On Massachusetts General Hospital, see Bowditch, *History of the Massachusetts General Hospital*. See also Vogel, *Invention of the Modern Hospital*. On Boston City Hospital, see Vogel, *Invention of the Modern Hospital*, 290.

9. Zakrzewska, "Ueber Hospitäler" (4 February 1863). Zakrzewska returns to this theme in "Report of the Attending Physician," *AR*, 1868, 11.

10. Cheney, "Report," *AR*, 1864, 3–9. On Zakrzewska's discussion of "Häuslichkeit," see "Ueber Hospitäler" (11 February 1863).

11. "Hospital for Women and Children," 187.

12. *Annual Report of the Trustees of the Massachusetts General Hospital*, 1863, 15; *Annual Report of the Trustees of the Massachusetts General Hospital*, 1864, 9. See also Kass, *Midwifery and Medicine*, 95.

13. Katz, *In the Shadow of the Poorhouse*, chap. 4.

14. See Chapter 7.

15. Regina Kunzel has written in particular of Christian evangelical reformers' belief in the "redemptive power of domesticity." See Kunzel, *Fallen Women, Problem Girls*, 28. See also Deutsch, *Women and the City*, 54–77, on the middle-class link between domesticity and morality.

16. Zakrzewska, "Ueber Hospitäler" (18 February 1863).

17. Zakrzewska, "Ueber Hospitäler" (4 February 1863). On the difficulties of distinguishing between the worthy and unworthy poor, see Katz, *In the Shadow of the Poorhouse*, 10. Sickness, unemployment, widowhood, and the like could reduce a "worthy" working-class family to paupers overnight. I mention Zakrzewska's derogatory comments about the French and the Irish in Chapter 6.

18. Zakrzewska, "Ueber Hospitäler" (11 February 1863).

19. Rosenberg, *Care of Strangers*.

20. Michael Katz was describing Josephine Shaw Lowell when he made this comment. See Katz, *In the Shadow of the Poorhouse*, 71.

21. Zakrzewska, "Ueber Hospitäler" (11 February 1863).

22. Zakrzewska, "Ueber Hospitäler" (4 February 1863). On the belief of some evangelical Christians that poverty was necessary, see Huggins, *Protestants against Poverty*, especially his introduction.

23. Zakrzewska, "Ueber Hospitäler" (4 February 1863). In the same speech, she criticized large public institutions for failing to offer a "home to the homeless in which the friendless are assured of friends." On the sentimentalism of evangelical reformers, see Kunzel, *Fallen Women, Problem Girls*, 25–35.

24. Zakrzewska, "Ueber Hospitäler" (4 March 1863). Zakrzewska's discussion of the foreign population was published in the same issue.

25. Ibid.

26. The quotation from Massachusetts General Hospital is cited in Kass, *Midwifery and Medicine*, 103. On Philadelphia, see Peitzman, *New and Untried Course*, 26, and Wells, *Out of the Dead House*, 19. Notably, when Boston City Hospital opened its doors in 1864, it too chose not to care for women in childbirth. See Vogel, *Invention of the Modern Hospital*, 35. The New York Asylum for Lying-In Women was more lenient, but it helped only first-time mothers. As I discuss in the next chapter, Zakrzewska defended single mothers of multiple births as well. On New York, see Quiroga, *Poor Mothers and Babies*, esp. chap. 2, and Stansell, *City of Women*, 70–72. On antebellum reform societies' interest in redeeming "fallen women," see Ginzberg, *Women and the Work of Benevolence*; Hewitt, *Women's Activism and Social Change*; and Ryan, *Cradle of the Middle Class*.

27. Kunzel, *Fallen Women, Problem Girls*, 20–21; Morton, *And Sin No More.*

28. No date; cited in *WQ,* 315.

29. The elite Boston physician Walter Channing, who consulted at the New England Hospital, shared Zakrzewska's view. See Kass, *Midwifery and Medicine*, 198–204. In contrast, the dominant view in antebellum America, best exemplified by reformers such as Lemuel Shattuck, held individual behavior to be the primary determinant of disease. See Rosenkrantz, *Public Health and the State*, 14–36.

30. Zakrzewska mentioned this strategy in "Annual Meeting of the 'Hospital for Women and Children,'" 182. See also Cheney, "Secretary's Report," *AR*, 1863, 5, and *History and Description of the New England Hospital*, 25.

31. Zakrzewska, "Ueber Hospitäler" (18 February 1863).

32. Zakrzewska, "Ueber Hospitäler" (25 February 1863).

33. Ibid.; "Ueber Hospitäler" (4 March 1863).

34. The bylaws can be found in *Fiftieth Anniversary of the New England Hospital*, 17. Also, the annual reports of the hospital did not fail to emphasize this point. See, for example, Cheney, "Report," *AR*, 1864, 3–9.

35. Zakrzewska, "Report of the Attending Physician," *AR*, 1865, 18. According to Wells (*Out of the Dead House*, 65), Ann Preston shared Zakrzewska's sentiment about male physicians attending female patients. On Horatio Storer's experience at the New England Hospital, see Drachman, *Hospital with a Heart*, 56–57; *WQ,* 310, 338–44; and a slip of paper (undated) mentioning Zakrzewska's dealings with Storer, in the NEHWC Collection, box 6, folder 14, SS. Storer's appointment did not turn out well, and he resigned after only three years.

36. On women physicians' positive assessment of coeducation, see Morantz-Sanchez, *Sympathy and Science*, 66–67.

37. Zakrzewska, "Report of the Attending Physician," *AR*, 1865, 13.

38. The complete list of all nineteen members can be found in *WQ,* 487 n. 8. For a good analysis of the supporters of the New England Hospital, see Drachman, *Hospital with a Heart*, 44–70. Cheney, Sewall, Bowditch, and Channing will all be dealt with in greater detail below. For evidence of the other individuals' social activism, see Jensen, "Severance"; Merrill and Ruchames, *Letters of William Lloyd Garrison*, 1:41, 2:331, 3:450, 4:184, 331, 359–66, 624, 687, 5:269; Tiffany, *Samuel E. Sewall*, 53, 73; Garrison and Garrison, *William Lloyd Garrison*, 2:189; *History and Description of the New England Hospital*, 6–8; *WQ,* 293–94; and an obituary of the Hon. Thomas Russell, in the *Boston Transcript*, 2 February 1887.

39. "Paper Read by Dr. Zakrzewska at the Opening of the Sewall Maternity House," *AR*, 1892, 13. Clarke founded the Church of the Disciples in 1841 and continued as its minister until his death in 1888. See W. W. F., "James Freeman Clarke," and Hale, *James Freeman Clarke*. On links between Clarke's church and members of the New England's staff, see Hale, *James Freeman Clarke*, 193–94, 207, 328, and Kass, *Midwifery and Medicine*, 221, 348 n. 59. In 1887, the hospital celebrated its twenty-fifth anniversary at Clarke's Church of the Disciples. See *Fiftieth Anniversary of the New England Hospital*, 20.

40. James Freeman Clarke to his sister, 7 January 1841, in Hale, *James Freeman Clarke*, 155. On Clarke, Parker, and Emerson's influence on them, see Robinson, *Unitarians and the Univer-*

salists, 75–86, 102–6, 234–35, 302–3. Clarke's wife, Mrs. Anna H. Clarke, served on the Board of Directors of the New England Hospital for the first several decades of its existence.

41. The list of interconnections between these individuals includes the friendship between the Severances and the Garrisons, as well as that between the Garrisons and the Stephensons. Hale also wrote a biography of Clarke, and the Sewalls and the Mays were cousins.

42. For biographical information on Cheney, see Cheney, *Reminiscences*; Ingebritsen, "Ednah Dow Littlehale Cheney"; Drachman, *Hospital with a Heart*, 48; and Cheney, "Theodore Parker," 51.

43. The founding members of the New England Women's Club included Caroline M. Severance, Ednah D. Cheney, Lucia M. Peabody, Mrs. Jonathan A. Lane, Julia Ward Howe, Lucy Goddard, and Mrs. H. W. Sewall. On the meaning of the New England Hospital for women's rights advocates, see Drachman, *Hospital with a Heart*, 45–48. On "female institution building," see Freedman, "Separatism as Strategy," 513. On nineteenth-century women's networks, see also Cott, *Bonds of Womanhood*, and Ryan, "Power of Women's Networks."

44. Cheney, "Report," *AR*, 1866, 6; Cheney, *Memoir of Susan Dimock*, 38–39. See also Cheney, "Report," *AR*, 1865, 10, and "Report," *AR*, 1867, 6, and *History and Description of the New England Hospital*, 25–26. Weld's gift is mentioned in the *AR*, 1868, 8. On Weld, see Anderson, *Under the Black Horse Flag*, 30–39, and Merrill and Ruchames, *Letters of William Lloyd Garrison*, 6:54.

The Woman's Hospital of Philadelphia was also on record as accepting patients "without regard to their religious belief, nationality or color"; cited in Peitzman, *New and Untried Course*, 26.

45. Cheney, *Reminiscences*, 60.

46. On Sewall, see Tiffany, *Samuel E. Sewall*; Drachman, *Hospital with a Heart*, 50–51; and Waite, *History of the New England Female Medical College*, 116. The various slave cases are discussed in Tiffany, *Samuel E. Sewall*, 58–100; the quotation is from 99.

47. Sewall, *Legal Condition*.

48. Zakrzewska's comment is cited in Tiffany, *Samuel E. Sewall*, 132. For Zakrzewska's refusal to attend his funeral, see her letter to Garrison, 22 December 1888, Garrison Family Collection, Correspondence, box 61, SS.

49. On Bowditch, see Bowditch, *Life and Correspondence*; Scanlon, "Henry Ingersoll Bowditch"; Merrill and Ruchames, *Letters of William Lloyd Garrison*, 3:155–56, 542, 641–42; and Tiffany, *Samuel E. Sewall*, 70. It bears mention that Bowditch was also a Unitarian. See Kass, *Midwifery and Medicine*, 338 n. 46.

50. Bowditch, *Life and Correspondence*, 1:130–31.

51. *WQ*, 277, 393–95.

52. Bowditch, *Life and Correspondence*, 2:212, 215. On Bowditch's support of women's rights, see as well *WQ*, 336–37, and his article "Female Practitioners of Medicine."

53. On Jarvis, see *Dictionary of American Biography*, s.v. Jarvis, Edward. On Channing's *Address on the Prevention of Pauperism* (1843), see Kass, *Midwifery and Medicine*, chap. 10. On Channing's and Ware's vote to admit black students to Harvard Medical School, see Kass, *Midwifery and Medicine*, 208. On Ware's political and religious leanings, see Kass, *Midwifery and Medicine*, 338 n. 46, and Robinson, *Unitarians and the Universalists*, 331–32.

54. In 1860, in an exchange of letters with Zakrzewska, John Ware reiterated the objections he had articulated in his article "Success in the Medical Profession," but he also admitted that he "may be mistaken" and was "quite willing to find myself in the wrong." Perhaps the year he consulted at the New England Hospital marked his willingness to explore the foundation of his views. Unfortunately, he died the following year without returning to the question of women's medical education. See John Ware to Zakrzewska, 13 December 1860, reprinted in *WQ*, 255–56. See also John Ware to Zakrzewska, 11 February 1860, reprinted in ibid., 254–55.

55. Drachman, *Hospital with a Heart*, 54–56, discusses Clarke's affiliation with the New England Hospital. See also *WQ*, 254.

56. Clarke, "Recent Progress in Materia Medica," 320–21.

57. Warner discusses Clarke's embrace of physiological therapeutics in *Against the Spirit of System*, 336.

58. Ibid., 344–47.

59. *WQ*, 315.

60. Zakrzewska to Lucy Sewall, 20 February 1863, cited in *WQ*, 308–9. Zakrzewska did not mention which friend accompanied her to New York. See also her letter on 25 January 1863, cited in ibid., 306–8. On Breed, see ibid., 295, and Rochford, "New England Hospital."

61. Zakrzewska to Lucy Sewall, 7 May 1863, cited in *WQ*, 311; Elizabeth Blackwell to Emily and Kitty, 15 November 1865, Blackwell Family Papers, SL. See also Zakrzewska to Dall, 26 January 1865, in Dall Papers, box 4, folder 1.

62. Zakrzewska to Caroline Dall, 25 March 1866, Dall Papers, box 2, folder 15. On the Lowell Institute, see Story, *Forging of an Aristocracy*, 14–16.

63. Cheney, "Report," *AR*, 1869, 5.

CHAPTER NINE

1. Zakrzewska, "Report of the Attending Physician," *AR*, 1868, 9–21. Statistics are from the annual reports for the years ending 1863–65.

2. *AR*, 1900–1902. See also *WQ*, 293; Drachman, *Hospital with a Heart*, 136–40; and *Fiftieth Anniversary of the New England Hospital*, 21–22.

3. Bertha van Hoosen, "Report of the Resident Physician," *AR*, 1891, 11; Cheney, "Report," *AR*, 1865, 6; Cheney, "Report of the Secretary," *AR*, 1886, 5.

4. See Rosenberg, "Inward Vision and Outward Glance" and *Care of Strangers*; Rosner, *Once Charitable Enterprise*; Starr, *Social Transformation of American Medicine*; and Stevens, *In Sickness and in Wealth*.

5. Cheney, "Secretary's Report," *AR*, 1863, 5. Statistics are from the annual reports, 1863–68. On the desire for expansion, see Cheney, "Report," *AR*, 1868, 7–8.

6. Rosenberg, *Care of Strangers*, 109–15.

7. Sewall's comment is from "Report of the Resident Physician," *AR*, 12; statistics are on 19. On the New England Hospital's popularity because of its all-female staff, see Drachman,

Hospital with a Heart, 71–75. On "women's diseases," see Wood, " 'Fashionable Diseases,' " and Morantz, "Perils of Feminist History."

8. Kirschmann, *Vital Force*, 58; Morantz-Sanchez, *Sympathy and Science*, 73–80; Peitzman, *New and Untried Course*, 24–26.

9. Cheney, "Report," *AR*, 1866, 8; Zakrzewska, "Report of the Attending Physician," *AR*, 1865, 19. On policies at Massachusetts General Hospital, see Sewall, "Report of the Resident Physician," *AR*, 1867, 12, in which she explicitly contrasted the policies of this hospital with those of the New England Hospital. On the dispensary movement in the United States, see Rosenberg, "Social Class and Medical Care."

10. I have culled together the hospital's admissions policy from the following sources: Cheney, "Report," *AR*, 1864, 6–7; Zakrzewska, "Report of the Attending Physician," *AR*, 1865, 15–16; C. K. W., "New England Hospital for Women and Children," 35; *AR*, 1869, 3; "Circular," *AR*, 1873; *History and Description of the New England Hospital*, 40; "Communication from the Medical Board of the NEHWC," 25 May 1891, NEHWC Collection, box 6, folder 16, SS, reprinted in *WQ*, 449–50. On the medical staff's concern with the morality of those patients seeking admission, see Drachman, *Hospital with a Heart*, 60–64, 84–86. On policies at Massachusetts General Hospital and other hospitals, see Warner, *Therapeutic Perspective*, 103–5, and Rosenberg, *Care of Strangers*, 22–26.

11. Peitzman, *New and Untried Course*, 26; Wells, *Out of the Dead House*, 19.

12. Lucy Sewall, "Report of the Resident Physician," *AR*, 1867, 16; Zakrzewska, "Report of the Attending Physician," *AR*, 1868, 10–12. See also Zakrzewska, "Report of the Attending Physician," *AR*, 1865, 13.

13. Zakrzewska, "Report of the Attending Physician," *AR*, 1868, 10, 17; see also 12. On Mary Delafield DuBois, see Quiroga, *Poor Mothers and Babies*, 63–64.

14. This is roughly comparable to the 51.6 percent of the women giving birth at the Boston Lying-In Hospital in the 1870s who were also single. See the *Annual Reports of the Boston Lying-In Hospital*, 1875–79.

15. On Boston's racial makeup in these years, see U.S. Bureau of the Census, *Eighth Census*, 1860, 608; *Ninth Census*, 1870, 380, 386; *Tenth Census*, 1880, 419; and *Eleventh Census*, 1890, 534.

16. According to U.S. Census reports, the foreign-born made up 35.9 percent of Boston's total population in 1860 and 35.1 percent in 1870. The increased percentage of foreign-born attending the dispensary did not, therefore, reflect an increase in their representation in the population at large. See U.S. Bureau of the Census, *Eighth Census*, 1860, 608, and *Ninth Census*, 1870, 380–91.

17. See "Annual Meeting of the 'Hospital for Women and Children,' " 182, and C. K. W., "New England Hospital for Women and Children," 35.

18. Zakrzewska, "Report of the Attending Physician," *AR*, 1865, 13.

19. Rosenberg, *Care of Strangers*, 47–68. Physicians did not gain control over hospital affairs until the end of the century.

20. "Communication from the Medical Board of the NEHWC," 25 May 1891, NEHWC Collection, box 6, folder 16, SS, reprinted in *WQ*, 449–50.

21. On the funds from the Lying-In Hospital Corporation, see Cheney, "Secretary's Re-

port," *AR*, 1863, 8; Cheney, "Report," *AR*, 1865, 9; Zakrzewska, "Report of the Attending Physician," *AR*, 1865, 13; and Cheney, "Report," *AR*, 1866, 8. In 1868, hoping to bring some stability to its fund-raising strategies, the board of directors informed subscribers that an annual donation of $250 would fund a "free bed." This remained the hospital's policy until 1872, when it substituted a one-time donation of $5,000 as a way of permanently funding a free bed that would also bear the donor's name. See Sewall, "Report of the Resident Physician," *AR*, 1867, 13; Cheney, "Report," *AR*, 1868, 5; and Cheney, "Report," *AR*, 1872, 10.

22. Cheney, "Report," *AR*, 1868, 4–5; Zakrzewska to Caroline Dall, 6 March 1869, Dall Papers, box 5, folder 2. The 1866 resolution can be found in Cheney, "Report," *AR*, 1866, 9. The decision to charge for medicines is discussed in Cheney, "Report," *AR*, 1868, 4–5. On the hospital's expansion and the financial pressures that resulted, see Cheney, "Report," *AR*, 1865, 8; Cheney, "Report," *AR*, 1866, 7–9; and Lucy E. Sewall, "Report of the Resident Physician," *AR*, 1866, 14. Statistics on the numbers of people attending the dispensary are drawn from the annual reports for the years 1867–69.

23. Zakrzewska, "Report of the Attending Physician," *AR*, 1869, 9. A striking example of Zakrzewska's willingness to place her hospital before her principles was her recommendation that the application of an intern be refused solely because she was black. Zakrzewska's fear was that patients would refuse to be treated by this intern and that trouble would arise. The board of directors, however, overturned Zakrzewska's recommendation, and the intern spent a year at the hospital without any apparent difficulties. See Records of the Meetings of Physicians, 27 January 1878 and 28 April 1878, in NEHWC Collection, SS.

24. Zakrzewska, "Report of the Attending Physician," *AR* 1865, 19; C. A. Buckel, "Report of the Resident Physician," *AR*, 1871, 11; Zakrzewska, "Report of the Attending Physician," *AR*, 1869, 9–10.

25. See Chapter 6. The greater representation of Irish among the dispensary population was not matched by a proportional increase in Boston's population at large. Indeed, between 1860 and 1870 the Irish went from 25.9 percent of Boston's total population to 22.7 percent. By 1880, they accounted for 17.9 percent. See U.S. Bureau of the Census, *Eighth Census*, 1860, 608; *Ninth Census*, 1870, 380–91; *Tenth Census*, 1880, 450, 536–41.

26. Cheney, "Report," *AR*, 1870, 8, 9. The New England was by no means alone in trying to reach out to paying patients. See, for example, *Annual Report of the Trustees of the Massachusetts General Hospital*, 1866, 5, 39–48, in which the author assesses the hospital's financial state and concludes that more paying patients must be attracted to the institution. On the changing nature of the hospital, see Rosenberg, *Care of Strangers*; Starr, *Social Transformation of American Medicine*; and Stevens, *In Sickness and in Wealth*.

27. The dispensary operated at first out of a house on the corner of Tremont and Pleasant streets. It eventually moved to 33 Warrenton and then to 29 Fayette Street. See *Circular. The New England Hospital for Women and Children* (published together with the *AR* for 1873); Lucy E. Sewall, "Report of the Dispensary," *AR*, 1875, 27; "Dispensary Report," *AR*, 1880, 10; and *Fiftieth Anniversary of the New England Hospital*.

28. See, for example, Kraut, *Silent Travelers*, and Rosenberg, *Cholera Years*. See also Douglas, *Purity and Danger*, and Baldwin, *Contagion and the State*.

29. Kisacky, "Architecture of Light and Air."

30. Zakrzewska, "Report of the Attending Physician," *AR*, 1869, 10.

31. For an explicit link between class and cure rate, see Lucy Sewall, "Report of the Resident Physician," *AR*, 1866, 14.

32. The intern was Alice Hamilton; cited in Sicherman, *Alice Hamilton*, 73.

33. *History and Description of the New England Hospital*, 12; Cheney, "Report," *AR*, 1872, 6–7; Cheney, "Report," *AR*, 1873, 8; Call, "Evolution of Modern Maternity Technic," 395; Cheney, "Annual Report," *AR*, 1877, 5. The distribution of the beds is from Zakrzewska et al., "Report of the Furnishing Committee," *AR*, 1873, 16–17.

34. Beginning in 1897 they reported both on the number of free days and on the numbers who paid board.

35. For example, whereas the percentage of free days in 1897 was 57.7, the percentage of charity cases was 43.7. See *AR* for the years 1897–1901.

36. See Crumpacker, "Female Patients in Four Boston Hospitals"; Drachman, *Hospital with a Heart*, 88, 219 n. 45; and Morantz and Zschoche, "Professionalism, Feminism, and Gender Roles."

37. The first quotation is from Zakrzewska, "Report of the Attending Physician," *AR*, 1865, 17. The second is from an address she gave on the occasion of the opening of the new dispensary building, cited in Cheney, "Report of the Secretary," *AR*, 1897, 9. On the "Diet Kitchen," see Lucy Sewall, "Report of the Dispensary," *AR*, 1876, 29.

38. Emma L. Call, "Report of the Dispensary," *AR*, 1881, 21; E. B. Culbertson, "Dispensary Report," *AR*, 1886, 10–11; Adaline S. Whitney, "Report of the Dispensary," *AR*, 1887, 7. On the Associated Charities of Boston, see Watson, *Charity Organization Movement*, 197–201. On the general move on the part of hospitals to pay organizations to check the financial status of those applying for charity, see Rosenberg, "Inward Vision and Outward Glance," 375. Statistics on the dispensary populations are from the *Annual Reports*, 1886, 1893.

39. The first reference I found to this ruling was in *History and Description of the New England Hospital*, 26. However, in this report nothing was said about extenuating circumstances. Not until 1879 did the board add that an exception could be made if the medical staff determined that there were extenuating circumstances. See *Reference Book of Standing Rules. Rules for the Hospital*, 12 May 1879, 7, Countway.

40. Bertha van Hoosen, "Report of the Resident Physician," *AR*, 1891, 11–12; Zakrzewska, "Report of the Attending Physician," *AR*, 1865, 13; Zakrzewska to George A. Goddard, 6 June 1893, NEHWC Collection, box 8, folder 40, SS.

41. Cheney, "Secretary's Report," *AR*, 1880, 8. On the new payment scheme, see *Reference Book of Standing Rules*, 17. On the relationship between wealth and care in the modern hospital, see Stevens, *In Sickness and in Wealth*.

42. Cheney, "Report," *AR*, 1870, 5–8; *Circular. The New England Hospital for Women and Children* (published together with the *AR* for 1873).

43. Zakrzewska, "Ueber Hospitäler" (4 March 1863). Cheney confirmed this in 1876, when she wrote that "the plea that the soldier's wife and child were here sheltered and cared for, was then more powerful with the public than any claim for education." See *History and Description of the New England Hospital*, 25.

CHAPTER TEN

1. Zakrzewska's commitment to the standards of the elite medical community has been the subject of both Drachman, *Hospital with a Heart*, and Walsh, *"Doctors Wanted,"* 76–105. I build on both these studies, although I often diverge from the authors' evaluations of Zakrzewska's motivations.

2. Warner, *Against the Spirit of System*, 330–64.

3. Ludmerer, *Learning to Heal*, chaps. 2 and 3; Reiser, *Medicine and the Reign of Technology*; Rosenberg, *Care of Strangers*, 190–211; Warner, *Therapeutic Perspective*, 266–71.

4. Atwater, "Touching the Patient"; Ludmerer, *Learning to Heal*, 155–65.

5. "Annual Meeting of the 'Hospital for Women and Children,' " 182.

6. Morantz-Sanchez, *Sympathy and Science*, 64–89; Peitzman, *New and Untried Course*, 38–44. I discussed this briefly in Chapter 7 of this book.

7. On Philadelphia, see Peitzman, *New and Untried Course*, 14–15, and Wells, *Out of the Dead House*, 126–27. On Elizabeth Blackwell and Clemence Lozier, see Kirschmann, *Vital Force*, 58–61, and Morantz-Sanchez, *Sympathy and Science*, 73–74.

8. See Zakrzewska, "Report of the Resident Physician," *AR*, 1875, 12–13. On Sewall, see Ingebritsen, "Lucy Ellen Sewall"; Hurd-Mead, *Medical Women of America*, 32; and Todd, *Life of Sophia Jex-Blake*. On Morton, see Lovejoy, *Women Doctors of the World*, 86; Jacobi, "Woman in Medicine," 166; and Hurd-Mead, *Medical Women of America*, 33. The women, other than Sewall and Morton, were C. Annette Buckel, Emma Louise Call, Emma Culbertson, Susan Dimock, Augusta C. Pope, Emily F. Pope, Mary Almira Smith, and Adeline Whitney.

9. Cited in *WQ*, 393. On the foundation of this society, see Walsh, *"Doctors Wanted,"* 104, and Drachman, *Hospital with a Heart*, 125–27. The all-female Practitioners' Society of Rochester, New York, also excluded anyone who did not have regular training. See More, *Restoring the Balance*, 46.

10. *WQ*, 411. The requirement in 1880 was in many ways a formality. By 1876, students were almost always graduates of medical colleges. See *History and Description of the New England Hospital*, 19. Massachusetts General Hospital had already in 1873 restricted its appointment of house pupils to Harvard students who had completed a three-year course of study. See Ludmerer, *Learning to Heal*, 113. For other actions on the part of Zakrzewska and her staff to distinguish the New England Hospital from unorthodox institutions, see Drachman, *Hospital with a Heart*, 127–28.

11. Zakrzewska, "Report of Resident Physician," *AR*, 1875, 18. Zakrzewska might, however, have gone further than most when she advised women against seeking admission to the Female Medical College of Pennsylvania, arguing that to "have fully educated female physicians, they must study like men, and *with* men." See Zakrzewska to Sewall, 20 February 1863, reprinted in *WQ*, 310.

12. *WQ*, 381. On the offer in 1881 to Harvard, see ibid., 401–3, and Mosher, "Woman Doctor Who 'Stuck It Out.' " On Hopkins, see Harvey et al., *Model of Its Kind*, 137–56; *WQ*, 436; and "Open Letters." On Zurich, see *WQ*, 383.

13. Bittel, "Science of Women's Rights"; Morantz-Sanchez, *Sympathy and Science*, 184–202; Peitzman, *New and Untried Course*, 45–55; Wells, *Out of the Dead House*, 57–79.

14. See Drachman, *Hospital with a Heart*, 127.

15. Zakrzewska, "Report of the Attending Physician," *AR*, 1865, 13–15.

16. Ibid. Of course, one must wonder how happy any woman could have been who had spent three days in labor. Relieved and exhausted would probably have been more apt a description.

17. Zakrzewska, "Report of the Attending Physician," *AR*, 1868, 14. See also Zakrzewska to Dall, 27 February 1869, Dall Papers, box 5, folder 1.

18. Morantz and Zschoche, "Professionalism, Feminism, and Gender Roles." Specifically, they found that at the New England Hospital, either anesthetics or forceps or both were used 18 percent of the time, whereas at Boston Lying-In it was 20 percent of the time. (Forceps were used alone in 9.5 percent of the cases and with anesthetics in 13.5 percent of the cases). In support of their work, see Moscucci, *Science of Woman*, 128. For a challenge to their work (which I consider weak), see Drachman, *Hospital with a Heart*, 88–89.

19. Morantz and Zschoche, "Professionalism, Feminism, and Gender Roles," 583. The authors entertained the possibility that class differences played a role in the differential treatment, but they did not pursue it.

20. Peitzman, *New and Untried Course*, 24–44.

21. On Jacobi's advocacy of vivisection, see Bittel, "Science, Suffrage, and Experimentation."

22. Call, "Evolution of Modern Maternity Technic." The quotation is on 393, the statistics on 400. See also Zakrzewska, "Report of the Attending Physician," *AR*, 1868, 15.

23. Calculated from the *Annual Report of the Boston Lying-In Hospital* and the *Annual Report of the New England Hospital* for the years 1879–81, 1883.

24. Walsh, *"Doctors Wanted,"* 94–95. See also Crumpacker, "Female Patients in Four Boston Hospitals."

25. Cheney, *Memoir of Susan Dimock*. My analysis of the role gender played in the New England Hospital's control of puerperal fever builds on Morantz and Zschoche, "Professionalism, Feminism, and Gender Roles," 581.

26. Zakrzewska, "Report of the Attending Physician," *AR*, 1868, 12. Zakrzewska also discussed many of these measures in an article she published toward the end of her career. See "Report of One Hundred and Eighty-Seven Cases."

27. Zakrzewska instituted the same policy when dealing with serious surgical patients, isolating them as well. See Zakrzewska, "Report of the Attending Physician," *AR*, 1865, 16, and "Report of the Attending Physician," *AR*, 1869, 9. According to Emma Call, the hand washing and use of oil were for the protection of the physician, not the patient. See Call, "Evolution of Modern Maternity Technic," 394.

28. Susan Dimock, "Report of Resident Physician," *AR*, 1873, 11. On hygienic measures at the hospital, see Zakrzewska, "Report of the Attending Physician," *AR*, 1869, 10; "Report of the Furnishing Committee," *AR*, 1873, 16–17; *History and Description of the New England Hospital*, 13–14; and Mary Smith, "Annual Report of Resident Physician," *AR*, 1881, 12.

29. Kisacky, "Architecture of Light and Air."

30. *WQ*, 304.

31. I discuss this notion of disease in greater detail in Tuchman, *Science, Medicine, and the*

State, 60–63. Max von Pettenkoffer's views, developed later in the century, were quite similar. See Evans, *Death in Hamburg*, 257–84.

32. Call, "Evolution of Modern Maternity Technic," 396.

33. Cited in ibid., 393. On the history of reactions to the germ theory, see Rosenberg, *Care of Strangers*, chap. 5, and Tomes, *Gospel of Germs*.

34. The first two were the New York Infirmary for Women and Children (1857) and the Woman's Hospital of Pennsylvania (1861).

35. In contrast, the Woman's Hospital of Philadelphia had thirty-seven beds in 1875. See Peitzman, *New and Untried Course*, 26.

36. Numbers are gathered from the annual reports. Interns at the Woman's Hospital of Philadelphia saw a similar number of dispensary patients in 1875 (more than three thousand); the New York Infirmary saw a much larger number (about eight thousand new patients). See Peitzman, *New and Untried Course*, 25–26, and McNutt, "Medical Women," 136.

37. *History and Description of the New England Hospital*, 18–19; *Fiftieth Anniversary of the New England Hospital*, 29.

38. Susan Dimock, "Report of the Resident Physician," *AR*, 1874, 15.

39. Cited in Morantz-Sanchez, *Sympathy and Science*, 169. See also Mosher, "Woman Doctor Who 'Stuck It Out.'" I derived the information on the interns' activities from several sources. See Zakrzewska to Sewall, 25 January 1863, cited in *WQ*, 308; Jex-Blake to her mother, 24 November 1865 and 27 November 1865, reprinted in Todd, *Life of Sophia Jex-Blake*, 173–74; Cheney, "Report," *AR*, 1874, 6; Cheney, *Memoir of Susan Dimock*, 11; "Rules for Internes, September 1886," in NEHWC, *Rules for the Hospital. February 1874–February 1889*, 39, Countway; Drachman, *Hospital with a Heart*, 77–78. The experiences of the New England's interns seem to mirror those of house pupils in other hospitals. See Ludmerer, *Learning to Heal*, 17.

40. McNutt, "Medical Women," 137.

41. For a discussion of the stiff competition that men who sought hospital internships experienced, see Rosenberg, *Care of Strangers*, 179.

42. Helen Morton, "Report of the Dispensary," *AR*, 1874, 20. See also Cheney, "Report," *AR*, 1865, 6–7.

43. Jex-Blake to her mother, 27 November 1865, reprinted in Todd, *Life of Sophia Jex-Blake*, 174. On Jex-Blake, see also Roberts, *Sophia Jex-Blake*.

44. Lucy Sewall, "Report of the Dispensary," *AR*, 1875, 28; Emma Call, "Report of the Dispensary," *AR*, 1881, 20; C. Augusta Pope, "Dispensary Report," *AR*, 1885, 10.

45. Call, "Evolution of Modern Maternity Technic," 395.

46. Drachman, *Hospital with a Heart*, 77. On the significance of including such "objective" information in the patient record, see Risse and Warner, "Reconstructing Clinical Activities," esp. 191–92.

47. For some examples, see NEHWC, *Surgical Case Records*: vol. 1B (1872), #2; vol. 2 (1874), #4, #9; vol. 8 (1884), #34; *Medical Case Records*: vol. 16 (1884), #16; Countway.

48. Hurd-Mead, *Medical Women of America*, 34. On Hurd-Mead, see Miller, "Kate Campbell Hurd-Mead."

49. Sophia Jex-Blake to her mother, 18 August 1865, reprinted in Todd, *Life of Sophia Jex-Blake*, 164–66.

50. Ibid.

51. Zakrzewska to the interns, 30 March 1883, 6, NEHWC Collection, box 27, folder 1173, SS. The best analysis of this first generation of women physicians remains Morantz-Sanchez, *Sympathy and Science*, 47–231.

52. Zakrzewska to the interns, 1 April 1876, 1, NEHWC Collection, box 27, folder 1173, SS. The following account of this conflict is partly indebted to Drachman, *Hospital with a Heart*, chap. 4, although I do not always share her interpretation of the evidence.

53. Zakrzewska to the interns, 1 April 1876, 2, NEHWC Collection, box 27, folder 1173, SS.

54. Ibid., 4.

55. See, especially, Drachman, *Hospital with a Heart*, 112–13.

56. Zakrzewska to the interns, 1 April 1876, 4–5, 7, NEHW Collection, box 27, folder 1173, SS.

57. Zakrzewska's 1877 address to the New England Women's Club is reprinted in *WQ*, 378.

58. Zakrzewska to the interns, 1 April 1876, 4, NEHWC Collection, box 27, folder 1173, SS.

59. For a detailed discussion of the debates surrounding the reform of Harvard's medical school, see Ludmerer, *Learning to Heal*, 47–53.

60. Zakrzewska to the interns, 1 April 1876, 6–7, NEHWC Collection, box 27, folder 1173, SS.

61. Ibid., 4–5.

62. Drachman, *Hospital with a Heart*, 113. Zakrzewska's comment is mentioned in the Records of the Meetings of Physicians, 16 April 1876, SS.

63. Zakrzewska to the interns, 30 March 1883, 7–8, NEHWC Collection, box 27, folder 1173, SS.

64. Ibid.

65. Ludmerer, *Learning to Heal*, 53–57; Peitzman, *New and Untried Course*, 38–44.

66. Zakrzewska to the interns, 30 March 1883, 3–4, NEHWC Collection, box 27, folder 1173, SS.

67. Bonner, *To the Ends of the Earth*, chap. 7; Drachman, *Hospital with a Heart*, 108–9; Morantz-Sanchez, *Sympathy and Science*, 78, 164, 166; Jacobi, "Women in Medicine," 189. Blockley had actually allowed Elizabeth Blackwell to spend a summer as an intern in 1849 and Sarah Dolley to spend eleven months as an intern in 1851, but thereafter it did not hire another woman until 1883. See More, *Restoring the Balance*, 22–23. Bear in mind that some of these hospitals allowed women to walk the wards prior to this date; however, that is different from offering a clinical internship.

68. Emily Blackwell, "New York Infirmary," 79.

69. On the fate of other all-women's hospitals, see Morantz-Sanchez, *Sympathy and Science*, 178.

70. Ibid., 159–60, 234, 253–55; Walsh, *"Doctors Wanted,"* chap. 6.

71. Zakrzewska made her comment about Heinzen's imminent death in a letter to Mr. Schmemann, 14 November 1880, Schmemann Papers, LBC. On Minna's death, see "Wilhelmine J. Zakrzewska," 5.

72. In her autobiographical sketch, Zakrzewska suggests that she responded to her mother's death by throwing herself into her work. This may have been her way of dealing with her grief. See *PI*, 148–49.

73. Cited in *WQ*, 253.

74. Zakrzewska, "Report of Resident Physician," *AR*, 1875, 17.

75. Zakrzewska to Sewall, 29 November 1862, cited in *WQ*, 302. Thanks to Judith Walzer Leavitt for helping me to understand Zakrzewska's maternal feelings toward some of her interns.

76. Zakrzewska to the interns, 30 October 1891, 1–2, NEHWC Collection, box 27, folder 1173, SS.

77. For an analysis of the way medical debates in the nineteenth century frequently revolved around claims about a practitioner's character, see Morantz-Sanchez, *Conduct Unbecoming a Woman*; Rosenkrantz, "Search for Professional Order"; and Warner, *Against the Spirit of System*.

78. Interns to the Board of Physicians, 12 October 1891, in NEHWC Collection, box 27, folder 1173, SS.

79. Alice Hamilton to Agnes Hamilton, 29 October 1893 and 6 December 1893, in Sicherman, *Alice Hamilton*, 71–72, 75.

80. Bledstein, *Culture of Professionalism*; Haber, *Quest for Authority and Honor*; Starr, *Social Transformation of American Medicine*; Larson, *Rise of Professionalism*; Numbers, "Fall and Rise of the American Medical Profession."

81. Front page, *AR*, 1865, 3. The five physicians included two attending physicians, one resident physician, and two assistant physicians.

82. Front page, *AR*, 1891, 4. The sixteen physicians included one resident physician, two advisory physicians, twelve attending physicians and surgeons, and one director of electricity. To be sure, compared with an operation like Massachusetts General, the New England was still small, but the growth was significant nonetheless.

83. Morantz-Sanchez, *Sympathy and Science*, 232–33.

84. Cited in ibid., 60–61.

85. Deutsch, *Women and the City*, 148. See also Ginzberg, *Women and the Work of Benevolence*.

86. See More, "Blackwell Medical Society" and *Restoring the Balance*, 8–9. See also Morantz-Sanchez, *Sympathy and Science*, 144.

87. Barry, *Susan B. Anthony*, 200.

88. Sicherman, *Exploring the Dangerous Trades*, 267–70. See also Morantz-Sanchez, *Sympathy and Science*, 178.

89. On hospitals and the metaphor of the family, see Rosenberg, *Care of Strangers*, 42–43.

90. Zakrzewska to the interns, 30 October 1891, 4, NEHWC Collection, box 27, folder 1173, SS. See also *WQ*, 376, 395, 426.

91. One should refrain from romanticizing the former. As Kate Hurd-Mead, who interned at the New England Hospital in 1888, pointed out, Zakrzewska's notion of stewardship "led her to watch even the spare time of the young doctors, and to denounce what she considered harmful contemporary literature, especially the novels of Tolstoi." See Hurd-Mead, *Medical Women of America*, 34. I am not, moreover, suggesting that Hamilton lacked a sense of ethical

wrongdoing when she decided to leave the hospital. However, she was more concerned about what it would mean to break a contract than about what it might mean for the institution.

92. On competing understandings of professionalism among women physicians in the United States, see Morantz-Sanchez, *Sympathy and Science*, esp. chap. 6, and More, *Restoring the Balance*, esp. chap. 2.

93. Alice Hamilton to Agnes Hamilton, 6 December 1893, in Sicherman, *Alice Hamilton*, 73–74.

94. See, for example, Zakrzewska to Mr. Goddard (board of directors), 13 May 1891 and 6 June 1893, both in NEHWC Collection, box 8, folder 40, SS. For a detailed discussion of these disagreements, see Drachman, *Hospital with a Heart*, 132–39.

95. Zakrzewska admitted as much, although her comment is not dated; mentioned in "Communication from the Medical Board of the NEHWC, presented to the Board of Directors," 25 May 1891, NEHWC collection, box 6, folder 16, SS.

96. Rosenberg, "Inward Vision and Outward Glance."

97. Zakrzewska to Susan B. Anthony, 30 January 1893, National American Women's Suffrage Association, LC. See also Drachman, *Hospital with a Heart*, 105.

98. Zakrzewska to Paulina Pope, 28 October 1901, NEHWC Collection, box 1, folder 2, SS. I am grateful to Regina Morantz-Sanchez for sending me a transcription of this letter.

99. Drachman, *Hospital with a Heart*, 160–72.

100. Ibid., 186–95.

101. Zakrzewska mentioned this in a letter to George A. Goddard, 6 June 1893, NEHWC Collection, box 8, folder 40, SS.

102. Rosenberg, "Inward Vision and Outward Glance," 383.

103. According to the author of a 1900 article in the *Journal of the American Medical Association*: "Indeed, to a large extent, the hospital with its wards, outpatient department, its operating rooms, its dead-house, and its laboratories, is the medical school"; cited in Haber, *Quest for Authority*, 345.

CHAPTER ELEVEN

1. Rosenberg, "Therapeutic Revolution."

2. On Blackwell, see Morantz-Sanchez, *Sympathy and Science*, 184–202, and "Feminist Theory and Historical Practice." On other critics of laboratory medicine, see Geison, "Divided We Stand"; Maulitz, " 'Physician versus Bacteriologist' "; and Warner, "Ideals of Science and Their Discontents" and *Against the Spirit of System*, especially the last chapter.

3. Warner, *Against the Spirit of System*, 336.

4. Morantz-Sanchez, "Feminist Theory and Historical Practice," 61. See also Blackwell, "Influence of Women in the Profession of Medicine" and "Erroneous Method in Medical Education."

5. Had Zakrzewska at this point directly challenged these gendered meanings, I would argue that her philosophical position had not changed. She would simply have become an advocate for a different style of practice, insisting just as adamantly that the way one prac-

ticed medicine had nothing to do with one's sex. But Zakrzewska's silence on this score—in direct contrast to her outspoken attack on the gendering of these styles back in the 1860s—suggests that she had become ambivalent, and even somewhat conflicted, about the role that her gender played in shaping her outlook on care.

6. Zakrzewska, "Report of One Hundred and Eighty-Seven Cases."

7. Leavitt, *Brought to Bed*, chaps. 2 and 6.

8. Zakrzewska, "Report of One Hundred and Eighty-Seven Cases," 557, 559.

9. Ibid., 557.

10. See Chapter 7 of this book.

11. Zakrzewska, "Report of One Hundred and Eighty-Seven Cases," 558.

12. See Chapter 2 of this book.

13. Zakrzewska, "Report of One Hundred and Eighty-Seven Cases," 558.

14. On developments in nineteenth-century statistical methods, see Cassedy, *American Medicine and Statistical Thinking*, and Porter, *Rise of Statistical Thinking* and *Trust in Numbers*.

15. On the centrality of storytelling in mid-nineteenth-century medical practices, see Stowe, "Seeing Themselves at Work."

16. This story is reprinted in *WQ*, 322–27; quotation on 324.

17. Zakrzewska to Blackwell, 21 March 1891, Blackwell Family Papers, SL. Zakrzewska's comments almost make her sound like a disciple of Hahnemann, although a closer reading suggests less an embrace of homeopathic principles than skepticism about the efficacy of any drugs at all. Still, her assertion that she used most medicines—if at all—in "infinitessimal [*sic*] doses" signals a move toward homeopathic practices, if not principles. Whether she had always favored a more conservative therapeutic approach (as she asserted) is difficult to determine, since we know virtually nothing about her style of medical practice and how it might have changed over time. But once again, as in her discussion of childbirth, what is certain is Zakrzewska's decision to portray herself in a radically different way than she had in the past.

18. Geison, "Divided We Stand"; Maulitz, " 'Physician versus Bacteriologist' "; Rosenkrantz, "Search for Professional Order"; Warner, "Ideals of Science and Their Discontents."

19. Warner, "From Specificity to Universalism" and *Against the Spirit of System*. See also Chapter 7 of this book.

20. Warner, *Against the Spirit of System*, 291–364. See also Rosenkrantz, "Search for Professional Order."

21. This more nuanced critique of the laboratory was also true by and large of the Paris-trained physicians. See Warner, *Against the Spirit of System*, 348.

22. On Jacobi's comment about "bacteriomania," see Warner, "Hunting the Yellow Fever Germ." A concise explanation of Virchow's position can be found in Evans, *Death in Hamburg*, 272–75. See also Goschler, *Rudolf Virchow*, 286–95.

23. On Mary Putnam Jacobi, see Bittel, "Science of Women's Rights"; Morantz-Sanchez, *Sympathy and Science*, 184–202; and Wells, *Out of the Dead House*, 146–92. On Mary Dixon-Jones, see Morantz-Sanchez, *Conduct Unbecoming a Woman*.

24. Morantz-Sanchez, "Gendering of Empathic Expertise"; More, " 'Empathy' Enters the Profession of Medicine" and *Restoring the Balance*.

25. Zakrzewska to Blackwell, 21 March 1891, Blackwell Family Papers, SL. Zakrzewska made several references to the golden rule throughout her lifetime. See *WQ*, 315, 316, 417, 422.

26. Zakrzewska to Blackwell, 21 March 1891, Blackwell Family Papers, SL. For Blackwell's comments on ovariotomies, see her "Scientific Method in Biology," 119–20.

27. Morantz-Sanchez, *Conduct Unbecoming a Woman*. On the controversies over gynecologic surgery, see Chapter 4. See also McGregor, *Sexual Surgery and the Origins of Gynecology*; Moscucci, *Science of Woman*; and Theriot, "Women's Voices in Nineteenth-Century Medical Discourse."

28. Cited in Morantz-Sanchez, *Sympathy and Science*, 195.

29. Blackwell, "Influence of Women in the Profession of Medicine," 9. See also Morantz-Sanchez, "Feminist Theory and Historical Practice," 59–60.

30. On Blackwell, see especially Morantz-Sanchez, "Gendering of Empathic Expertise."

31. Zakrzewska's comment about Booth is from "Mary L. Booth," 106. Her comment about the year is from Zakrzewska to Severance, 14 February 1890, Severance Papers.

32. Zakrzewska to Severance, 8 September 1889, Severance Papers. The letter from 10 September was a continuation of this letter.

33. Zakrzewska to Severance, 10 September 1889, Severance Papers. Although Haeckel eventually transformed monism into a quasi-religious philosophy, in the late 1880s he was still promoting his ideas as a pro-Darwinian scientific movement that drew heavily on the German scientific materialists in its anti-Christian stance. See Holt, "Ernst Haeckel's Monistic Religion."

34. Zakrzewska to Severance, 10 September 1889, Severance Papers.

35. Zakrzewska to Severance, 11 September, no year but probably 1890, Severance Papers.

36. Zakrzewska to Blackwell, undated but probably 1900, National American Women's Suffrage Association, LC.

37. Zakrzewska to Blackwell, 21 March 1891, Blackwell Family Papers, SL.

38. Ibid.

39. Bittel, "Science of Women's Rights."

40. See Morantz-Sanchez, "Gendering of Empathic Expertise," and More, *Restoring the Balance*, 8–9. More builds on the work of Judith Walzer Leavitt, who argues that the values that became female-gendered at the end of the century were once shared by male physicians as well, especially those practicing in rural settings where the distinction between public and private often made little sense. See Leavitt, " 'Worrying Profession.' "

41. "Paper Read by Dr. Zakrzewska," *AR*, 1892, 11–12.

42. Zakrzewska to Mr. Goddard, 13 May 1891, NEHWC Collection, SS.

43. Cited in *Marie Elizabeth Zakrzewska: A Memoir*, 24.

CHAPTER TWELVE

1. On Zakrzewska's involvement with the New England Women's Club, see the New England Women's Club Records, box 1, vols. 3 and 4, SL. On her involvement with the

Roxbury Women's Suffrage League, see her letter to Susan B. Anthony, 30 January 1893, National American Women's Suffrage Association, LC.

2. The first quotation is cited in *WQ,* 221; it is undated, and the source is not mentioned. The second quotation is from Zakrzewska to Sprague, 6 September 1896, New England Women's Club Records, vol. 1, Scrapbook, SL.

3. Sprague to Severance, 9 August 1892; Zakrzewska to Severance, 31 August 1890; Zakrzewska to Severance, 8 September 1889; Zakrzewska to Severance, 2 August 1891, all in Severance Papers; Sprague to Kitty Blackwell, 25 August 1899, Blackwell Family Papers, LC.

4. Zakrzewska to Blackwell, 29 October 1895, Blackwell Family Papers, LC.

5. Ibid. On earlier tensions in their relationship, see Elizabeth Blackwell to Emily and Kitty Blackwell, 15 November 1865; Elizabeth Blackwell to Kitty Barry, 27 May 1881; and Kitty Barry to Alice Stone Blackwell, 18 January 1886, all in Blackwell Family Papers, LC.

6. Sprague to Kitty Blackwell, 28 December 1896, Blackwell Family Papers, LC. On Zakrzewska's realization that this was her last trip to Europe, see Sprague to Severance, 9 November 1905, Severance Papers.

7. Zakrzewska to Cheney, undated, cited in *Marie Elizabeth Zakrzewska: A Memoir,* 24–25.

8. Sprague to Severance, 7 June 1901, Severance Papers.

9. Zakrzewska to Blackwell, 6 July 1901, Blackwell Family Papers, HL.

10. Zakrzewska to Elizabeth and Kitty Barry Blackwell, 24 January 1902, Blackwell Family Papers, LC.

11. Sprague to Severance, 2 February 1902; see also Sprague to Severance, 8 July 1902; both in Severance Papers.

12. Sprague mentions this diagnosis in a letter to Severance, 22 February, no year but probably 1905, Severance Papers. The physician who attended Zakrzewska during her final illness was Dr. Fanny Berlin.

13. Sprague to Severance, 8 July 1901, Severance Papers.

14. Sprague to Kitty Barry, 16 November 1902, Blackwell Family Papers, SL.

15. Sprague discusses her inheritance in two letters, one to Severance, 8 July 1902, Severance Papers, and the other to Kitty Barry, 16 November 1902, Blackwell Family Papers, SL. I have been unable to determine Sprague's exact date of death, but her last letter to Severance was written around 1909 or 1910, and since Severance lived on until 1914, that may have marked the approximate time of Sprague's death.

16. Sprague to Severance, 13 July, no year but probably around 1909, Severance Papers.

17. "Farewell Message. Words by Dr. Zakrzewska Read at Her Funeral," *Boston Herald,* 16 May 1902, 10, reprinted in *WQ,* 474–78.

18. Sprague to Kitty Blackwell, 28 December 1896, Blackwell Family Papers, LC.

19. Cited in *Marie Elizabeth Zakrzewska: A Memoir,* 24. Interestingly, Vietor, who also cites this letter, omits this sentence. See *WQ,* 473.

20. Most telling is the letter in which Sprague discussed how she allowed Zakrzewska to turn down invitations by claiming (falsely) that Sprague was feeling unwell. See Sprague to Kitty Barry, 28 December 1896, Blackwell Family Papers, LC. I discuss this comment in Chapter 5 of this book.

21. Sprague to Severance, 22 February, no year but probably 1905, Severance Papers.

22. On the cover page of a memorial published one year after Zakrzewska's death the following sentence was cited: "I prefer to be remembered only as a woman who was willing to work for the elevation of Woman." The source of this comment is not mentioned. See *Marie Elizabeth Zakrzewska: A Memoir*, cover page.

23. Tighe, "Lesson in the Political Economics of Medical Education"; Hudson, "Abraham Flexner in Perspective"; Ludmerer, *Learning to Heal*, 166–90; More, *Restoring the Balance*, 95–121.

24. Morantz-Sanchez, *Sympathy and Science*, 249.

25. Moldow, *Women Doctors in Gilded-Age Washington*; Morantz-Sanchez, *Sympathy and Science*; Walsh, *"Doctors Wanted."* See also Blackwell, "New York Infirmary," 79, for her assessment of the problems facing women in 1900.

26. Vietor, afterword to *WQ*, 479.

27. Ibid., 480.

28. Vietor, foreword to *WQ*, ix, and afterword to *WQ*, 482.

29. More, *Restoring the Balance*, 182–86.

30. "That They Might Live," Archives and Special Collections on Women in Medicine and Homeopathy, Drexel University College of Medicine, Philadelphia, Pa. On the "Cavalcade of America" series, see Grams, *History of the Cavalcade of America*; Grams, "Cavalcade of America"; and Riley, Lucas, and Pettit, "Cavalcade of America." "Cavalcade of America" aired weekly. Each half-hour-long episode featured one "hero," meant to inspire the nation. Many of the names would have been familiar to listeners: George Washington, Abraham Lincoln, Thomas Edison, James Fenimore Cooper, Noah Webster, Oliver Wendell Holmes. But others were less well known, and Zakrzewska was clearly among them.

31. "That They Might Live."

32. Ibid.

33. See, for example, Alcoff, "Cultural Feminism versus Poststructuralism," and Fraser, "Structuralism or Pragmatics?"

34. The literature is quite extensive. See, however, Schiebinger, *Has Feminism Changed Science?*; Creager, Lunbeck, and Schiebinger, *Feminism*; Haraway, "Situated Knowledges"; Harding, *Whose Science?*; Keller, "Developmental Biology as a Feminist Cause?"; Kohlstedt, "Women in the History of Science"; and Kohlstedt and Longino, "Women, Gender, and Science Questions."

BIBLIOGRAPHY

Unpublished Primary Sources

GERMANY

Berlin

Geheimes Staatsarchiv Preussischer
  Kulturbesitz. Files of the Ministry of
  Culture
Rep. 76 I, Sekt. 31, Litt. S, Nr. 55 (Joseph
  Hermann Schmidt's personnel file)
Rep. 76 I, Sekt. 31, Lit. Z, Nr. 2 (Martin
  Ludwig Zakrzewski's personnel file)
Rep. 76 Va, Sekt. 2, Tit. X, Nr. 8, Bd. V
  (University of Berlin, obstetrics clinic,
  1835–41)
Rep. 76 Va, Sekt. 2, Tit. X, Nr. 8, Bd. VI
  (University of Berlin, obstetrics clinic,
  1841–53)
Rep. 76 VIIIA, Nr. 896 (quackery and
  swaddling women, 1847–48)

Rep. 76 VIIIA, Nr. 1002 (midwifery in
  Berlin, 1815–22)
Rep. 76 VIIIA, Nr. 1004 (midwifery in
  Berlin, 1846–59)
Universitätsarchiv der Humboldt Universität
  zu Berlin. Charité Direktion
Nr. 192 (appointment of the professor of
  midwifery, 1821–1907)
Nr. 199 (training of midwives and swaddling
  women, 18??–1839)
Nr. 200 (training of midwives and swad-
  dling women, 1840–1904)
Nr. 802 (midwifery institute and obstetrics
  institute, 1818–51)

Potsdam

Potsdam-Brandenburgisches Landeshauptarchiv
Rep. 30 Berlin, C-Polizei Präsidium, Tit.
  50

Nr. 2232 (swaddling women, 1841–71)
Nr. 2234 (register of city midwives; com-
  plaints of quackery, 1822)
Nr. 2236 (midwifery teaching institute)

UNITED STATES

Ann Arbor, Michigan

Labadie Collection
  Karl Heinzen Papers

Karl Schmemann Papers
George Schumm Papers

Boston, Massachusetts

Boston Medical Library in the Francis A.
Countway Library of Medicine
New England Hospital for Women and
Children
Maternity Case Records [B MS b19.3]
Medical Case Records [B MS b19.2]
Misc [B MS misc]

Records of Patients Who Received Prescriptions [B MS b19.5]
Reference Book of Standing Rules. Rules for the Hospital [B MS b19.6.]
Surgical Case Records [B MS b19.1]
Massachusetts Historical Society
Caroline Healey Dall Papers

Cambridge, Massachusetts

Schlesinger Library, Radcliffe
Blanche Ames Ames Papers

Blackwell Family Papers
New England Women's Club Collection

Cleveland, Ohio

Archives, Allen Memorial Medical
Library, Case Western Reserve
University

Marie E. Zakrzewska, "Thesis. The Organ
of Parturition" (medical thesis), Cleveland Medical College, 1855–56

Northampton, Massachusetts

Sophia Smith Collection, Smith College
Garrison Family Collection

New England Hospital for Women and
Children Collection

Philadelphia, Pennsylvania

Drexel University College of Medicine,
Archives and Special Collections on
Women in Medicine and Homeopathy

"That They Might Live." Part of "The
Cavalcade of America" Du Pont Radio
Series, October 1942

San Marino, California

Huntington Library
Caroline Maria Seymour Severance Papers

Washington, D.C.

Library of Congress
Blackwell Family Papers

National American Women's Suffrage
Association

Published Primary Sources

"An Address by Mrs. Clara Neymann." *The Index*, 16 March 1882.
"Annual Meeting of the 'Hospital for Women and Children.'" *Liberator*, 14 November 1862.
Annual Report of the Boston Lying-In Hospital. Boston: Boston Lying-In Hospital, 1875–93.
Annual Report of the New-England Hospital for Women and Children. Boston: Prentiss and
Deland, 1863–1902.

Annual Report of the Trustees of the Massachusetts General Hospital. Boston, 1863–93.

An Appeal in Behalf of the Medical Education of Women. New York, 1856.

Augustin, F. L. *Die Königlich Preußische Medicinalverfassung.* Potsdam, Germany: Karl Christian Horvath, 1818.

Austin, John Mather. *A Voice to the Married.* Utica, New York: 1841.

"Biographical. Sketches of the Life and Work of the Pioneer Women in Medicine. Marie E. Zakrzewska, M.D. From Berlin to Life in New York." *Woman's Medical Journal* 11 (April 1901): 135–38.

Blackwell, Elizabeth. "Erroneous Method in Medical Education." In Elizabeth Blackwell, *Essays in Medical Sociology,* 2 vols. in 1, 2:35–45. New York: Arno Press, 1972.

——. "The Influence of Women in the Profession of Medicine." In Elizabeth Blackwell, *Essays in Medical Sociology,* 2 vols. in 1, 2:1–32. New York: Arno Press, 1972.

——. *Pioneer Work in Opening the Medical Profession to Women.* New York: Schocken Books, 1977.

——. "Scientific Method in Biology." In Elizabeth Blackwell, *Essays in Medical Sociology,* 2 vols. in 1, 2:87–196. New York: Arno Press, 1972.

Blackwell, Emily. "The New York Infirmary and Medical College for Women." *Transactions of the . . . Annual Meeting of the Alumnae Association of the Woman's Medical College of Pennsylvania* (1900): 76–80.

"Bostoner Heilanstalt für Frauen und Kinder." *Der Pionier,* 28 March 1861.

"The Boston 'Pionier.'" *Liberator,* 16 January 1863, 10.

Bowditch, Henry I. "Female Practitioners of Medicine." *Boston Medical and Surgical Journal* 76 (1867): 272–75.

Bowditch, N. I. *A History of the Massachusetts General Hospital.* Boston: J. Wilson, 1851.

Bowditch, Vincent Yardley. *Life and Correspondence of Henry Ingersoll Bowditch.* 2 vols. Boston: Houghton, Mifflin and Co., 1902.

Call, Emma L. "The Evolution of Modern Maternity Technic." *American Journal of Obstetrics and Diseases of Women and Children* 58, no. 3 (1908): 392–404.

Cheney, Ednah Dow. *Memoir of Susan Dimock.* Cambridge, Mass.: J. Wilson, 1875.

——. *Reminiscences of Ednah Dow Cheney (born Littlehale).* Boston: Lee and Shepard, 1902.

——. "Theodore Parker." In *West Roxbury Magazine.* Hudson, Mass.: E. F. Worcester Press, 1900, 51.

C. K. W. "New England Hospital for Women and Children." *Liberator,* 3 March 1865.

Clarke, Edward H. "Recent Progress in Materia Medica." *Boston Medical and Surgical Journal* 71 (1864): 309–23.

Credé, C. S. F. *Die Preußischen Hebammen, ihre Stellung zum Staate und zur Geburtshülfe.* Berlin: August Hirschwald, 1855.

C. W. "Dr. Zakrzewska's Funeral." *Woman's Journal,* 24 May 1902.

Dall, Caroline H. *"Woman's Right to Labor"; or, Low Wages and Hard Work: In Three Lectures delivered in Boston, November, 1859.* Boston: Walker, Wise, and Co., 1860.

"Das Hospital für Frauen und Kinder." *Der Pionier,* 6 August 1862.

"Die teutsche Organisation." *Der Pionier,* 4 January 1865.

"Erörterungen der bisherigen Verhältnisse der Hebammen und Wickelfrauen zu Berlin." *Verhandlungen der Gesellschaft für Geburtshülfe in Berlin* 6 (1852): 53–54.

Fiftieth Anniversary of the New England Hospital for Women and Children. Boston: Geo. H. Ellis, 1913.

Garrison, Wendell Phillips, and Francis Jackson Garrison. *William Lloyd Garrison, 1805–1879: The Story of His Life Told by His Children.* 4 vols. 1885–89. Reprint, New York: Arno Press, 1969.

Gregory, Samuel. "Female Physicians." *Little's Living Age,* 3rd ser., 17 (May 1862): 243–49.

———. *Letter to Ladies, in Favor of Female Physicians for Their Own Sex.* 2nd ed. Boston: Female Medical Education Society, 1854.

———. *Man-Midwifery Exposed and Corrected.* Boston: George Gregory, 1848.

Hale, Edward Everett, ed. *James Freeman Clarke: Autobiography, Diary and Correspondence.* New York: Negro Universities Press, 1891.

Heinzen, Karl. *Communism and Socialism.* Indianapolis: Association for the Propagation of Radical Principles, 1881.

———. *Die Helden des teutschen Kommunismus: Dem Herrn Karl Marx gewidmet.* Bern, Switzerland: Jenni, Sohn, 1848.

———. "Die Ungenügsamkeit der 'Rechts'-Weiber." In Karl Heinzen, *Teutscher Radikalismus in Amerika: Ausgewählte Vorträge,* 4:409. Boston: Verein zur Verbreitung radikaler Prinzipien, 1867–79.

———. *The Rights of Women and the Sexual Relations: An Address to an Unknown Lady Reader.* Translated by Mrs. Emma Heller Schumm. Boston: Benj. R. Tucker, 1891.

———. *Separation of State and Church.* Indianapolis: Association for the Propagation of Radical Principles, 1882.

———. *Six Letters to a Pious Man.* Translated from the German by an American Lady. Indianapolis: Association for the Diffusion of Radical Principles, 1869.

———. "Ueber die 'Liebe.'" In Karl Heinzen, *Teutscher Radikalismus in Amerika: Ausgewählte Vorträge,* 1:28–38. Boston: Verein zur Verbreitung radikaler Prinzipien, 1867–79.

———. "Verlegung des 'Pionier' nach Boston." *Der Pionier,* 17 October 1858.

———. "Was ist Humanität?" In Karl Heinzen, *Teutscher Radikalismus in Amerika: Ausgewählte Vorträge,* 2:274–312. Boston: Verein zur Verbreitung radikaler Prinzipien, 1867–79.

———. "Weiberrecht und Liebe vor dem Richterstuhl der Moral." In Karl Heinzen, *Teutscher Radikalismus in Amerika: Ausgewählte Vorträge,* 4:237–48. Boston: Verein zur Verbreitung radikaler Prinzipien, 1867–79.

———. "Wer and was ist, das Volk." In Karl Heinzen, *Teutscher Radikalismus in Amerika: Ausgewählte Vorträge,* 2:192–221. Boston: Verein zur Verbreitung radikaler Prinzipien, 1867–79.

———. *What Is Real Democracy? Answered by an Exposition of the Constitution of the United States.* Indianapolis: Association for the Propagation of Radical Principles, 1871.

———. "Zur Moral des Radikalismus." In Karl Heinzen, *Teutscher Radikalismus in Amerika: Ausgewählte Vorträge,* 1:5–27. Boston: Verein zur Verbreitung radikaler Prinzipien, 1867–79.

History and Description of the New England Hospital for Women and Children. Boston: W. L. Deland, 1876. Reprinted as an appendix to the *Annual Report of the NEH for the year ending September 30, 1876.*

"Hospital for Women and Children." *Liberator*, 20 November 1863.

Hunt, Harriot K. *Glances and Glimpses; or Fifty Years Social, including Twenty Years Professional Life*. Boston: John P. Jewett and Co., 1856.

Hurd-Mead, Kate Campbell. *Medical Women of America*. New York: Froben Press, 1933.

Jacobi, Mary Putnam. "Women in Medicine." In *Woman's Work in America*, edited by Annie Nathan Meyers, 139–205. New York: Henry Holt, 1891.

"Lecture on Hospitals." *Liberator*, 30 January 1863.

Marie Elizabeth Zakrzewska: A Memoir. Boston, 1903.

McNutt, Sarah J. "Medical Women, Yesterday and To-Day." *Medical Record* 94 (July 1918): 135–39.

Mosher, Eliza. "A Woman Doctor Who 'Stuck It Out.' " *Literary Digest*, 4 April 1925, 68.

"Notizen." *Der Pionier*. 4 June 1862.

"Obituary. Mary L. Booth," *New York Times*, 6 March 1889, 2.

"Open Letters. On the Opening of the Johns Hopkins Medical School to Women." *Century Illustrated Monthly Magazine* 41 (November 1890–April 1891): 632–37.

"Organisation der freisinnigen Teutschen." *Der Pionier*, 15 July 1863.

"Postponement of the Woman's Journal." *Der Pionier*, 3 September 1862.

"Postponement of the Woman's Journal." *Liberator*, 5 September 1862.

Robinson, Harriet Jane. *Massachusetts in the Woman Suffrage Movement: A General, Political, Legal and Legislative History from 1774 to 1881*. Boston: Roberts Bros., 1881.

Ruddy, Ella Giles, ed. *The Mother of Clubs: Caroline M. Seymour Severance. An Estimate and an Appreciation*. Los Angeles: Baumgardt Publishing Co., 1906.

Schmidt, Joseph Hermann. "Die geburtshülflich-klinischen Institute der Königlichen Charité." *Annalen des Charité-Krankenhauses* 1, no. 3 (1850): 485–523.

——. *Die Reform der Medizinalverfassung Preußens*. Berlin: Enslin, 1846.

——. *Lehrbuch der Geburtskunde für die Hebammen in den königlichen Preussischen Staaten*. 2nd ed. Berlin: August Hirschwald, 1850.

Sewall, Samuel E. *Legal Condition of Women in Massachusetts*. 4th ed. Boston: A. C. Getchell, 1886.

Sprague, Julia. *History of the New England Women's Club from 1868 to 1893*. Boston: Lee and Shepard, 1894.

"Stadt Boston." *Der Pionier*, 27 February 1862; 2 July 1872.

Stanton, Elizabeth Cady, Susan B. Anthony, and Matilda Joslyn Gage, eds. *History of Woman Suffrage*. 6 vols. New York: Fowler and Wells, 1881–[1922].

Todd, Margaret. *The Life of Sophia Jex-Blake*. London: Macmillan, 1918.

U.S. Bureau of the Census. *Eighth Census of the United States*. Washington: Government Printing Office, 1864.

——. *Eleventh Census of the United States*. Washington: Government Printing Office, 1895.

——. *Ninth Census of the United States*. Vol. 1, *Statistics of the Population*. Washington: Government Printing Office, 1872.

——. *Tenth Census of the United States*. Washington: Government Printing Office, 1883–88.

Ware, John. "Success in the Medical Profession." *Boston Medical and Surgical Journal* 43 (1851): 496–504, 509–22.

"Wilhelmine J. Zakrzewska." Obituary. *Der Pionier*, 3 October 1877.

"Woman and the Press." *Liberator*, 13 June 1862, 95.

Wunderlich, Carl. "Einleitung." *Archiv für physiologische Heilkunde* 1 (1842): xvi.

[Zakrzewska, Marie E.] Eine "Aerztinn." "Weibliche Aerzte." *Der Pionier*, 19 March 1859, 6.

Zakrzewska, Marie E. *Introductory Lecture delivered Wednesday, November 2, before the New England Female Medical College, at the opening of the term of 1859–60.* Boston: J. M. Hewes, 1859.

———. "Mary L. Booth." *Woman's Journal*, 6 April 1889, 105–6.

———. *A Practical Illustration of "Woman's Right to Labor"; or, A Letter from Marie E. Zakrzewska, M.D.* Edited by Caroline H. Dall. Boston: Walker, Wise, and Co., 1860.

———. "Report of One Hundred and Eighty-Seven Cases of Midwifery in Private Practice." *Boston Medical and Surgical Journal* 121 (1889): 557–60. Reprinted in the *Woman's Medical Journal* 1 (December 1893): 225–30.

———. "Sind Hebammenschulen wünschenswerth?" *Der Pionier*, 16 April 1859, 6.

———. "Ueber Hospitäler." *Der Pionier*, 4 February 1863, 3, 6; 11 February 1863, 2; 18 February 1863, 2; 25 February 1863, 2; 4 March 1863, 2.

Secondary Sources

Abir-Am, Pnina G., and Dorinda Outram, eds. *Uneasy Careers and Intimate Lives: Women in Science, 1789–1979.* New Brunswick, N.J.: Rutgers University Press, 1987.

Abram, Ruth J., ed. *"Send Us a Lady Physician": Women Doctors in America, 1835–1920.* New York: Norton, 1985.

Ackerknecht, Erwin H. "Beiträge zur Geschichte der Medizinalreform von 1848." *Sufhoffs Archiv* 25 (1932): 61–109, 113–83.

———. *Rudolf Virchow: Doctor, Statesman, Anthropologist.* Madison: University of Wisconsin Press, 1953.

Albisetti, James C. *Schooling German Girls and Women: Secondary and Higher Education in the Nineteenth Century.* Princeton, N.J.: Princeton University Press, 1988.

Alcoff, Linda. "Cultural Feminism versus Poststructuralism: The Identity Crisis in Feminist Theory." *Signs* 13 (1988): 405–36.

Anderson, Isabel. *Under the Black Horse Flag: Annals of the Weld Family and Some of Its Branches.* Boston: Houghton Mifflin, 1926.

Apple, Rima D., ed. *Women, Health, and Medicine in America: A Historical Handbook.* New Brunswick, N.J.: Rutgers University Press, 1992.

Atwater, Edward C. "Touching the Patient: The Teaching of Internal Medicine in America." In *Sickness and Health in America*, 2nd ed., edited by Judith Walzer Leavitt and Ronald L. Numbers, 129–47. Madison: University of Wisconsin Press, 1985.

Baker, Robert B. "The American Medical Ethics Revolution." In *The American Medical Ethics Revolution: How the AMA's Code of Ethics Has Transformed Physicians' Relationships to Patients,*

Professionals, and Society, edited by Robert B. Baker, Arthur L. Caplan, Linda L. Emanuel, and Stephen R. Latham, 17–51. Baltimore: Johns Hopkins University Press, 1999.

Baldwin, Peter. *Contagion and the State in Europe, 1830–1930.* Cambridge: Cambridge University Press, 1999.

Barney, William L. *The Passage of the Republic: An Interdisciplinary History of Nineteenth-Century America.* Lexington, Mass.: D. C. Heath, 1987.

Barry, Kathleen. *Susan B. Anthony: A Biography of a Singular Feminist.* New York: New York University Press, 1988.

Benjamin, Marina, ed. *Science and Sensibility: Gender and Scientific Enquiry, 1780–1945.* Oxford, England: Blackwell, 1991.

Bittel, Carla. "The Science of Women's Rights: The Medical and Political Worlds of Mary Putnam Jacobi." Ph.D. diss., Cornell University, 2003.

——. "Science, Suffrage, and Experimentation: Mary Putnam Jacobi and the Controversy over Vivisection in Late Nineteenth-Century America." *Bulletin of the History of Medicine* 79 (2005): 664–94.

Blackbourn, David. "The German Bourgeoisie: An Introduction." In *The German Bourgeoisie: Essays on the Social History of the German Middle Class from the Late Eighteenth to the Early Twentieth Century*, edited by David Blackbourn and Richard J. Evans, 1–45. London: Routledge, 1991.

Blackbourn, David, and Richard J. Evans, eds. *The German Bourgeoisie: Essays on the Social History of the German Middle Class from the Late Eighteenth to the Early Twentieth Century.* London: Routledge, 1991.

Blake, John B. "Women and Medicine in Ante-Bellum America." *Bulletin of the History of Medicine* 39 (1965): 99–123.

Bledstein, Burton J. *The Culture of Professionalism: The Middle Class and the Development of Higher Education in America.* New York: Norton, 1976.

Bleker, Johanna. *Die naturhistorische Schule, 1825–1845: Ein Beitrag zur Geschichte der klinischen Medizin in Deutschland.* Stuttgart, Germany: G. Fischer, 1981.

Bonner, Thomas Neville. *American Doctors and German Universities: A Chapter in International Intellectual Relations, 1870–1914.* Lincoln: University of Nebraska Press, 1963.

——. *Becoming a Physician: Medical Education in Great Britain, France, Germany, and the United States, 1750–1945.* New York: Oxford University Press, 1995.

——. *To the Ends of the Earth: Women's Search for Education in Medicine.* Cambridge, Mass.: Harvard University Press, 1992.

Borst, Charlotte. *Catching Babies: The Professionalization of Childbirth, 1870–1920.* Cambridge, Mass.: Harvard University Press, 1995.

——. "The Training and Practice of Midwives: A Wisconsin Study." In *Women and Health in America: Historical Readings*, 2nd ed., edited by Judith Walzer Leavitt, 425–43. Madison: University of Wisconsin Press, 1999.

Bowman, Nancy. "Caroline Healey Dall: Her Creation and Reform Career." In *Women of the Commonwealth: Work, Family, and Social Change in Nineteenth-Century Massachusetts*, edited by Susan L. Porter, 121–46. Amherst: University of Massachusetts Press, 1996.

Boyer, Paul. *Urban Masses and Moral Order in America, 1820–1920*. Cambridge, Mass.: Harvard University Press, 1978.

Brancaforte, Charlotte L., ed. *The German Forty-Eighters in the United States*. New York: Peter Lang, 1989.

Bullough, Vern, and Martha Voght. "Women, Menstruation, and Nineteenth-Century Medicine." *Bulletin of the History of Medicine* 47 (1973): 66–82.

Butler, Judith. *Gender Trouble: Feminism and the Subversion of Identity*. New York: Routledge, 1990.

Carter, Codell. "Puerperal Fever." In *The Cambridge World History of Human Disease*, edited by Kenneth F. Kipple, 955–57. New York: Cambridge University Press, 1993.

Cassedy, James H. *American Medicine and Statistical Thinking, 1800–1860*. Cambridge, Mass.: Harvard University Press, 1984.

Cayleff, Susan E. *Wash and Be Healed: The Water-Cure Movement and Women's Health*. Philadelphia: Temple University Press, 1987.

Conze, Werner, and Jürgen Kocka, eds. *Bildungsbürgertum im 19. Jahrhundert*. 4 vols. Stuttgart, Germany: Klett-Cotta, 1985–92.

Cott, Nancy F. *The Bonds of Womanhood: "Woman's Sphere" in New England, 1780–1835*. New Haven, Conn.: Yale University Press, 1977.

———. "Passionless: An Interpretation of Victorian Sexuality, 1790–1850." *Signs* 4 (1978): 219–36.

———. *Public Vows: A History of Marriage and the Nation*. Cambridge, Mass.: Harvard University Press, 2000.

Creager, Angela N. H., Elizabeth Lunbeck, and Londa Schiebinger, eds. *Feminism in Twentieth-Century Science, Technology, and Medicine*. Chicago: University of Chicago Press, 2001.

Crumpacker, Laurie. "Female Patients in Four Boston Hospitals of the 1890's." Paper delivered at the 3rd Berkshire Conference on the History of Women, October 1974. Copy on deposit at the Schlesinger Library.

Davies, Norman. *God's Playground: A History of Poland*. 2 vols. New York: Columbia University Press, 1982.

Davis, Asa J. "The George Latimer Case: A Benchmark in the Struggle for Freedom." <http://edison.rutgers.edu/latimer/glatcase.htm>. April 2005.

Davis, Natalie Zemon. *Fiction in the Archives: Pardon Tales and Their Tellers in Sixteenth-Century France*. Stanford, Calif.: Stanford University Press, 1987.

Deutsch, Sarah. *Women and the City: Gender, Space, and Power in Boston, 1870–1940*. Oxford: Oxford University Press, 2000.

di Leonardo, Micaela. "Warrior Virgins and Boston Marriages: Spinsterhood in History and Culture." *Feminist Issues* 5, no. 2 (1985): 47–68.

Diepgen, Paul, and Edith Heischkel. *Die Medizin an der Berliner Charité bis zur Gründung der Universität*. Berlin: Verlag von Julius Springer, 1935.

Donegan, Jane B. *"Hydropathic Highway to Health": Women and Water-Cure in Antebellum America*. Westport, Conn.: Greenwood Press, 1986.

——. *Women and Men Midwives: Medicine, Morality, and Misogyny in Early America*. Westport, Conn.: Greenwood Press, 1978.

Donnison, Jean. *Midwives and Medical Men: A History of Inter-Professional Rivalries and Women's Rights*. New York: Schocken Books, 1977.

Douglas, Ann. *The Feminization of American Culture*. New York: Knopf, 1977.

Douglas, Mary. *Purity and Danger: An Analysis of Concepts of Pollution and Taboo*. London: Routledge, 2000.

Drachman, Virginia G. "Female Solidarity and Professional Success: The Dilemma of Women Doctors in Late Nineteenth-Century America." *Journal of Social History* 15 (1982): 607–19.

——. *Hospital with a Heart: Women Doctors and the Paradox of Separatism at the New England Hospital, 1862–1969*. Ithaca, N.Y.: Cornell University Press, 1984.

Dudenhausen, Joachim Wolfram, Manfred Stürzbecher, and Michael Engel. *Die Hebamme im Spiegel der Hebammen-Lehrbücher*. Berlin: Universitätsbibliothek der Freien Universität Berlin, 1985.

Ehrenreich, Barbara, and Deirdre English. *Complaints and Disorders: The Sexual Politics of Sickness*. Old Westbury, N.Y.: Feminist Press, 1973.

——. *For Her Own Good: 150 Years of the Expert's Advice to Women*. Garden City, N.Y.: Anchor Books, 1978.

——. *Witches, Midwives and Nurses*. 2nd ed. Old Westbury, N.Y.: Feminist Press, 1973.

Evans, Richard J. *Death in Hamburg: Society and Politics in the Cholera Years, 1830–1910*. New York: Penguin Books, 1987.

Evans, Sara M. *Born for Liberty: A History of Women in America. With a New Chapter and Preface by the Author*. New York: Free Press Paperbacks, 1997.

Faderman, Lillian. *Odd Girls and Twilight Lovers: A History of Lesbian Life in Twentieth-Century America*. New York: Columbia University Press, 1991.

——. *Surpassing the Love of Men: Romantic Friendship and Love between Women from the Renaissance to the Present*. New York: William Morrow, 1981.

Fassbender, Heinrich. *Geschichte der Geburtshilfe*. Hildesheim, Germany: Georg Olms, 1964.

Fischer, Alfons. *Geschichte des deutschen Gesundheitswesens*. 2 vols. Berlin: F. A. Herbig, 1933.

Fischer, W., J. Krengel, and J. Wietog, eds. *Sozialgeschichtliches Arbeitsbuch I. Materialien zur Statistik des Deutschen Bundes 1815–1870*. Munich: Verlag C. H. Beck, 1982.

Fraatz, Paul. *Der Paderborner Kreisarzt Joseph Hermann Schmidt*. Abhandlungen zur Geschichte der Medizin und der Naturwissenschaften, vol. 29. Berlin: Verlag Dr. Emil Ebering, 1939.

Fraser, Angus. *The Gypsies*. 2nd ed. Oxford, England: Blackwell, 1995.

Fraser, Nancy. "Structuralism or Pragmatics? On Discourse Theory and Feminist Politics." In *The Second Wave: A Reader in Feminist Theory*, edited by Linda Nicholson, 379–95. New York: Routledge, 1997.

Freedman, Estelle B. *Maternal Justice: Miriam Van Waters and the Female Reform Tradition*. Chicago: Chicago University Press, 1996.

——. "Separatism as Strategy: Female Institution Building and American Feminism, 1870–1930." *Feminist Studies* 5 (1979): 512–39.

Frevert, Ute. *Women in German History: From Bourgeois Emancipation to Sexual Liberation.* Translated by Stuart McKinnon-Evans, in association with Terry Bond and Barbara Norden. Oxford, England: Berg, 1988.

Fricke, Dieter, ed. *Lexikon zur Parteiengeschichte: Die Bürgerlichen und Kleinbürgerlichen Parteien und Verbände in Deutschland (1789–1945).* 4 vols. Leipzig, Germany: VEB Bibliographisches Institut Leipzig, 1983–86.

Gamble, Douglas Andrew. "Moral Suasion in the West: Garrisonian Abolitionism, 1831–1861." Ph.D. diss., Ohio State University, 1973.

Gardner, Martha N. "Midwife, Doctor, or Doctress? The New England Female Medical College and Women's Place in Nineteenth-Century Medicine and Society." Ph.D. diss., Brandeis University, 2002.

Geison, Gerald L. "Divided We Stand: Physiologists and Clinicians in the American Context." In *The Therapeutic Revolution: Essays in the Social History of American Medicine,* edited by Morris J. Vogel and Charles E. Rosenberg, 67–90. Philadelphia: University of Pennsylvania Press, 1979.

Gevitz, Norman, ed. *Other Healers: Unorthodox Medicine in America.* Baltimore: Johns Hopkins University Press, 1988.

Gienapp, William E. "Nativism and the Creation of a Republican Majority in the North before the Civil War." *Journal of American History* 72, no. 3 (1985): 529–59.

Ginzberg, Lori D. *Women and the Work of Benevolence: Morality, Politics, and Class in the Nineteenth-Century United States.* New Haven, Conn.: Yale University Press, 1990.

Goldstein, Linda Lehmann. "Roses Bloomed in Winter: Women Medical Graduates of Western Reserve College, 1852–1856." Ph.D. diss., Case Western Reserve University, 1989.

Gordon, Linda. *Pitied but Not Entitled: Single Mothers and the History of Welfare, 1890–1935.* New York: Free Press, 1994.

———. "Voluntary Motherhood: The Beginnings of Feminist Birth Control Ideas in the United States." *Feminist Studies* 1 (1973): 5–22.

Goschler, Constantin. *Rudolf Virchow: Mediziner—Anthropologe—Politiker.* Cologne, Germany: Böhlau Verlag, 2002.

Grams, Martin, Jr. "Cavalcade of America: The Lost Episodes." <http://www. old-time.com/otrlogs/cavalcade—mg.html>. January 2005.

———. *The History of the Cavalcade of America.* Delta, Pa.: M. Grams, 1998.

Gregory, Frederick. "Kant, Schelling, and the Administration of Science in the Romantic Era." *Osiris,* 2nd ser., 5 (1989): 17–35.

———. *Scientific Materialism in Nineteenth Century Germany.* Dordrecht, Holland: D. Reidel Publishing Co., 1977.

Grodzins, Dean. *American Heretic: Theodore Parker and Transcendentalism.* Chapel Hill: University of North Carolina Press, 2002.

Haber, Samuel. *The Quest for Authority and Honor in the American Professions, 1750–1900.* Chicago: University of Chicago Press, 1991.

Habermas, Rebekka. *Frauen und Männer des Bürgertums: Eine Familiengeschichte (1750–1850).* Göttingen, Germany: Vandenhoeck and Ruprecht, 2000.

Hachtmann, Rüdiger. *Berlin 1848: Eine Politik- und Gesellschaftsgeschichte der Revolution.* Bonn, Germany: J. H. W. Dietz, 1997.

Haller, John S., Jr. *American Medicine in Transition, 1840–1910.* Urbana: University of Illinois Press, 1981.

Hamerow, Theodore S. "The Two Worlds of the Forty-Eighters." In *The German Forty-Eighters in the United States,* edited by Charlotte L. Brancaforte, 19–35. New York: Peter Lang, 1989.

Hancock, Ian. "Gypsy History in Germany and Neighboring Lands: A Chronology Leading to the Holocaust and Beyond." In *The Gypsies of Eastern Europe,* edited by David Crow and John Kolsti, 11–30. New York: M. E. Sharpe, 1991.

——. Introduction to *The Gypsies of Eastern Europe,* edited by David Crow and John Kolsti, 3–9. New York: M. E. Sharpe, 1991.

Handlin, Oscar. *Boston's Immigrants: A Study in Acculturation.* Cambridge, Mass.: Harvard University Press, 1959.

Haraway, Donna. "Situated Knowledges: The Science Question in Feminism and the Privilege of Partial Perspective." In Donna Haraway, *Simians, Cyborgs, and Women: The Reinvention of Nature,* 183–201. New York: Routledge, 1991.

Harding, Sandra. *Whose Science? Whose Knowledge? Thinking from Women's Lives.* Ithaca, N.Y.: Cornell University Press, 1991.

Harvey, A. McGehee, Gert H. Brieger, Susan L. Abrams, and Victor A. McKusick. *A Model of Its Kind.* 2 vols. Baltimore: Johns Hopkins University Press, 1989.

Harvey, Joy. "*La Visite*: Mary Putnam Jacobi and the Paris Medical Clinics." In *French Medical Culture in the Nineteenth Century,* edited by Ann La Berge and Mordechai Feingold, 350–71. Amsterdam: Rodopi, 1994.

——. "Medicine and Politics: Dr. Mary Putnam Jacobi and the Paris Commune." *Dialectical Anthropology* 15 (1992): 107–17.

Hausen, Karin. "Family and Role Division: The Polarisation of Sexual Stereotypes in the Nineteenth Century." In *The German Family: Essays on the Social History of the Family in Nineteenth- and Twentieth-Century Germany,* edited by Richard J. Evans and W. Robert Lee, 51–83. London: Croom Helm, 1981.

Heilbrun, Carolyn G. *Writing a Woman's Life.* New York: Norton, 1988.

Hewitt, Nancy A. *Women's Activism and Social Change, Rochester, New York, 1822–1872.* Ithaca, N.Y.: Cornell University Press, 1984.

Hirsch, August, ed. *Biographisches Lexikon der hervorragenden Ärzte aller Zeiten und Völker.* Munich: Verlag von Urban and Schwarzenberg, 1962.

Holt, Niles R. "Ernst Haeckel's Monistic Religion." *Journal of the History of Ideas* 32 (1971): 265–80.

Hudson, Robert P. "Abraham Flexner in Perspective: American Medical Education, 1865–1910." In *Sickness and Health in America,* 2nd ed., edited by Judith Walzer Leavitt and Ronald L. Numbers, 147–58. Madison: University of Wisconsin Press, 1985.

Huerkamp, Claudia. *Der Aufstieg der Ärzte im 19. Jahrhundert.* Göttingen, Germany: Vandenhoeck and Ruprecht, 1985.

Huggins, Nathan Irvin. *Protestants against Poverty: Boston's Charities, 1870–1900*. Westport, Conn.: Greenwood Press, 1971.

Ingebritsen, Shirley Phillips. "Ednah Dow Littlehale Cheney." In *Notable American Women, 1607–1950: A Biographical Dictionary*, edited by Edward T. James, Janet Wilson James, and Paul S. Boyer, 1:325–27. Cambridge, Mass., Harvard University Press, Belknap Press, 1971.

———. "Lucy Ellen Sewall." In *Notable American Women, 1607–1950: A Biographical Dictionary*, edited by Edward T. James, Janet Wilson James, and Paul S. Boyer, 3:268–69. Cambridge, Mass., Harvard University Press, Belknap Press, 1971.

Irving, Frederick C. *Safe Deliverance*. Boston: Houghton Mifflin, 1942.

Jelinek, Estelle C. *The Tradition of Women's Autobiography: From Antiquity to the Present*. Boston: Twayne Publishers, 1986.

Jensen, Joan M. "Severance, Carolina Maria Seymour." In *Notable American Women, 1607–1950: A Biographical Dictionary*, edited by Edward T. James, Janet Wilson James, and Paul S. Boyer, 3:265–68. Cambridge, Mass.: Harvard University Press, Belknap Press, 1971.

Jordanova, Ludmilla. *Sexual Visions: Images of Gender in Science and Medicine between the Eighteenth and Twentieth Centuries*. Madison: University of Wisconsin Press, 1989.

Kass, Amalie M. *Midwifery and Medicine in Boston: Walter Channing, M.D., 1786–1876*. Boston: Northeastern University Press, 2002.

Katz, Michael B. *In the Shadow of the Poorhouse: A Social History of Welfare in America*, 10th ed. New York: Basic Books, 1996.

Kaufman, Martin. "The Admission of Women to Nineteenth-Century American Medical Societies." *Bulletin of the History of Medicine* 50 (1976): 251–60.

———. *Homeopathy in America: The Rise and Fall of a Medical Heresy*. Baltimore: Johns Hopkins University Press, 1971.

Keller, Evelyn Fox. "Developmental Biology as a Feminist Cause?" *Osiris*, 2nd ser., 12 (1997): 16–28.

———. "Gender and Science: Origin, History, and Politics." *Osiris*, 2nd ser., 10 (1995): 27–38.

———. *Reflections on Gender and Science*. New Haven, Conn.: Yale University Press, 1985.

Kirschmann, Anne Taylor. *A Vital Force: Women in American Homeopathy*. New Brunswick, N.J.: Rutgers University Press, 1999.

Kisacky, Jeanne Susan. "An Architecture of Light and Air: Theories of Hygiene and the Building of the New York Hospital." Ph.D. diss, Cornell University, 2000.

Kobrin, Frances E. "The American Midwife Controversy: A Crisis of Professionalization." *Bulletin of the History of Medicine* 40 (1966): 350–63.

Kohlstedt, Sally Gregory. "Women in the History of Science: An Ambiguous Place." *Osiris*, 2nd ser., 10 (1995): 39–58.

Kohlstedt, Sally Gregory, and Helen E. Longino. "The Women, Gender, and Science Questions." *Osiris*, 2nd ser., 12 (1997): 3–15.

Koselleck, Reinhart. *Preussen zwischen Reform und Revolution: Allgemeines Landrecht, Verwaltung und soziale Bewegung von 1791–1848*. Stuttgart, Germany: Klett, 1967.

Kraut, Alan M. *Silent Travelers: Germs, Genes, and the "Immigrant Menace."* New York: Basic Books, 1994.

Kunzel, Regina G. *Fallen Women, Problem Girls: Unmarried Mothers and the Professionalization of Social Work, 1890–1945*. New Haven, Conn.: Yale University Press, 1993.

Larson, Magali Sarfatti. *The Rise of Professionalism: A Sociological Analysis*. Berkeley: University of California Press, 1977.

La Vopa, Anthony J. *Prussian Schoolteachers: Profession and Office, 1763–1848*. Chapel Hill: University of North Carolina Press, 1980.

Leavitt, Judith Walzer. *Brought to Bed: Childbearing in America, 1750–1950*. New York: Oxford University Press, 1986.

——, ed. *Women and Health in America: Historical Readings*. Madison: University of Wisconsin Press, 1984.

——, ed. *Women and Health in America: Historical Readings*. 2nd ed. Madison: University of Wisconsin Press, 1999.

——. "'A Worrying Profession': The Domestic Environment of Medical Practice in Mid-Nineteenth-Century America." *Bulletin of the History of Medicine* 69 (1995): 1–29.

Leavitt, Judith Walzer, and Ronald L. Numbers, eds. *Sickness and Health in America*, 2nd ed. Madison: University of Wisconsin Press, 1985.

——, eds. *Sickness and Health in America*. 3rd ed. Madison: University of Wisconsin Press, 1997.

Lenoir, Timothy. *The Strategy of Life: Teleology and Mechanics in Nineteenth-Century German Biology*. Dordrecht, Holland: D. Reidel, 1982.

Lerner, Gerda. *The Grimké Sisters from South Carolina: Pioneers for Woman's Rights and Abolition*. New York: Oxford University Press, 1998.

L'Esperance, Elise S. "Influence of the New York Infirmary on Women in Medicine." *Journal of the American Medical Women's Association* 4 (June 1949): 255–61.

Levine, Bruce. *The Spirit of 1848: German Immigrants, Labor Conflict, and the Coming of the Civil War*. Urbana: University of Illinois Press, 1992.

Lindemann, Mary. *Health and Healing in Eighteenth-Century Germany*. Baltimore: Johns Hopkins University Press, 1996.

Litoff, Judy Barrett. *American Midwives: 1860 to the Present*. Westport, Conn.: Greenwood Press, 1978.

Loetz, Francisca. *Vom Kranken zum Patienten: "Medikalisierung" und medizinische Vergesellschaftung am Beispiel Badens 1750–1850*. Stuttgart, Germany: Franz Steiner Verlag, 1993.

Loudon, Irvine, ed. *Childbed Fever: A Documentary History*. New York: Garland, 1995.

Lovejoy, Esther Pohl. *Women Doctors of the World*. New York: Macmillan, 1957.

Lüdicke, Reinhard. *Die Preußischen Kultusminister und ihre Beamten im ersten Jahrhundert des Ministeriums 1817–1917*. Stuttgart, Germany: J. S. Cotta'sche, 1918.

Ludmerer, Kenneth M. *Learning to Heal: The Development of American Medical Education*. New York: Basic Books, 1985.

Marland, Hilary, ed. *The Art of Midwifery: Early Modern Midwives in Europe*. London: Routledge, 1993.

——, ed. *Midwives, Society and Childbirth: Debates and Controversies in the Modern Period*. London: Routledge, 1997.

"Mary Louis Booth." In *Encyclopedia Britannica's Women in American History*, <http://www.search.eb.com/women/articles/Booth—Mary—Louise.html>. February 2005.

Maulitz, Russell C. " 'Physician versus Bacteriologist': The Ideology of Science in Clinical Medicine." In *The Therapeutic Revolution: Essays in the Social History of American Medicine*, edited by Morris J. Vogel and Charles E. Rosenberg, 91–107. Philadelphia: University of Pennsylvania Press, 1979.

McClelland, Charles E. *The German Experience of Professionalization: Modern Learned Professions and Their Organizations from the Early Nineteenth Century to the Hitler Era*. Cambridge: Cambridge University Press, 1991.

McCormick, E. Allen, ed. *Germans in America: Aspects of German-American Relations in the Nineteenth Century*. New York: Columbia University Press, 1983.

McGregor, Deborah Kuhn. *Sexual Surgery and the Origins of Gynecology: J. Marion Sims, His Hospital, and His Patients*. New York: Garland, 1989.

Merrill, Walter M., and Louis Ruchames, eds. *The Letters of William Lloyd Garrison*. 6 vols. Cambridge, Mass.: Harvard University Press, 1971–81.

Miller, Carol Poh, and Robert Wheeler. *Cleveland: A Concise History, 1796–1990*. Bloomington: Indiana University Press, 1990.

Miller, Genevieve. "Kate Campbell Hurd-Mead." *Notable American Women, 1607–1950: A Biographical Dictionary*, edited by Edward T. James, Janet Wilson James, and Paul S. Boyer, 2:241–42. Cambridge, Mass.: Harvard University Press, Belknap Press, 1971.

Mohr, James C. *Abortion in America: The Origins and Evolutions of National Policy, 1800–1900*. New York: Oxford University Press, 1978.

Moldow, Gloria. *Women Doctors in Gilded-Age Washington: Race, Gender and Professionalization*. Urbana: University of Illinois Press, 1987.

Morantz, Regina Markell. "The 'Connecting Link': The Case for the Woman Doctor in Nineteenth-Century America." In *Sickness and Health in America*, 2nd ed., edited by Judith Walzer Leavitt and Ronald L. Numbers, 161–72. Madison: University of Wisconsin Press, 1985.

———. "The Perils of Feminist History." In *Women and Health in America: Historical Readings*, edited by Judith Walzer Leavitt, 239–45. Madison: University of Wisconsin Press, 1984.

Morantz, Regina Markell, Cynthia Stodola Pomerleau, and Carol Hansen Fenichel, eds. *In Her Own Words: Oral Histories of Women Physicians*. Westport, Conn.: Greenwood Press, 1982.

Morantz, Regina Markell, and Sue Zschoche. "Professionalism, Feminism, and Gender Roles: A Comparative Study of Nineteenth-Century Medical Therapeutics." *Journal of American History* 67, no. 3 (1980): 568–88.

Morantz-Sanchez, Regina. *Conduct Unbecoming a Woman: Medicine on Trial in Turn-of-the-Century Brooklyn*. New York: Oxford University Press, 1999.

———. "Feminist Theory and Historical Practice: Rereading Elizabeth Blackwell." *History and Theory* 31 (1992): 50–69.

———. "The Gendering of Empathic Expertise: How Women Physicians Became More Empathic than Men." In *The Empathic Practitioner: Empathy, Gender, and Medicine*, edited by Ellen Singer More and Maureen A. Milligan, 40–58. New Brunswick, N.J.: Rutgers University Press, 1994.

———. *Sympathy and Science: Women Physicians in American Medicine*. New York: Oxford University Press, 1985.

———. *Sympathy and Science: Women Physicians in American Medicine*. 2nd ed. Chapel Hill: University of North Carolina Press, 2000.

More, Ellen S. "The Blackwell Medical Society and the Professionalization of Women Physicians." *Bulletin of the History of Medicine* 67 (1987): 603–28.

———. " 'Empathy' Enters the Profession of Medicine." In *The Empathic Practitioner: Empathy, Gender, and Medicine*, edited by Ellen Singer More and Maureen A. Milligan, 19–39. New Brunswick, N.J.: Rutgers University Press, 1994.

———. *Restoring the Balance: Women Physicians and the Profession of Medicine, 1850–1995*. Cambridge, Mass.: Harvard University Press, 1999.

Morton, Marian J. *And Sin No More: Social Policy and Unwed Mothers in Cleveland, 1855–1990*. Columbus: Ohio State University Press, 1993.

Moscucci, Ornella. *The Science of Woman: Gynecology and Gender in England, 1800–1929*. Cambridge: Cambridge University Press, 1990.

Nadel, Stanley. *Little Germany: Ethnicity, Religion, and Class in New York City, 1845–80*. Urbana: University of Illinois Press, 1990.

Nicholson, Linda, ed. *The Second Wave: A Reader in Feminist Theory*. New York: Routledge, 1997.

Nipperdey, Thomas. *Deutsche Geschichte 1866–1918*. Munich: C. H. Beck, 1990.

Numbers, Ronald L. "The Fall and Rise of the American Medical Profession." In *Sickness and Health in America*, 3rd ed., edited by Judith Walzer Leavitt and Ronald L. Numbers, 225–36. Madison: University of Wisconsin Press, 1997.

Numbers, Ronald L., and Rennie B. Schoepflin. "Ministries of Healing: Mary Baker Eddy, Ellen G. White, and the Religion of Health." In *Women and Health in America: Historical Readings*, 2nd ed., edited by Judith Walzer Leavitt, 579–95. Madison: University of Wisconsin Press, 1999.

Paschen, Joachim. *Demokratische Vereine und Preußischer Staat: Entwicklung und Unterdrückung der demokratischen Bewegung während der Revolution von 1848/49*. Munich: Oldenbourg, 1977.

Peitzman, Steven J. *A New and Untried Course: Woman's Medical College and Medical College of Pennsylvania, 1850–1998*. New Brunswick, N.J.: Rutgers University Press, 2000.

Pellauer, Mary D. *Toward a Tradition of Feminist Theology: The Religious Social Thought of Elizabeth Cady Stanton, Susan B. Anthony, and Anna Howard Shaw*. Brooklyn, N.Y.: Carlson Publishing, 1991.

Perry, Lewis. *Radical Abolitionism: Anarchy and the Government of God in Antislavery Thought*. Ithaca, N.Y.: Cornell University Press, 1973.

Porter, Theodore M. *The Rise of Statistical Thinking, 1820–1900*. Princeton, N.J.: Princeton University Press, 1986.

———. *Trust in Numbers: The Pursuit of Objectivity in Science and Public Life*. Princeton, N.J.: Princeton University Press, 1995.

Quiroga, Virginia A. Metaxas. *Poor Mothers and Babies: Social History of Childbirth and Child Care Hospitals in Nineteenth-Century New York City*. New York: Garland, 1989.

Randers-Pehrson, Justine Davis. *Adolf Douai, 1819–1888: The Turbulent Life of a German Forty-Eighter in the Homeland and in the United States*. New York: Peter Lang, 2000.

Reagan, Leslie J. *When Abortion Was a Crime: Women, Medicine, and Law in the United States, 1867–1973*. Berkeley: University of California Press, 1997.

Reiser, Stanley Joel. *Medicine and the Reign of Technology*. Cambridge: Cambridge University Press, 1978.

Riley, Anne, Will Lucas, and Bryan Pettit. "The Cavalcade of America: Examining the Myth and Reality of Hero Worship in American Radio. Editor's Introduction." <http://xroads.virginia.edu/~UG03/radio/content.html>. January 2005.

Risse, Guenter B., and John Harley Warner. "Reconstructing Clinical Activities: Patient Records in Medical History." *Society for the Social History of Medicine* 5 (1992): 183–205.

Roberts, Shirley. *Sophia Jex-Blake: A Woman Pioneer in Nineteenth Century Medical Reform*. London: Routledge, 1993.

Robertson, David A. "Mayo, Amory Dwight." In *Dictionary of American Biography*, edited by Dumas Malone, 6:461–62. New York: Charles Scribner's Sons, 1933.

Robinson, David. *The Unitarians and the Universalists*. Westport, Conn.: Greenwood Press, 1985.

Rochford, Grace E. "The New England Hospital for Women and Children." *Journal of the American Medical Women's Association* 5 (December 1950): 497–99.

Rogers, Naomi. *An Alternative Path: The Making and Remaking of Hahnemann Medical College and Hospital of Philadelphia*. New Brunswick, N.J.: Rutgers University Press, 1998.

———. "American Homeopathy Confronts Scientific Medicine." In *Culture, Knowledge, and Healing: Historical Perspectives of Homeopathic Medicine in Europe and North America*, edited by Robert Jütte, Guenter B. Risse, and John Woodward, 31–64. Sheffield, England: European Association for the History of Medicine and Health Publications, 1998.

———. "Women and Sectarian Medicine." In *Women, Health, and Medicine in America: A Historical Handbook*, edited by Rima D. Apple, 281–310. New Brunswick, N.J.: Rutgers University Press, 1992.

Rosenberg, Charles E. *The Care of Strangers: The Rise of America's Hospital System*. New York: Basic Books, 1987.

———. *The Cholera Years: The United States in 1832, 1849, and 1866*. Chicago: University of Chicago Press, 1962.

———. "Inward Vision and Outward Glance: The Shaping of the American Hospital, 1880–1914." *Bulletin of the History of Medicine* 53 (1979): 356–91.

———. "Social Class and Medical Care in Nineteenth-Century America: The Rise and Fall of the Dispensary." *Journal of the History of Medicine and Allied Sciences* 29 (1974): 32–54.

———. "The Therapeutic Revolution: Medicine, Meaning, and Social Change in Nineteenth-Century America." In *The Therapeutic Revolution: Essays in the Social History of American Medicine*, edited by Morris J. Vogel and Charles E. Rosenberg, 3–25. Philadelphia: University of Pennsylvania Press, 1979.

Rosenberg, Hans. *Bureaucracy, Aristocracy, and Autocracy: The Prussian Experience, 1660–1815.* Cambridge, Mass.: Harvard University Press, 1958.

Rosenkrantz, Barbara Gutman. *Public Health and the State: Changing Views in Massachusetts, 1842–1936.* Cambridge, Mass.: Harvard University Press, 1972.

———. "The Search for Professional Order in Nineteenth-Century American Medicine." In *Sickness and Health in America*, 2nd ed., edited by Judith Walzer Leavitt and Ronald L. Numbers, 219–32. Madison: University of Wisconsin Press, 1985.

Rosner, David. *A Once Charitable Enterprise: Hospital and Health Care in Brooklyn and New York, 1885–1915.* Cambridge: Cambridge University Press, 1982.

Rossiter, Margaret W. *Women Scientists in America: Before Affirmative Action.* Baltimore: Johns Hopkins University Press, 1995.

———. *Women Scientists in America: Struggles and Strategies to 1940.* Baltimore: Johns Hopkins University Press, 1982.

Rothstein, William G. *American Physicians in the Nineteenth Century: From Sects to Science.* Baltimore: Johns Hopkins University Press, 1985.

Rupp, Leila J. " 'Imagine My Surprise': Women's Relationships in Historical Perspective." *Frontiers* 5, no. 3 (1980): 61–70.

Ryan, Mary P. *Cradle of the Middle Class: The Family in Oneida County, New York, 1790–1865.* Cambridge: Cambridge University Press, 1981.

———. "The Power of Women's Networks: A Case Study of Female Moral Reform in Antebellum America." *Feminist Studies* 5 (1979): 66–85.

———. *Women in Public: Between Banners and Ballots, 1825–1880.* Baltimore: Johns Hopkins University Press, 1990.

Sahli, Nancy A. *Elizabeth Blackwell, M.D. (1821–1910): A Biography.* New York: Arno Press, 1982.

———. "Smashing: Women's Relationships before the Fall." *Chrysalis* 8 (1979): 17–27.

Scanlon, Dorothy T. "Henry Ingersoll Bowditch." In *Biographical Dictionary of Social Welfare in America*, edited by Walter I. Trattner, 107–11. New York: Greenwood Press, 1976.

Schiebinger, Londa. *Has Feminism Changed Science?* Cambridge, Mass.: Harvard University Press, 1999.

———. *The Mind Has No Sex? Women in the Origins of Modern Science.* Cambridge, Mass.: Harvard University Press, 1989.

———. *Nature's Body: Gender in the Making of Modern Science.* Boston: Beacon, 1993.

Schoepflin, Rennie B. *Christian Science on Trial: Religious Healing in America.* Baltimore: Johns Hopkins University Press, 2003.

Schöler, Walter. *Geschichte des naturwissenschaftlichen Unterrichts im 17. bis 19. Jahrhundert.* Berlin: de Gruyter, 1970.

Sczibilanski, Klaus. "Von der Prüfungs- und Vorprüfungsordnung (1883) bis zur Approbationsordnung 1970 für Aerzte der Bundesrepublik Deutschland: Die Entwicklung der medizinischen Prüfungsordnungen, darg. an Aufsätzen aus der deutschen ärztlichen Standespresse." Medical diss., University of Münster, 1977.

Sheehan, James J. *German History, 1770–1866.* Oxford, England: Clarendon Press, 1989.

Shryock, Richard Harrison. *The Development of Modern Medicine: An Interpretation of the Social and Science Factors Involved*. 1936. Reprint, Madison: University of Wisconsin, 1979.

———. "Women in American Medicine." *Journal of the American Medical Women's Association* 5 (1950): 371–79.

Sicherman, Barbara. *Alice Hamilton, a Life in Letters*. Cambridge, Mass.: Harvard University Press, 1984.

———. *Exploring the Dangerous Trades: The Autobiography of Alice Hamilton, M.D.* Boston: Northeastern University Press, 1985.

Siemann, Wolfram. *Gesellschaft im Aufbruch: Deutschland 1849–1871*. Frankfurt am Main, Germany: Suhrkamp, 1990.

Silver-Isenstadt, Jean L. *Shameless: The Visionary Life of Mary Gove Nichols*. Baltimore: Johns Hopkins University Press, 2002.

Sklar, Kathryn Kish. *Catherine Beecher: A Study in American Domesticity*. New Haven, Conn.: Yale University Press, 1973.

Smith, Helmut Walser. *German Nationalism and Religious Conflict: Culture, Ideology, Politics, 1870–1914*. Princeton, N.J.: Princeton University Press, 1995.

———, ed. *Protestants, Catholics, and Jews in Germany, 1800–1914*. Oxford, England: Berg, 2001.

Smith, Susan L. "Medicine, Midwifery, and the State: Japanese Americans and Health Care in Hawai'i, 1885–1945." *Journal of Asian American Studies* 4, no. 1 (2001): 57–75.

Smith-Rosenberg, Carroll. *Disorderly Conduct: Visions of Gender in Victorian America*. New York: Knopf, 1985.

———. "The Female World of Love and Ritual: Relationships between Women in Nineteenth-Century America." *Signs* 1 (1975): 1–29.

———. "The Hysterical Woman: Sex Roles and Role Conflict in Nineteenth-Century America." *Social Research* 39 (1972): 652–78.

Smith-Rosenberg, Carroll, and Charles E. Rosenberg. "The Female Animal: Medical and Biological Views of Woman and Her Role in Nineteenth-Century America." In *Women and Health in America: Historical Readings*, 2nd ed., edited by Judith Walzer Leavitt, 111–30. Madison: University of Wisconsin Press, 1999.

Stansell, Christine. *City of Women: Sex and Class in New York, 1789–1860*. Urbana: University of Illinois Press, 1982.

Starr, Paul. *The Social Transformation of American Medicine*. New York: Basic Books, 1982.

Stevens, Rosemary. *In Sickness and in Wealth: American Hospitals in the Twentieth Century*. New York: Basic Books, 1989.

Stewart, James Brewer. *Holy Warriors: The Abolitionists and American Slavery*. New York: Hill and Wang, 1976.

Story, Ronald. *The Forging of an Aristocracy: Harvard and the Boston Upper Class, 1800–1870*. Middletown, Conn.: Wesleyan University Press, 1980.

Stowe, Steven M. "Seeing Themselves at Work: Physicians and the Case Narrative in the Mid-Nineteenth-Century American South." In *Sickness and Health in America*, 3rd ed., edited by Judith Walzer Leavitt and Ronald L. Numbers, 161–86. Madison: University of Wisconsin Press, 1997.

Sudhoff, Karl. "Aus der Geschichte des Charite-Krankenhauses zu Berlin." *Muenchener medizinische Wochenschrift* 57 (1910): 1015–18.

Theriot, Nancy M. "Women's Voices in Nineteenth-Century Medical Discourse: A Step toward Deconstructing Science." *Signs* 19 (1993): 1–31.

Thernstrom, Stephan. *The Other Bostonians: Poverty and Progress in the American Metropolis, 1880–1970.* Cambridge, Mass.: Harvard University Press, 1973.

Tiffany, Nina Moore. *Samuel E. Sewall, a Memoir.* Boston: Houghton, Mifflin & Co., 1898.

Tighe, Janet A. "A Lesson in the Political Economics of Medical Education." In *Major Problems in the History of American Medicine and Public Health*, edited by John Harley Warner and Janet A. Tighe, 309–15. Boston: Houghton Mifflin, 2001.

Tomes, Nancy. *The Gospel of Germs: Men, Women, and the Microbe in American Life.* Cambridge, Mass.: Harvard University Press, 1998.

Tuchman, Arleen Marcia. " 'Only in a Republic Can It Be Proved That Science Has No Sex': Marie Elizabeth Zakrzewska (1829–1902) and the Multiple Meanings of Science in the Nineteenth-Century United States." *Journal of Women's History* 11 (1999): 121–42.

——. *Science, Medicine, and the State in Germany: The Case of Baden, 1815–1871.* New York: Oxford University Press, 1993.

——. "Situating Gender: Marie E. Zakrzewska and the Place of Science in Women's Medical Education." *Isis* 95 (2004): 34-57.

——. " 'The True Assistant to the Obstetrician': The Legal Protection of Midwives in Nineteenth-Century Prussia." *Social History of Medicine* 18, no. 1 (2005): 23–38.

Ulrich, Laurel Thatcher. *A Midwife's Tale: The Life of Martha Ballard, Based on Her Diary, 1785–1812.* New York: Vintage Books, 1990.

Vietor, Agnes, ed. *A Woman's Quest: The Life of Marie E. Zakrzewska, M.D.* 1924. Reprint, New York: Arno Press, 1972.

Viner, Russell. "Abraham Jacobi and German Medical Radicalism in Antebellum New York." *Bulletin of the History of Medicine* 72 (1998): 434–63.

——. "Healthy Children for a New World: Abraham Jacobi and the Making of American Pediatrics." Ph.D. diss., University of Cambridge, 1997.

Vogel, Morris J. *The Invention of the Modern Hospital: Boston, 1870–1930.* Chicago: University of Chicago Press, 1980.

——. "Patrons, Practitioners, and Patients: The Voluntary Hospital in Mid-Victorian Boston." In *Sickness and Health in America*, 2nd ed., edited by Judith Walzer Leavitt and Ronald L. Numbers, 287–97. Madison: University of Wisconsin Press, 1985.

Wach, Howard M. "A Boston Feminist in the Victorian Public Sphere: The Social Criticism of Caroline Healey Dall." *New England Quarterly* 68, no. 3 (1995): 429–50.

Waddington, Ivan. "The Role of the Hospital in the Development of Modern Medicine." *Sociology* 7, no. 2 (1973): 211–24.

Wagner-Martin, Linda. *Telling Women's Lives: The New Biography.* New Brunswick, N.J.: Rutgers University Press, 1994.

Waite, Frederick Clayton. *History of the New England Female Medical College, 1848–1874.* Boston: Boston University School of Medicine, 1950.

——. *Western Reserve University: The Hudson Era. A History of Western Reserve College and Academy at Hudson, Ohio, from 1826 to 1882.* Cleveland: Western Reserve University Press, 1943.

Walsh, Mary Roth. *"Doctors Wanted—No Women Need Apply": Sexual Barriers in the Medical Profession, 1835–1975.* New Haven, Conn.: Yale University Press, 1977.

——. "Feminist Showplace." In *Women and Health in America: Historical Readings,* edited by Judith Walzer Leavitt, 392–405. Madison: University of Wisconsin Press, 1984.

Warner, John Harley. *Against the Spirit of System: The French Impulse in Nineteenth-Century American Medicine.* Princteon, N.J.: Princeton University Press, 1998.

——. "From Specificity to Universalism in Medical Therapeutics: Transformation in the Nineteenth-Century United States." In *Sickness and Health in America,* 3rd ed., edited by Judith Walzer Leavitt and Ronald L. Numbers, 87–101. Madison: University of Wisconsin Press, 1997.

——. "Ideals of Science and Their Discontents in Late Nineteenth-Century American Medicine." *Isis* 82 (1991): 454–78.

——. "Orthodoxy and Otherness: Homeopathy and Regular Medicine in Nineteenth-Century America." In *Culture, Knowledge, and Healing: Historical Perspectives of Homeopathic Medicine in Europe and North America,* edited by Robert Jütte, Guenter B. Risse, and John Woodward, 5–29. Sheffield, England: European Association for the History of Medicine and Health Publications, 1998.

——. "The Selective Transport of Medical Knowledge: Antebellum American Physicians and Parisian Medical Therapeutics." *Bulletin of the History of Medicine* 59 (1985): 213–31.

——. *The Therapeutic Perspective: Medical Practice, Knowledge, and Identity in America, 1820–1885.* Cambridge, Mass.: Harvard University Press, 1986.

Warner, Margaret. "Hunting the Yellow Fever Germ: The Principle and Practice of Etiological Proof in Late Nineteenth-Century America." *Bulletin of the History of Medicine* 59 (1985): 361–82.

Warner, Sam B., Jr. *Streetcar Suburbs: The Process of Growth in Boston, 1870–1900.* Cambridge, Mass.: Harvard University Press and MIT Press, 1962.

Watson, Frank Dekker. *The Charity Organization Movement in the United States: A Study in American Philanthropy.* New York: Macmillan, 1922.

Wells, Susan. *Out of the Dead House: Nineteenth-Century Women Physicians and the Writing of Medicine.* Madison: University of Wisconsin Press, 2001.

Welter, Barbara. "The Cult of True Womanhood: 1820–1860." *American Quarterly* 18, no. 2, pt. 1 (1966): 151–74.

Wertz, Richard W., and Dorothy C. Wertz, *Lying-in: A History of Childbirth in America.* Expanded ed. New Haven, Conn.: Yale University Press, 1989.

White, Haydn. *The Content of the Form: Narrative Discourse and Historical Representation.* Baltimore: Johns Hopkins University Press, 1987.

Williams, Peter W. "Unitarianism and Universalism." In *Encyclopedia of the American Religious Experience: Studies of Traditions and Movements,* edited by Charles H. Lippy and Peter W. Williams, 1:579–93. New York: Charles Scribner's Sons, 1988.

Wilson, Adrian. *The Making of Man-Midwifery: Childbirth in England, 1660–1770.* Cambridge, Mass.: Harvard University Press, 1995.

Wittke, Carl. *Against the Current: The Life of Karl Heinzen (1809–80).* Chicago: University of Chicago Press, 1945.

Wood, Ann Douglas. " 'The Fashionable Diseases': Women's Complaints and Their Treatment in Nineteenth-Century America." In *Women and Health in America: Historical Readings*, edited by Judith Walzer Leavitt, 222–38. Madison: University of Wisconsin, 1984.

W. W. F. "James Freeman Clarke." In *Dictionary of American Biography*, edited by Dumas Malone, 4:153–54. New York: Charles Scribner's Sons, 1930.

INDEX

Alpha (women's association), 84

American Medical Association (AMA), 60, 61, 140, 173

American Medical Women's Association, 257

American Woman Suffrage Association, 170, 235

Anthony, Susan B., 71–72, 121–22, 201, 203, 284 (n. 61)

Anti-Catholicism. *See* German radicals: on religion; Heinzen, Karl: on religion; Zakrzewska, Marie—views: on religion

Apprenticeship, 59, 138, 223

Associated Charities of Boston, 157, 195

Association for the Advancement of Women, 170

Autobiography, 122, 125

"Bacteriomania," 238

Barringer, Emily Dunning, 257

Bellevue Hospital (New York), 218

Berlin Society of Obstetricians, 39

Bigelow, Henry Jacob, 215

Bildungsbürgertum. See German bourgeoisie

Blackwell, Elizabeth, 3, 104, 176, 236, 242, 243, 249, 250, 300 (n. 67); and New York Infirmary, 2, 74–75, 79, 81–88, 156; on coeducation, 12; on orthodox medicine, 12, 61, 201; as student at Geneva Medical College, 59, 69; supports Zakrzewska's career, 62–63, 124, 129; *An Appeal in Behalf of the Medical Education of Women*, 81–84; on gender differences in medical practice, 94, 151, 206, 230, 239; and spiritual power of maternity, 94, 241; and tensions with Zakrzewska, 98; and medical standards, 154; as critic of vivisec-

tion, 229; on ovariotomies, 240; on science, 263 (n. 17)

Blackwell, Emily: and New York Infirmary, 2, 75, 79, 81, 86, 98; on coeducation, 12, 218–19; on orthodox medicine, 12, 61; and medical standards, 154; and generational tensions, 224

Blackwell, Henry, 81, 102

Blackwell, Kitty Barry, 104, 115, 249, 250

Blockley Hospital (Philadelphia), 218, 300 (n. 67)

Boivin, Marie Anne Victorine, 91, 146, 152, 288 (n. 27)

Bond, George W., 168

Bond, Louisa C., 168

Booth, Mary L., 84–85, 86, 99–100, 115, 120, 123–24, 125–26, 135, 136, 241

Boston City Hospital, 157, 198, 218; and patients' class, 193–95; and policy on unwed mothers, 290 (n. 26)

Boston Lying-In Hospital, 157, 187, 198; and patients' class, 192–93, 195; and patients' marital status, 196, 294 (n. 14); obstetrics practices at, 205; and puerperal fever, 206

Boston marriages, 9, 115, 116, 118. *See also* Same-sex relationships

Bowditch, Henry Ingersoll, 144, 168, 172–73, 174, 246

Breed, Mary E., 175

Brown, Charlotte Blake, 180

Büchner, Ludwig, 109, 118

Buckel, C. Annette, 176

Busch, Dietrich Wilhelm Heinrich, 25

Butler, Emma Merrill, 251

Butler, Judith, 7